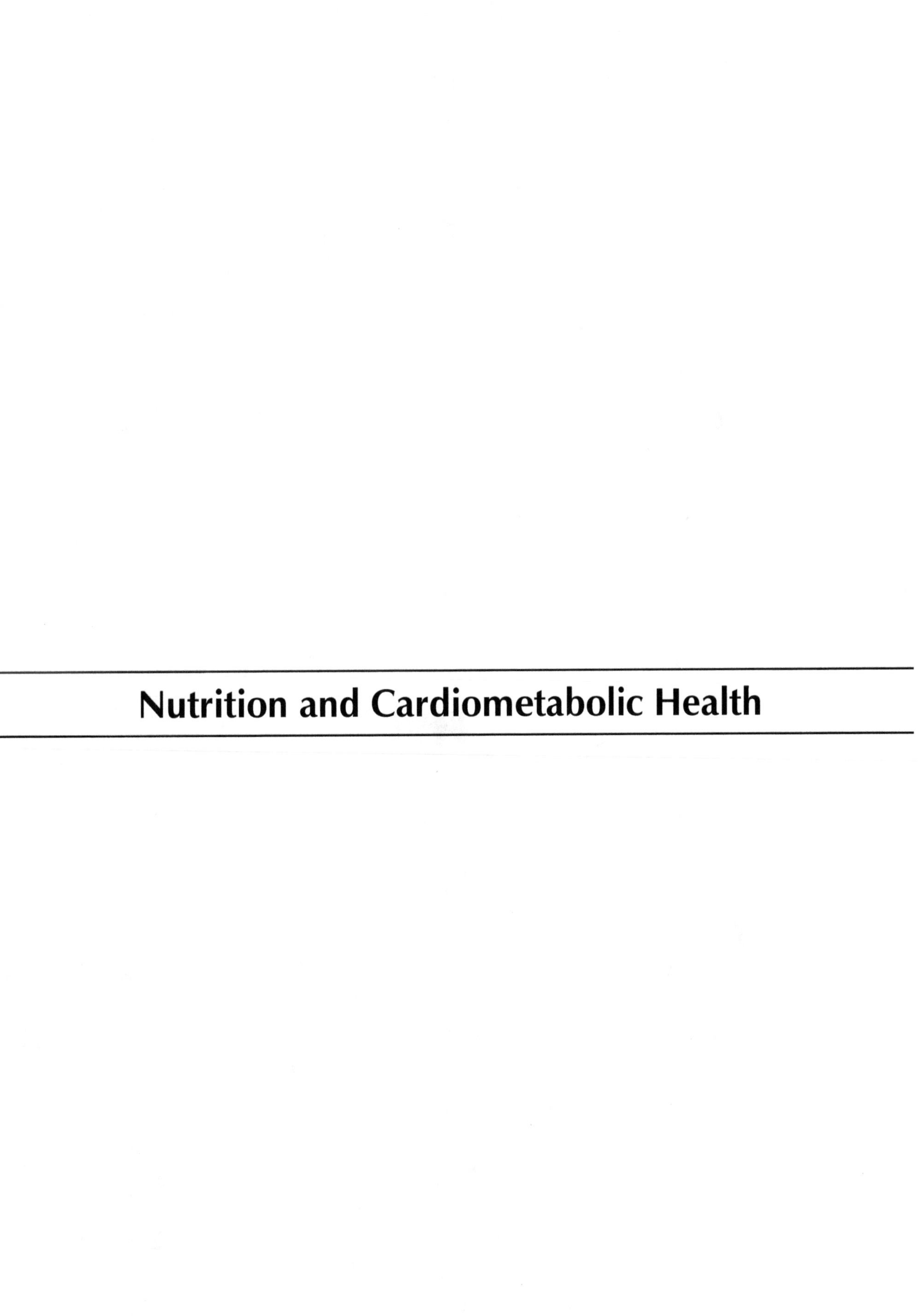

Nutrition and Cardiometabolic Health

Nutrition and Cardiometabolic Health

Editor: Jesse Adley

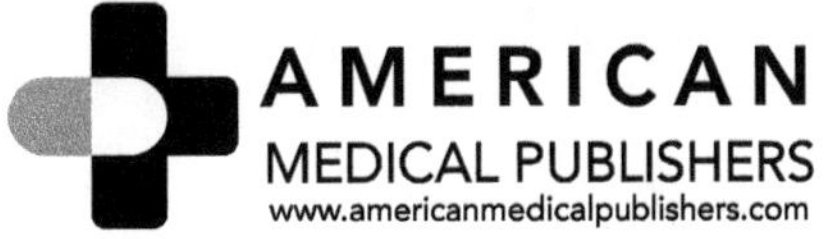

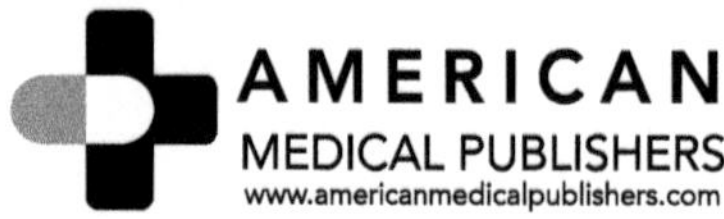

Cataloging-in-Publication Data

Nutrition and cardiometabolic health / edited by Jesse Adley.
p. cm.
Includes bibliographical references and index.
ISBN 978-1-63927-758-2
1. Cardiovascular system--Diseases--Nutritional aspects. 2. Cardiovascular system--Diseases--Prevention.
3. Reducing diets. 4. Diet therapy. I. Adley, Jesse.
RC669 .N88 2023
616.1--dc23

American Medical Publishers,
41 Flatbush Avenue,
1st Floor, New York,
NY 11217, USA

ISBN 978-1-63927-758-2 (Hardback)

Contents

Preface

Every book is initially just a concept; it takes months of research and hard work to give it the final shape in which the readers receive it. In its early stages, this book also went through rigorous reviewing. The notable contributions made by experts from across the globe were first molded into patterned chapters and then arranged in a sensibly sequential manner to bring out the best results.

Nutrition is the consumption of a balanced and healthy diet. It is the process by which the body absorbs and utilizes food, as well as other nourishing materials. Poor nutrition can play a significant role in increasing the risk of cardiometabolic diseases but a nutrient-rich and well-balanced diet can assist in significantly lowering or preventing the risk of these diseases. Various risk factors affecting the cardiometabolic health are influenced by diet, most notably dyslipidemia, high blood pressure, excessive body fat and poor glucose metabolism. A balanced diet that includes necessary omega-3 and omega-6 fatty acids, plant-based meals, non-nutritive bioactive compounds, and lean meats lower the cardiometabolic risks. Various other important nutrients, such as soluble fibers like oat beta-glucan, as well as vitamins C and E have also been discovered to boost heart function. Thus, improving diet quality and dietary intake becomes crucial for maintaining cardiometabolic health. This book unravels the recent studies on the role of nutrition in cardiometabolic health. The readers would gain knowledge that would broaden their perspective in this area of study.

It has been my immense pleasure to be a part of this project and to contribute my years of learning in such a meaningful form. I would like to take this opportunity to thank all the people who have been associated with the completion of this book at any step.

Editor

Preface

Non-Energy-Restricted Low-Carbohydrate Diet Combined with Exercise Intervention Improved Cardiometabolic Health in Overweight Chinese Females

Shengyan Sun [1,2], Zhaowei Kong [2], Qingde Shi [3], Mingzhu Hu [2], Haifeng Zhang [4], Di Zhang [2] and Jinlei Nie [3,*]

1 Institute of Physical Education, Huzhou University, Huzhou 313000, China; sysun@zjhu.edu.cn
2 Faculty of Education, University of Macau, Macao 999078, China; zwkong@um.edu.mo (Z.K.); mb74811@um.edu.mo (M.H.); mb74812@um.edu.mo (D.Z.)
3 School of Health Sciences and Sports, Macao Polytechnic Institute, Macao 999078, China; qdshi@ipm.edu.mo
4 College of Physical Education, Hebei Normal University, Shijiazhuang 050000, China; hbnuzhanghaifeng@sina.com
* Correspondence: jnie@ipm.edu.mo

Abstract: This study aimed to examine the effects of four weeks of a low-carbohydrate diet (LC) and incorporated exercise training on body composition and cardiometabolic health. Fifty-eight overweight/obese Chinese females (age: 21.2 ± 3.3 years, body mass index (BMI): 25.1 ± 2.8 kg/m^2) were randomly assigned to the control group (CON, $n = 15$), the LC control group (LC-CON, $n = 15$), the LC and high-intensity interval training group (LC-HIIT, $n = 15$), or the LC and moderate-intensity continuous training group (LC-MICT, $n = 13$). Subjects consumed a four week LC, whereas LC-HIIT and LC-MICT received extra training 5 d/week (LC-HIIT: 10 × 6 s cycling interspersed with 9 s rest, MICT: 30 min continuous cycling at 50–60% VO_{2peak}). After intervention, the three LC groups demonstrated significant reductions in body weight (−2.85 kg in LC-CON, −2.85 kg in LC-HIIT, −2.56 kg in LC-MICT, $p < 0.001$, $\eta^2 = 0.510$), BMI ($p < 0.001$, $\eta^2 = 0.504$) and waist-to-hip ratio ($p < 0.001$, $\eta^2 = 0.523$). Groups with extra training (i.e., LC-HIIT and LC-MICT) improved VO_{2peak} by 14.8 and 17.3%, respectively. However, fasting glucose and blood lipid levels remained unchanged in all groups. Short-term LC is a useful approach to improve body composition in overweight/obese Chinese females. Incorporated exercise training has no additional effects on weight loss, but has additional benefits on cardiorespiratory fitness, and HIIT is more time efficient than the traditional MICT (2.5 min vs. 30 min).

Keywords: ketogenic diet; short term; exercise; body composition; cardiorespiratory fitness; blood lipids

---

1. Introduction

The obesity pandemic is a major health challenge faced by both developed and developing nations [1]. This is due to its close association with multiple comorbidities which are among the top causes of mortality, such as type 2 diabetes (T2D), cardiovascular diseases (CVDs), and cancer [2]. The beneficial health effects of weight loss are well recognized [3–5], and diet and exercise remain the most common strategies to fight obesity.

The conventional dietary guidelines for weight loss (i.e., low-fat, high-carbohydrate, reduced-calorie diets) [6] have been challenged, especially by supporters of low-carbohydrate diets

(LCs). Emerging evidence mainly derived from western countries has clearly shown that LCs could be effective dietary strategies for weight loss and the management of several common and rare pathological conditions [7–13]. A meta-analysis has revealed that LCs had greater long-term effects on weight loss when compared to the traditional low-fat diets; furthermore, triglycerides, high-density lipoprotein cholesterol (HDL-C), and blood pressure values were also more favorably altered in LCs [7]. Additionally, LC-induced weight loss is generally accompanied with several positive metabolic changes, including improvements in blood pressure, glycaemic control, insulin sensitivity, and serum concentrations of C-reactive protein and certain lipids [8–12], which may have the potential to alleviate the features of metabolic disorder and reduce the risk factors associated with developing CVD and T2D. However, limited studies have tested whether LCs are also useful and feasible for the large Chinese overweight/obese population [11,13] given that people in China and in Western countries have distinct dietary patterns and preferences [14,15], which may lead to different levels of acceptance toward LCs. Furthermore, previous LC trials were invariably administered ad libitum without fixed daily energy intakes, or had an overemphasis on energy restriction [8,10–12,16,17]. Undeniably, this approach is more effective and easier to implement in public practice, where researchers are unable to provide strict controls and intensive monitors on diet as compared to the clinical setting. Yet, it is difficult to evaluate whether the beneficial cardiometabolic health outcomes resulting from these LCs should be attributed to the reduction in calorie intake or the tested dietary pattern. Therefore, with potential confounding factors being controlled, it is necessary to provide initial evidence regarding the effects of LC with a fixed or unchanged calorie intake on cardiometabolic health in the Chinese overweight/obese population.

In addition to diet, exercise is the main outlet for excessive energy, thus leading to weight reduction, although exercise and LC may work through different metabolic pathways. High-intensity interval training (HIIT) protocols have been developed in the past decade as time-saving replacements of the traditional moderate-intensity continuous training (MICT) to improve fitness and health. With less time commitment and a lower overall exercise amount, previous studies have shown that HIIT programs have the potential to improve cardiorespiratory fitness (CRF), body composition, and cardiometabolic risk factors to a similar extent as MICT programs [18–21]. Thus, combining HIIT or MICT intervention with LC may induce additional benefits on weight loss and cardiometabolic health. Furthermore, during LC intervention with minimal carbohydrate supplements, muscle glycogen stores and glycolytic enzyme activity are typically lowered if there is no preadaptation [22]. As a result, short-term LC has been reported to reduce CRF [17,23], whereas regular exercise is considered the most effective approach to improve CRF. Therefore, combined LC with HIIT or MICT may potentially compensate or even reverse the CRF-lowering effects of LC. Until now, no study has examined whether collaborate LC with time-saving HIIT or MICT have additional benefits for weight loss and cardiometabolic health, and for this reason, this is one of the research interests of the present study.

Given the above, we adopted an extremely brief HIIT protocol, involving only 1 min of intense exercise (i.e., 10 × 6 s sprint cycling interspersed with 9 s rest periods, 2.5 min in total), and combined it with LC. Our objectives were as follows: (1) To examine the efficacy of four weeks of non-energy-restricted LC on body composition and cardiometabolic health-related profiles in overweight/obese Chinese females; (2) to evaluate whether LC combined with brief HIIT or traditional MICT (i.e., continuous cycling at 50–60% peak oxygen uptake (VO_{2peak}) for 30 min) would trigger additional effects on weight loss and cardiometabolic health. We hypothesized that the short-term, non-energy-restricted LC intervention alone could effectively improve body composition and cardiometabolic health in overweight/obese Chinese females, and groups incorporated with extra HIIT or MICT would have additional benefits in terms of weight loss and CRF.

2. Materials and Method

2.1. Participants

This study was approved by the Research Ethics Committee of the University of Macau (RC Ref. no. MYRG2017-00199-FED) and carried out according to the Declaration of Helsinki. A power calculation was conducted to estimate the sample size using G * Power (Version 3.1). Under the assumptions of a correlation of 0.8 between pre–post intervention measurements and an effect size of 0.32 based on a meta-analysis for the primary outcome of VO_{2peak} resulting from HIIT [24], we would need to enroll 12 subjects for the HIIT group with a power of 0.8 at a significance level of 5%. When a potential dropout rate of 25% is considered, we aimed to recruit a total of 60 subjects. Public recruitment notices, including research intention and inclusion criteria, were released through the university bulletin board and e-mail to recruit eligible overweight or obese young females. The inclusion criteria were as follows: (1) between the age of 18 to 30 years old; (2) body mass index (BMI) $\geq$ 23 kg/m^2 [25]; (3) maintenance of a stable body weight in the past six months (variation of less than 2 kg); (4) sedentary lifestyle, not involved in any regular or structured exercise programs in the past 6 months; and (5) healthy (no endocrine, metabolic, osteoarticular, or heart diseases). Smokers, alcoholics, and subjects who were taking prescribed medication of any kind, regularly consuming nutritional supplements, adhering to specific diet programs, suffering from respiratory problems or eating disorders were excluded. After screening, a total of 70 eligible overweight/obese young females (19–25 years old) were included. Written informed consent was obtained from all participants before they were randomly allocated to either one of the four groups, namely the normal diet control group (CON, n = 17), the low-carbohydrate diet control group (LC-CON, n = 18), the low-carbohydrate diet and HIIT group (LC-HIIT, n = 18), and the low-carbohydrate diet and MICT group (LC-MICT, n = 17). Twelve participants discontinued the intervention for different reasons, 58 participants completed the intervention and all measurements were included in the data analysis (Figure 1).

2.2. Experimental Design

This interventional study used a four-arm pre- and post-test comparison design. The experimental procedure was composed of a preparation period, preintervention measurements (including blood assay, anthropometric assessments, and a maximal incremental exercise test to determine VO_{2peak}), a 4 week (28 days) diet intervention with or without exercise training, and postintervention measurements (Figure 1).

During the preparation period, all subjects took nutrition classes and received detailed diet instructions and individual counselling from registered dietitians. Moreover, subjects were instructed to record their normal diet and daily activities for 2 weeks before intervention as baseline, and provided self-reported menstrual phases for the past 3 months. After the preparation period, subjects undertook preintervention measures of anthropometric indices, CRF levels, and blood profiles, which finished within 3–5 days prior to intervention. For the 4 week intervention period, subjects in the CON group served as controls remaining on a normal diet, and subjects in the LC-CON group were switched to LC, but with no exercise training. Besides of changing from normal diet to LC, subjects in the LC-HIIT and LC-MICT groups performed additional supervised HIIT or MICT exercise 5 days/week. The postintervention measurements were carried out in the same way as the preintervention measurements and were completed within 72–96 h following the last intervention day. All pre–post intervention measurements were performed within the same phase of each subject's menstrual cycle (i.e., the luteal phase), which was estimated according to the self-reported menstrual phase obtained in the preparation period.

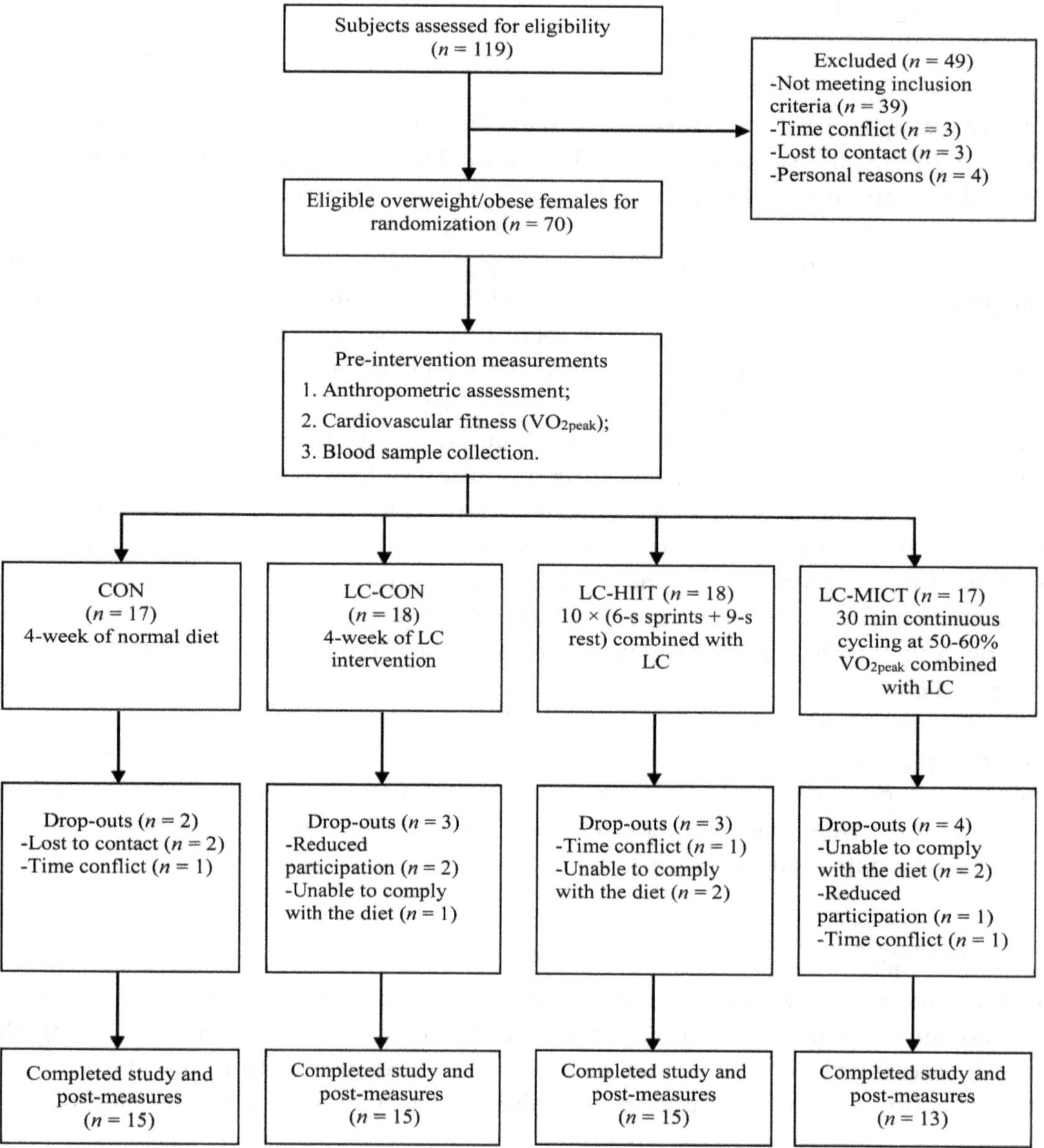

Figure 1. Flow-chart of the study.

2.3. *Diet Intervention*

Except for the CON group, subjects in the LC-CON, LC-HIIT, and LC-MICT groups were instructed to consume LC, in which carbohydrates comprised approximately 10% of the calories (~50 g/d), and about 65% of the calories were obtained from fats, with the remaining ~25% from proteins. During the preparation periods, subjects received nutrition education, and individual dietary instructions regarding how to consume meals within the targeted nutrition goals from registered dietitians. Handouts outlining the main aspects of a LC and specific lists of suitable foods, drinks, cooking recipes, and sample meals for LC were also provided to all subjects. They were free to choose food with low carbohydrate contents according to their own preferences, but were required to not change the daily energy intake as measured in the normal diet (2 weeks before the intervention). The appropriate foods for LC comprised pork, beef, fish, fowl (e.g., chickens, ducks), eggs, seafoods, cheese, all kinds of fat, oils, nonstarchy and green vegetables, nuts/seeds, water and drinks with low carbohydrate contents (e.g., green/red tea, black coffee). Although the types of fat from saturated or unsaturated sources were not restricted, subjects were encouraged to add five tablespoons of olive oil to their diet each day. Foods with high carbohydrate contents were avoided during the study period, including rice, noodles, bread, desserts, cereals, sweets, honey, beans, corns, starchy vegetables, fruits (with the exception of blueberry, lemon, and avocado), milk, yoghourt, juices, soft drinks, and alcoholic beverages.

To ensure compliance with LC, all subjects took urinary ketone assessments daily and kept 3 day food records (2 weekdays and 1 weekend day). Subjects received self-testing reagent strips (UROPAPER, Suzhou First Pharmaceutical Co. Ltd., Suzhou, China) to measure their urinary ketones daily in the early morning or after dinner [26], and the results were recorded in the offered logbook. In addition, subjects were instructed to keep 3 day food records, 2 weeks before intervention and 4 weeks during intervention. Thorough instructions on how to report food/beverage items in food records were given to the subjects in the preparation period, and they were also provided with digital scales and food measuring utensils to assure that the amounts and weights of the food/beverages ingested were documented accurately. Subjects were required to return to the laboratory each week to hand in food diaries, measure body weight, and evaluate dietary compliance. Food records were analyzed for energy intake and macronutrient content by the same dietician using the nutrition analysis and management software (NRISM, version 3.1, Beijing, China). On the basis of these results, the dieticians would offer the subjects individualized follow-up counselling and dietary suggestions. Any questions related to the experiment would be answered via WeChat, phone, e-mail, or face-to-face meetings throughout the study period.

Besides dietary and/or training intervention, subjects were required to maintain their normal daily routines and not to participate in any additional exercises throughout the study period. Their physical activities were assessed daily using validated pedometers (Yamax Digi-Walker SW-200, Tokyo, Japan). A logbook with calendar was provided to the subjects to record the results of daily urinary ketone tests, daily activities, any adverse effects or symptoms, and to document food intakes.

2.4. Exercise Intervention

Besides consuming LC, subjects in the LC-HIIT and LC-MICT groups took extra exercise training at the Kinesiology lab at a strictly controlled room temperature (22 °C) and humidity (50–60%). The training intervention was performed 5 days/week for a duration of 4 weeks under the supervision of two trained research assistants. For the LC-HIIT group, subjects performed intermittent sprint cycling on a cycle ergometer (Monark 894E, Varberg, Sweden). Each training session comprised 10 bouts of 6 s cycling sprints followed by 9 s passive recoveries (a total of 2.5 min/session). Subjects pedaled as fast as possible during the 6 s sprint phases and rested on the seat during the 9 s recovery periods. The initial workload was set at 1 kg. If the cycling speed of all exercise bouts exceeded 100 rpm for two consecutive training sessions, the workload was increased by 0.5 kg until arriving at a workload equivalent to 5% of the subject's body weight. Ratings of perceived exertion (RPE, Borg 6–20 scale) [27] were recorded before and immediately after the 5th and 10th exercise bouts. The power output and heart rate (HR) for each exercise bout were recorded automatically by the Monark Anaerobic Test software. For the LC-MICT group, subjects cycled continuously for 30 min on a Monark cycle ergometer (839E, Varberg, Sweden). The exercise intensity was 50% of VO_{2peak} for the first 10 training sessions and increased to 60% of VO_{2peak} for the last 10 training sessions. The cycling speed was maintained at 50 ± 5 rpm throughout each training session. RPE and HR were recorded for every 5 min.

To assess the exercise energy expenditure of HIIT and MICT, oxygen uptake (VO_2) during exercise was measured breath-by-breath using a gas analyzer (Vmax Encore, CareFusion Corp., San Diego, CA, USA) in the 1st, 10th, and 20th training sessions. The exercise energy expenditure was computed as 4.8 ($Kcal \cdot L^{-1}$) × VO_2 ($L \cdot min^{-1}$) × exercise time (min), where VO_2 was the mean oxygen consumption value throughout the training session, and the exercise time was 2.5 min for HIIT and 30 min for MICT.

2.5. Pre- and Post-Intervention Measurements

2.5.1. Blood Profiles

Blood samples were collected before and 72 h after the last intervention by a certificated nurse. Strenuous physical activity, caffeine, and alcohol were confined 48 h prior to blood sampling. The subjects were required to arrive at the laboratory before 7:30 a.m. after a 12 h overnight fast, and 5 mL blood samples were extracted from the cubital vein using serum separation tubes. The blood samples were set aside clotting for 1 h at room temperature and subsequently centrifuged at 3000 rpm for 5 min, separated for serum and frozen immediately at −80 °C for further analysis.

An automatic biochemical analyzer (Olympus AU400, Olympus, Tokyo, Japan) was used to assay blood glucose, total cholesterol (CHOL), total triglyceride (TG), HDL-C, and low-density lipoprotein cholesterol (LDL-C) profiles. The coefficients of variations for intra-assay and inter-assay were all below 3%. All blood samples were assayed in standard procedures in accordance with the manufacturer's instructions (KingMed Diagnostics Co., Ltd., Guangzhou, China).

2.5.2. Anthropometric Assessments

After blood sampling, each subject underwent anthropometric assessments in the same morning. Height and weight were measured via standard methods (without shoes and in light clothing), using a wall-mounted stadiometer and an electronic scale, and the values were accurate to 0.1 cm and 0.1 kg, respectively. The BMI (in kg/m^2) was calculated as weight (kg) divided by height squared (m^2). Waist circumference (WC) was measured at the level midway between the rib cage and the iliac crest when the participant was gently breathing out. Hip circumference (HC) was determined as the maximum circumference over the buttocks; the WC and HC values were recorded to the nearest 0.5 cm. Waist-to-hip ratio (WHR) was calculated as WHR = WC/HC (in cm). The pre–post intervention anthropometric assessments were performed by the same research staff.

2.5.3. Maximal Incremental Exercise Test

All subjects undertook two maximal incremental exercise tests before and 72 h after the last intervention session to determine their VO_{2peak} and CRF levels. After warming-up at 25 W for 3 min, subjects began to pedal on a computer-controlled cycle ergometer (Monark 839E, Varberg, Sweden) with the starting workload of 50 W. The workload during exercise would be increased by 25 W for every 3 min until the subjects reached their endurance limit, followed by a 3 min recovery period at 25 W. Throughout the test, the cycling cadence was maintained at 60 ± 5 rpm, and the respiratory gases were continuously analyzed by the Vmax Encore System (CareFusion Corp., San Diego, CA, USA). The highest oxygen consumption value averaged over 15 s of the final stage was considered as the VO_{2peak} [28].

2.6. Statistical Analysis

The PASW software (Release 22.0; IBM, New York, NY, USA) was used to perform statistical analyses. Prior to the main statistical analyses, the normality assumption of outcome variables was confirmed using the Shapiro–Wilk test. Analysis of covariance (ANCOVA) with the preintervention values as covariate was used to examine the group differences of main outcome variables among the four groups. One-way ANOVA tests were computed to assess the differences of changes in outcome variables after intervention and the daily activities, energy intake and macronutrient proportion among the four groups. Independent samples *T*-test was used to detect the differences of exercise training data between LC-HIIT and LC-MICT. Partial η^2 values were used to assess effect sizes of the main and interaction effects; η^2 was considered small if <0.06 and large if >0.14 [29]. Cohen's *d* values were also calculated to evaluate the effect sizes for the difference between variables, which was considered small when *d* was 0.2–0.3, medium when *d* was around 0.5 and large when $d > 0.8$ [30]. The outcome variables are shown as means (standard deviations, SDs), and the statistical significance level was set at $p < 0.05$.

3. Results

3.1. Compliance, Diet Compositions, and Daily Physical Activities

Approximately 3 days after LC consumption, subjects were able to detect ketone bodies in the urine. When the data of the three initial transition days were excluded, urinary ketosis was detected on 97.6 ± 4.5%, 96.2 ± 8.3%, and 96.9 ± 6.0% of the days in the LC-CON, LC-HIIT, and LC-MICT groups, respectively, whereas the percentage was only 2.6 ± 9.2% in the CON group, indicating that subjects in LC dietary groups had good compliance with LC.

At baseline, the reported normal dietary energy intake and nutrient compositions were similar among the three LC groups. Average energy intake in the habitual diet was 2057 ± 437 kcal, with carbohydrates, proteins, and fats accounting for 45.9 ± 8.0% (236 ± 59 g), 15.0 ± 2.7% (77 ± 23 g), and 36.9 ± 6.9% (84 ± 25 g) of the total energy intake, respectively. During the intervention period, mean energy intake and the proportion of energy intake derived from carbohydrate, protein, and fat were 1776 ± 284 kcal, 9.3 ± 5.5% (41 ± 24 g), 22.8 ± 3.2% (100 ± 21 g), and 68.1 ± 4.6% (135 ± 25 g) in the LC-CON group; 1871 ± 246 kcal, 10.5 ± 3.2% (49 ± 17 g), 23.3 ± 4.7% (109 ± 28 g), and 66.1 ± 6.1% (137 ± 17 g) in the LC-HIIT group; and 2028 ± 284 kcal, 10.3 ± 2.9% (52 ± 15 g), 23.5 ± 3.2% (119 ± 23 g), and 66.3 ± 3.1% (149 ± 23 g) in the LC-MICT group; whereas the CON group remained at 1990 ± 345 kcal, 43.1 ± 7.9% (216 ± 48 g), 15.9 ± 3.6% (78 ± 23 g), and 40.2 ± 5.7% (88 ± 20 g) (Figure 2A–D). Daily energy intakes were not changed from the habitual diet in all groups ($p > 0.05$), whereas macronutrient intakes were changed significantly, with higher protein ($p < 0.05$) and fat ($p < 0.01$) consumptions and lower carbohydrate consumption ($p < 0.01$) as compared to the normal diet and the CON group (data are presented in Supplementary Materials Table S1).

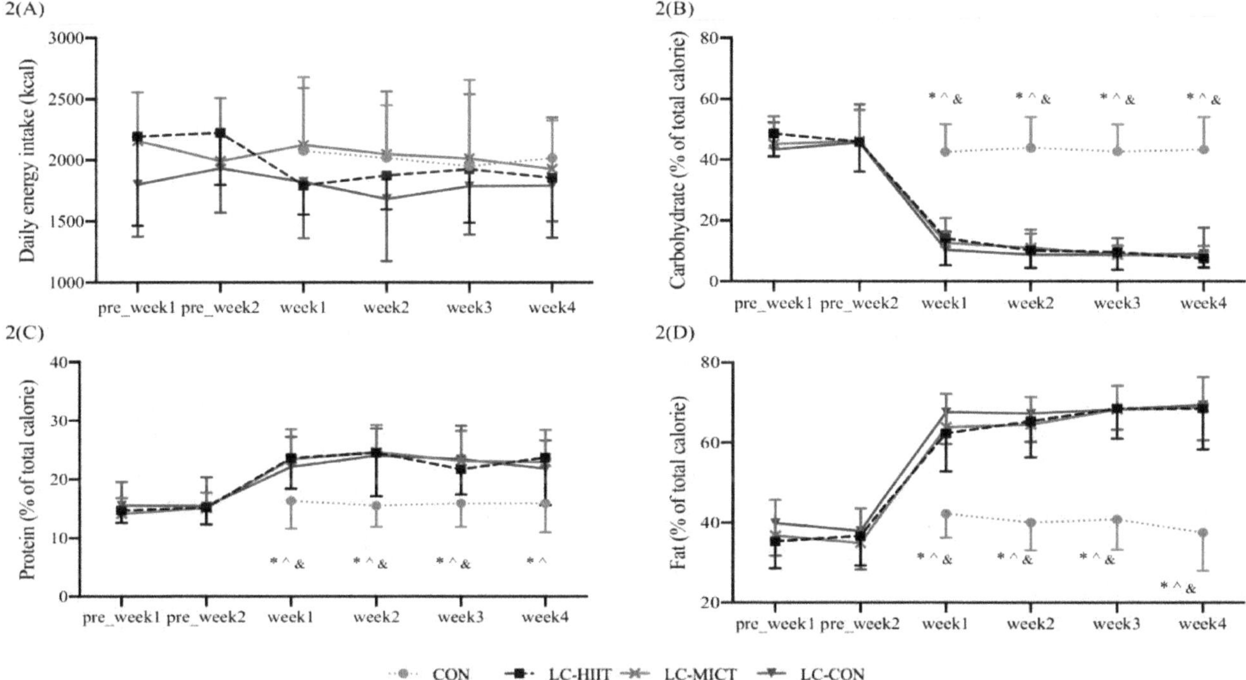

Figure 2. Daily dietary intake (**A**), and proportions of carbohydrate (**B**), protein (**C**), and fat (**D**) in energy intake before and during the intervention. * $p < 0.05$ compared to LC-HIIT, ^ $p < 0.05$ compared to LC-MICT, and $p < 0.05$ compared to LC-CON.

There were no statistical differences in terms of daily physical activities among the CON group (7770–8867 steps), the LC-HIIT group (7779–9156 steps), the LC-MICT group (8028–9317 steps), and the LC-CON group (7694–8852 steps) at baseline or any subsequent time point (data are presented in Supplementary Materials Table S2).

3.2. Training Data

For the two groups with additional exercise training (i.e., LC-HIIT and LC-MICT), the total training time spent in MICT (600 min) was 12 times that spent in HIIT (50 min). Similarly, the exercise energy expenditure of MICT (148.6 ± 15.5 kcal/session) was significantly larger than that of HIIT (17.6 ± 2.2 kcal/session, $p < 0.01$). The exercise intensity corresponded to 86.8 ± 9.5% and 59.5 ± 6.6% of VO_{2peak} for the LC-HIIT group and the LC-MICT group, respectively. During exercise training, subjects in the LC-HIIT group maintained a higher mean HR level (146 ± 5 bpm) than those of the LC-MICT group (139 ± 8 bpm, $p < 0.01$), and HIIT training was perceived to be harder than MICT training, as reflected by the self-reported RPE value (14 ± 1 in the LC-HIIT group vs. 11 ± 1 in the LC-MICT group, $p < 0.01$) (Table 1).

Table 1. Training data during exercise intervention.

	LC-HIIT	LC-MICT
Weekly training time (min)	12.5	150
Total training time (min)	50	600
Energy expenditure (kcal)	17.6 (2.2) **	148.6 (15.5)
Training power (W)	248.7 (34.1) **	53.8 (9.7)
Intensity (% VO_{2peak})	86.8 (9.5) **	59.5 (6.6)
Training HR (bpm)	146 (5) **	139 (8)
Training HR/HRmax (%)	81.7 (3.5) **	74.9 (3.1)
Training RPE	14 (1) **	11 (1)

All values are presented as means (standard deviations). LC-HIIT: low-carbohydrate diet combined with high-intensity interval training, LC-MICT: low-carbohydrate diet combined with moderate- intensity continuous training, HR: heart rate, RPE: ratings of perceived exertion. Comparison with LC-MICT at ** $p < 0.01$.

3.3. Anthropometric Parameters

After intervention, all three LC groups (i.e., LC-CON, LC-HIIT, and LC-MICT) experienced remarkable reductions in body weight ($p < 0.01$, $\eta^2 = 0.510$) and BMI ($p < 0.01$, $\eta^2 = 0.504$), whereas no change in body weight or BMI was found in the CON group (Table 2). On post-test, body weight was reduced by 2.85 ± 1.5, 2.85 ± 1.1, and 2.56 ± 1.3 kg in the LC-CON group, LC-HIIT group, and LC-MICT group, respectively (Table 3). Correspondingly, postintervention BMI was decreased by 1.09 ± 0.56, 1.07 ± 0.41, and 0.98 ± 0.49 kg/m^2 in the groups of LC-CON, LC-HIIT, and LC-MICT, respectively (Table 3). The LC intervention also significantly lowered WC ($p < 0.01$, $\eta^2 = 0.523$), HC ($p < 0.01$, $\eta^2 = 0.338$), and WHR ($p < 0.01$, $\eta^2 = 0.313$) in all three LC groups, while it remained unchanged in the CON group (Table 2). The decrements of body weight, BMI, WC, HC, and WHR of the three LC groups were significantly more than that of the CON group ($p < 0.05$); however, there was no group difference among the three groups consuming LC ($p > 0.05$, Table 3).

Table 2. Outcome variables before and after four weeks of intervention.

	CON (n = 15)		LC-CON (n = 15)		LC-HIIT (n = 15)		LC-MICT (n = 13)		Group Effect	
	Pre	Post	Pre	Post	Pre	Post	Pre	Post	p	*Partial* η^2
Age (y)	21.6 (3.9)		20.9 (3.7)		20.8 (2.7)		21.5 (3.1)			
Height (cm)	163 (5.6)		161.3 (4.7)		162.9 (6.2)		160.9 (4.3)			
Weight (kg)	66.0 (10.2)	66.1 (10.8)	65.1 (7.3)	62.3 (6.7) *	67.9 (10.3)	65.0 (9.7) *	64.5 (6.4)	61.9 (6.0) *	0.000	0.510
BMI ($kg \cdot m^{-2}$)	24.8 (3.2)	24.8 (3.4)	25.0 (2.9)	24.0 (2.7) *	25.5 (3.1)	24.4 (2.9) *	24.9 (1.9)	23.9 (1.8) *	0.000	0.504
WC (cm)	77.7 (9.0)	78.5 (9.2)	78.0 (6.9)	74.0 (6.2) *	79.5 (9.4)	75.7 (9.5) *	75.5 (6.3)	71.2 (4.8) *	0.000	0.523
HC (cm)	100.5 (6.1)	100.4 (6.9)	100.7 (3.9)	98.2 (3.9) *	100.3 (4.8)	98.5 (5.3) *	101.0 (5.1)	97.7 (5.3) *	0.000	0.338
WHR	0.77 (0.1)	0.78 (0.1)	0.77 (0.0)	0.75 (0.0) *	0.79 (0.1)	0.77 (0.1) *	0.75 (0.0)	0.73 (0.0) *	0.000	0.313
VO_{2peak} ($mL \cdot min^{-1} \cdot kg^{-1}$)	25.6 (4.0)	25.4 (4.2)	25.2 (4.3)	24.8 (2.4)	23.3 (2.5)	26.7 (3.4) *#	23.4 (4.4)	27.1 (3.8) *#	0.009	0.193
FG ($mmol \cdot L^{-1}$)	4.6 (0.5)	4.7 (0.3)	4.7 (0.4)	4.6 (0.4)	4.9 (0.5)	4.7 (0.6)	4.8 (0.3)	4.8 (0.3)	0.307	0.065
CHOL ($mmol \cdot L^{-1}$)	4.6 (0.8)	4.9 (0.7)	5.1 (1.0)	6.1 (1.3)	4.5 (0.7)	5.3 (1.0)	4.5 (0.6)	5.1 (1.0)	0.087	0.115
HDL-C ($mmol \cdot L^{-1}$)	1.6 (0.4)	1.6 (0.4)	1.7 (0.3)	1.7 (0.3)	1.5 (0.3)	1.5 (0.4)	1.5 (0.3)	1.7 (0.4)	0.470	0.046
LDL-C ($mmol \cdot L^{-1}$)	2.7 (0.7)	3.0 (0.6)	3.3 (1.0)	4.2 (1.2)	2.8 (0.6)	3.6 (0.8)	2.8 (0.5)	3.4 (0.9)	0.084	0.117
TG ($mmol \cdot L^{-1}$)	1.1 (1.0)	1.1 (1.0)	1.0 (0.5)	1.1 (0.6)	1.2 (0.4)	0.9 (0.3)	0.9 (0.4)	0.8 (0.2)	0.229	0.077

Outcome variables are presented as means (standard deviations). Significant difference from CON at * $p < 0.01$, significant difference from LC-CON at # $p < 0.01$. Partial η^2 value for effect size (ES). CON: control group, LC-CON: low-carbohydrate diet control group, LC-HIIT: low-carbohydrate diet combined with high-intensity interval training, LC-MICT: low-carbohydrate diet combined with moderate-intensity continuous training, BMI: body mass index, WC: waist circumference, HC: hip circumference, WHR: waist-to-hip ratio, VO_{2peak}: peak oxygen uptake, FG: fasting glucose, CHOL: total cholesterol, HDL-C: high-intensity lipoprotein cholesterol, LDL-C: low-intensity lipoprotein cholesterol, TG: triglycerides.

Table 3. Changes in outcome variables after intervention.

	CON (n = 15)	LC-CON (n = 15)	LC-HIIT (n = 15)	LC-MICT (n = 13)	ES (d)		
					LC-CON	LC-HIIT	LC-MICT
Δ Weight (kg)	0.09 (1.25)	−2.85 (1.50) **	−2.85 (1.12) **	−2.56 (1.31) **	2.12	2.48	2.07
Δ BMI ($kg \cdot m^{-2}$)	0.02 (0.48)	−1.09 (0.56) **	−1.07 (0.41) **	−0.98 (0.49) **	2.14	2.45	2.08
Δ WC (cm)	0.8 (1.47)	−4.02 (2.36) **	−3.81 (1.98) **	−4.36 (2.87) **	2.45	2.65	2.32
Δ HC (cm)	−0.13 (1.52)	−2.51 (1.93) **	−1.83 (1.78) *	−3.27 (1.40) **	1.37	1.03	2.14
Δ WHR	0.01 (0.01)	−0.02 (0.03) **	−0.02 (0.02) **	−0.02 (0.03) **	1.35	1.96	1.41
Δ VO_{2peak} ($ml \cdot min^{-1} \cdot kg^{-1}$)	−0.21 (2.46)	−0.37 (3.75)	3.41 (2.22) **#	3.67 (3.00) **#	0.05	1.55	1.43
Δ VO_{2peak}%	−0.62 (9.26)	−0.37 (14.06)	14.76 (9.62) **#	17.32 (14.24) **#	0.08	1.63	1.52
Δ FG ($mmol \cdot L^{-1}$)	0.11 (0.31)	−0.13 (0.41)	−0.21 (0.42)	−0.07 (0.30)	0.68	0.86	0.60
Δ CHOL ($mmol \cdot L^{-1}$)	0.31 (0.64)	0.98 (1.07)	0.77 (0.84)	0.61 (0.63)	0.75	0.62	0.47
Δ HDL-C ($mmol \cdot L^{-1}$)	0.01 (0.17)	0.04 (0.25)	0.09 (0.18)	0.13 (0.16)	0.14	0.48	0.70
Δ LDL-C ($mmol \cdot L^{-1}$)	0.31 (0.52)	0.89 (0.98)	0.78 (0.72)	0.58 (0.54)	0.74	0.74	0.50
Δ TG ($mmol \cdot L^{-1}$)	−0.03 (0.24)	0.09 (0.65)	−0.23 (0.43)	−0.16 (0.28)	0.25	0.55	0.49

Outcome variables are presented as mean ± standard deviation. Significant difference from CON at * $p < 0.05$, ** $p < 0.01$, significant difference from LC-CON at # $p < 0.01$. Cohen's d value for effect size (ES) when compared to the CON group. Delta (Δ): change from pre–post intervention, CON: control group, LC-CON: low-carbohydrate diet control group, LC-HIIT: low-carbohydrate diet combined with high-intensity interval training, LC-MICT: low-carbohydrate diet combined with moderate-intensity continuous training, BMI: body mass index, WC: waist circumference, HC: hip circumference, WHR: waist-to-hip ratio, VO_{2peak}: peak oxygen uptake, FG: fasting glucose, CHOL: total cholesterol, HDL-C: high-intensity lipoprotein cholesterol, LDL-C: low-intensity lipoprotein cholesterol, TG: triglycerides.

3.4. Cardiorespiratory Fitness Levels

We observed that only the two groups with extra training (i.e., LC-HIIT, LC-MICT) improved CRF, as reflected by VO_{2peak}, which remained unchanged in the control groups of CON and LC-CON. The VO_{2peak} was increased by 14.8% (+3.40 ± 2.22 mL·min^{-1}·kg^{-1}) and 17.3% (+3.70 ± 3.00 mL·min^{-1}·kg^{-1}) in the LC-HIIT group and LC-MICT group, respectively, which was significantly larger than that of the CON group (−0.21 ± 2.46 mL·min^{-1}·kg^{-1}) and the LC-CON group (−0.37 ± 3.75 mL·min^{-1}·kg^{-1}, $p < 0.05$, $\eta^2 = 0.193$) (Table 3).

3.5. Blood Lipids and Fasting Glucose

Blood lipid and fasting glucose levels did not differ among the four groups at baseline and postintervention ($p > 0.05$, Tables 2 and 3).

3.6. Adverse Events

During the study period, we received a total of 20 complaints from 16 subjects in the LC-CON (seven complaints), LC-HIIT (seven complaints) and LC-MICT (six complaints) groups, whereas no feedback of adverse events was offered by subjects in the CON group. Luckily, none of them were adverse clinical events. The main symptoms experienced were similar to those reported in previous studies [8,12,17], including fatigue (7, or 35%), reduced appetite (4, or 20%), constipation (6, or 30%), diarrhea (2, or 10%), and headache (1, or 5%).

4. Discussion

This study proved that using a four week non-calorie-restricted LC intervention, with or without extra exercise, is able to rapidly improve a series of anthropometric profiles in overweight/obese Chinese young females. In particular, we observed significant reductions in body weight, BMI, WC, HC, and WHR, which are related to the risks of developing CVD and T2D. Moreover, this study firstly combined a brief HIIT or traditional MICT with LC. Although the collaborated training had no synergistic effects on anthropometric and blood parameters, groups with extra training (i.e., LC-HIIT and LC-MICT) showed additional improvements in CRF as compared to LC intervention alone (i.e., LC-CON). Most importantly, the LC-HIIT group obtained the same improvement in CRF to that of the LC-MICT group in less time and with a lower training amount. Thus, LC in combination with HIIT may represent an optimal choice for weight loss and CRF improvement.

Unlike the majority of previous studies which evaluated the effects of LC dietary patterns when delivered with ad libitum eating patterns or with energy restriction, this study was designed to assess whether short-term LC is also effective in the overweight/obese Chinese population without changing their habitual calorie intake. The present data showed that with professional support, the overweight/obese Chinese females in all three LC groups lost more than 2.5 kg of body weight, or ~1 unit of BMI following four weeks of LC administration. The amount of weight reduction was similar to that of other non-energy-restricted studies which reported ~2.0 kg weight losses in western adults after adopting LC for six weeks [17,31], but smaller than ~8.0 kg weight reductions in obese Chinese adults following eight weeks [11] and 12 weeks [13] of calorie-reduced LCs. With unchanged calorie intake, the weight-loss effects of the present study should be interpreted as resulting from changes in macronutrient composition. In addition to weight loss, significant reductions in WC and WHR were also detected in the overweight/obese females. As surrogate markers of visceral adipose tissue [32], decrements in WC and WHR are meaningful to reduce cardiac and metabolic risks [33]. The plausible mechanisms responsible for body composition improvements following non-caloric-restricted LC may include a decrease in lipogenesis and an increase in lipolysis, as regulated by LC-induced changes in insulin and other hormones [34], as well as an increased reliance on gluconeogenesis for energy production under high-fat, low-carbohydrate conditions, which is an energy-demanding process costing ~400–600 kcal/day of extra energy [35,36]. Nonetheless, we found no collaborative weight-loss effects of exercise training in either the LC-HIIT group or the LC-MICT group. This finding was consistent with our previous observation that short-term exercise training was unlikely to result in weight loss [37,38].

Many studies, varying in intervention length, have shown that LC dietary approaches were beneficial to blood glucose and lipid regulation [8,9,11,12,31], whereas several other studies have reported elevated LDL-C and/or TC levels in response to LC [16,17,39]. However, the present study did not detect any changes in circulating levels of glucose and blood lipids, even in the groups with extra training. The reasons for the diverse results of blood profiles among studies remain unknown, but may include differences in LC dietary approaches, intervention durations, subjects' health status and the baseline blood glucose and lipid values. The current study illustrated that the four week LC had no adverse effects on blood profiles in the overweight/obese, otherwise healthy females with an initially normal baseline level.

The CRF, as measured during incremental exercise to exhaustion, is a strong and independent marker for CVD and all-cause mortality [40,41]. However, with an insufficient energy supply, the LC-induced changes in energy metabolism have been reported to subsequently impair CRF [17,23]. In contrast, the present study found an unchanged CRF level in the LC-CON group, which was supported by other studies [39,42]. These findings indicate that LC dietary interventions are unlikely to improve CRF, if not reduce it. Therefore, the significant increments of CRF observed in the LC-HIIT group and the LC-MICT group could be attributed to the additional exercise training, despite having no additional effects on weight loss and other cardiometabolic profiles. As revealed by meta-analysis, every 1 metabolic equivalent (MET) increment in CRF was associated with a 13% and 15% risk reduction in all-cause and CVD mortality, respectively [40]. Thus, the ~3.5 $mL \cdot min^{-1} \cdot kg^{-1}$ (corresponding to ~1 MET) increment of CRF yielded in the LC-HIIT and LC-MICT groups may lower the risks of all-cause and CVD mortality with important clinical significance. Surprisingly, the brief HIIT improved CRF to the same extent as MICT, but with only 1/12 of the time commitment and less than 1/8 of the exercise energy expenditure, indicating that HIIT is more efficient than the traditional MICT in improving CRF.

Nonetheless, our study has a few limitations. First, subjects in the CON group only recorded their normal diet and physical activity data for four weeks during the study period. From the perspective of study design, it would be better to evaluate their baseline values two weeks prior to intervention, just like the other three groups. Second, given that body composition was not assessed via dual-energy X-ray absorptiometry (DXA) or other techniques, we are unable to specify which composition (e.g., body water, fat mass) was associated with the main weight loss induced by LC. Third, considering that the Chinese population is scarcely involved in LC studies, with an unknown acceptance level, we chose a short-term intervention to start with. Despite the successful weight loss, the longer effects of LC on weight loss and weight maintenance are unclear. In this sense, more randomized controlled trials with longer periods are expected to reveal the long-term weight-loss effects and the underlying mechanisms of LC in the overweight/obese Chinese population.

5. Conclusions

Collectively, the four week non-energy-restricted LC program led to significant weight loss and visceral fat mass loss without adverse clinical events, indicating that the LC dietary patterns could also be effective and feasible for the overweight/obese Chinese population. The strength of this study is combined LC with extra exercise training, and we report, for the first time, that the collaborated HIIT and MICT would result in a marked improvement in CRF, which cannot be attained through LC intervention, despite having no additional effects on weight loss. Such an increment in CRF could be clinically beneficial to the overweight/obese population who are at a higher risk of developing CVD and T2D [2]. Given that the same CRF increment was yielded within much less time when using HIIT (2.5 min/session in HIIT vs. 30 min/session in MICT), we believe that combining LC with brief HIIT is able to trigger additional cardiometabolic health benefits beyond weight reduction, thus representing a better and time-efficient combination for health promotion in people with insufficient time.

Supplementary Materials:
Table S1: Dietary energy intake and nutrient compositions before and during intervention, Table S2: Daily physical activities before and during intervention.

Author Contributions: Conceptualization, S.S., Z.K., Q.S., and J.N.; data curation, S.S., Z.K., M.H., and J.N.; formal analysis, S.S. and Q.S.; funding acquisition, Z.K.; investigation, S.S., M.H., and D.Z.; methodology, S.S., Z.K., Q.S., H.Z., and J.N.; project administration, Z.K. and D.Z.; resources, Z.K.; software, S.S. and Z.K.; supervision, Z.K. and J.N.; validation, S.S. and J.N.; visualization, S.S., Q.S., and J.N.; writing—original draft preparation, S.S., Z.K., and J.N.; writing—review and editing, S.S., Z.K., Q.S., M.H., H.Z., and J.N. All authors read and approved the final version of the manuscript.

Acknowledgments: We are appreciated for the generous support from Grace Chau, Director of Office of Sports Affairs at the University of Macau, and we would like to thank participants of this study for their time.

References

1. Ng, M.; Fleming, T.; Robinson, M.; Thomson, B.; Graetz, N.; Margono, C.; Mullany, E.C.; Biryukov, S.; Abbafati, C.; Abera, S.F. Global, regional, and national prevalence of overweight and obesity in children and adults during 1980–2013: A systematic analysis for the Global Burden of Disease Study 2013. *Lancet* **2014**, *384*, 766–781. [CrossRef]
2. Guh, D.P.; Zhang, W.; Bansback, N.; Amarsi, Z.; Birmingham, C.L.; Anis, A.H. The incidence of co-morbidities related to obesity and overweight: A systematic review and meta-analysis. *BMC Public Health* **2009**, *9*, 88. [CrossRef] [PubMed]
3. Wing, R.R.; Lang, W.; Wadden, T.A.; Safford, M.; Knowler, W.C.; Bertoni, A.G.; Hill, J.O.; Brancati, F.L.; Peters, A.; Wagenknecht, L. Benefits of modest weight loss in improving cardiovascular risk factors in overweight and obese individuals with type 2 diabetes. *Diabetes Care* **2011**, *34*, 1481–1486. [CrossRef] [PubMed]
4. Lindstrom, J.; Ilanneparikka, P.; Peltonen, M.; Aunola, S.; Eriksson, J.G.; Hemio, K.; Hämäläinen, H.; Härkönen, P.; Keinänen-Kiukaanniemi, S.; Laakso, M. Sustained reduction in the incidence of type 2 diabetes by lifestyle intervention: Follow-up of the Finnish Diabetes Prevention Study. *Lancet* **2006**, *368*, 1673–1679. [CrossRef]
5. Espeland, M.A.; Pisunyer, X.; Blackburn, G.L.; Brancati, F.L.; Bray, G.A.; Bright, R. Reduction in weight and cardiovascular disease risk factors in individuals with type 2 diabetes: One-year results of the look AHEAD trial. *Diabetes Care* **2007**, *30*, 1374–1383.
6. Seagle, H.M.; Strain, G.W.; Makris, A.; Reeves, R.S. Position of the American Dietetic Association: Weight management. *J. Am. Diet. Assoc.* **2009**, *109*, 330–346.
7. Bueno, N.B.; de Melo, I.S.V.; de Oliveira, S.L.; da Rocha Ataide, T. Very-low-carbohydrate ketogenic diet v. low-fat diet for long-term weight loss: A meta-analysis of randomised controlled trials. *Br. J. Nutr.* **2013**, *110*, 1178–1187. [CrossRef]
8. Bazzano, L.A.; Hu, T.; Reynolds, K.; Yao, L.; Bunol, C.; Liu, Y.; Chen, C.S.; Klag, M.J.; Whelton, P.K.; He, J. Effects of Low-Carbohydrate and Low-Fat Diets: A Randomized Trial. *Ann. Intern. Med.* **2014**, *161*, 309–318. [CrossRef]
9. Cicero, A.F.G.; Benelli, M.; Brancaleoni, M.; Dainelli, G.; Merlini, D.; Negri, R. Middle and Long-Term Impact of a Very Low-Carbohydrate Ketogenic Diet on Cardiometabolic Factors: A Multi-Center, Cross-Sectional, Clinical Study. *Ann. Rev. Physiol.* **2015**, *22*, 389–394. [CrossRef]
10. Gardner, C.D.; Kiazand, A.; Alhassan, S.; Kim, S.; Stafford, R.S.; Balise, R.R.; Kraemer, H.C.; King, A.C. Comparison of the Atkins, Zone, Ornish, and LEARN diets for change in weight and related risk factors among overweight premenopausal women: The A TO Z Weight Loss Study: A randomized trial. *JAMA* **2007**, *297*, 969–977. [CrossRef]
11. Gu, Y.; Yu, H.; Li, Y.; Ma, X.; Lu, J.; Yu, W.; Xiao, Y.; Bao, Y.; Jia, W. Beneficial Effects of an 8-Week, Very Low Carbohydrate Diet Intervention on Obese Subjects. *Evid.-Based Complement. Altern. Med.* **2013**, *2013*, 760804. [CrossRef] [PubMed]

12. Westman, E.C.; Yancy, W.S.; Mavropoulos, J.C.; Marquart, M.; Mcduffie, J.R. The effect of a low-carbohydrate, ketogenic diet versus a low-glycemic index diet on glycemic control in type 2 diabetes mellitus. *Nutr. Metab.* **2008**, *5*, 36. [CrossRef] [PubMed]
13. Sun, J.; Xu, N.; Lin, N.; Wu, P.; Yuan, K.; An, S.; Zhang, Z.; Ruan, Y.; Zhang, Y.; Xu, G.; et al. 317-LB: Optimal Weight Loss Effect of Short-Term Low Carbohydrate Diet with Calorie Restriction on Overweight/Obese Subjects in South China—A Multicenter Randomized Controlled Trial. *Diabetes* **2019**, *68*. [CrossRef]
14. Popkin, B.M.; Gordon-Larsen, P. The nutrition transition: Worldwide obesity dynamics and their determinants. *Int. J. Obes.* **2004**, *28*, S2–S9. [CrossRef] [PubMed]
15. Zhai, F.; Wang, H.; Du, S.; He, Y.; Wang, Z.; Ge, K.; Popkin, B.M. Prospective study on nutrition transition in China. *Nutr. Rev.* **2009**, *67*, S56–S61. [CrossRef]
16. Brinkworth, G.D.; Noakes, M.; Buckley, J.D.; Keogh, J.B.; Clifton, P.M. Long-term effects of a very-low-carbohydrate weight loss diet compared with an isocaloric low-fat diet after 12 mo. *Am. J. Clin. Nutr.* **2009**, *90*, 23–32. [CrossRef]
17. Urbain, P.; Strom, L.; Morawski, L.; Wehrle, A.; Deibert, P.; Bertz, H. Impact of a 6-week non-energy-restricted ketogenic diet on physical fitness, body composition and biochemical parameters in healthy adults. *Nutr. Metab.* **2017**, *14*, 17. [CrossRef]
18. Sun, S.; Zhang, H.; Kong, Z.; Shi, Q.; Tong, T.K.; Nie, J. Twelve weeks of low volume sprint interval training improves cardio-metabolic health outcomes in overweight females. *J. Sports Sci.* **2019**, *37*, 1257–1264. [CrossRef]
19. Trapp, E.G.; Chisholm, D.J.; Freund, J.; Boutcher, S.H. The effects of high-intensity intermittent exercise training on fat loss and fasting insulin levels of young women. *Int. J. Obes.* **2008**, *32*, 684–691. [CrossRef]
20. Kessler, H.S.; Sisson, S.B.; Short, K.R. The potential for high-intensity interval training to reduce cardiometabolic disease risk. *Sports Med.* **2012**, *42*, 489–509. [CrossRef]
21. Martins, C.; Kazakova, I.; Ludviksen, M.; Mehus, I.; Wisloff, U.; Kulseng, B.; Morgan, L.; King, N. High-intensity interval training and isocaloric moderate-intensity continuous training result in similar improvements in body composition and fitness in obese individuals. *Int. J. Sport Nutr. Exerc. Metab.* **2016**, *26*, 197–204. [CrossRef] [PubMed]
22. Chang, C.; Borer, K.T.; Lin, P.J. Low-Carbohydrate-High-Fat Diet: Can it Help Exercise Performance? *J. Hum. Kinet.* **2017**, *56*, 81–92. [CrossRef] [PubMed]
23. Okeeffe, K.; Keith, R.E.; Wilson, G.D.; Blessing, D.L. Dietary carbohydrate intake and endurance exercise performance of trained female cyclists. *Nutr. Res.* **1989**, *9*, 819–830. [CrossRef]
24. Gist, N.H.; Fedewa, M.V.; Dishman, R.K.; Cureton, K.J. Sprint interval training effects on aerobic capacity: A systematic review and meta-analysis. *Sports Med.* **2014**, *44*, 269–279. [CrossRef]
25. World Healt Organization. *The Asia-Pacific Perspective: Redefining Obesity and Its Treatment*; Health Commurhoadsnications Austrbya: Sydney, Australia, 2000.
26. Urbain, P.; Bertz, H. Monitoring for compliance with a ketogenic diet: What is the best time of day to test for urinary ketosis? *Nutr. Metab.* **2016**, *13*, 77. [CrossRef]
27. Borg, G. Simple Rating Methods for Estimation of Perceived Exertion. In *Physical Work and Effort*; Pergamon Press: Oxford, UK, 1976; pp. 39–46.
28. Rossiter, H.B.; Kowalchuk, J.M.; Whipp, B.J. A test to establish maximum O_2 uptake despite no plateau in the O_2 uptake response to ramp incremental exercise. *J. Appl. Physiol.* **2006**, *100*, 764–770. [CrossRef]
29. Kirk, R.E. Practical significance: A concept whose time has come. *Educ. Psychol. Meas.* **1996**, *56*, 746–759. [CrossRef]
30. Cohen, J. *Statistical Power Analysis for the Behavioral Sciences*; Routledge: London, UK, 2013.
31. Sharman, M.J.; Kraemer, W.J.; Love, D.M.; Avery, N.G.; Gomez, A.L.; Scheett, T.P.; Volek, J.S. A Ketogenic Diet Favorably Affects Serum Biomarkers for Cardiovascular Disease in Normal-Weight Men. *J. Nutr.* **2002**, *132*, 1879–1885. [CrossRef]
32. Nazare, J.; Smith, J.B.; Borel, A.; Aschner, P.; Barter, P.; Van Gaal, L.; Tan, C.E.; Wittchen, H.U.; Matsuzawa, Y.; Kadowaki, T. Usefulness of measuring both body mass index and waist circumference for the estimation of visceral adiposity and related cardiometabolic risk profile (from the INSPIRE ME IAA study). *Am. J. Cardiol.* **2015**, *115*, 307–315. [CrossRef]

33. Neeland, I.J.; Ayers, C.R.; Rohatgi, A.; Turer, A.T.; Berry, J.D.; Das, S.R. Associations of visceral and abdominal subcutaneous adipose tissue with markers of cardiac and metabolic risk in obese adults. *Obesity* **2013**, *21*, E439–E447. [CrossRef]
34. Paoli, A.; Rubini, A.; Volek, J.; Grimaldi, K. Beyond weight loss: A review of the therapeutic uses of very-low-carbohydrate (ketogenic) diets. *Eur. J. Clin. Nutr.* **2013**, *67*, 789. [CrossRef] [PubMed]
35. Veldhorst, M.A.; Westerterp-Plantenga, M.S.; Westerterp, K.R. Gluconeogenesis and energy expenditure after a high-protein, carbohydrate-free diet. *Am. J. Clin. Nutr.* **2009**, *90*, 519–526. [CrossRef] [PubMed]
36. Fine, E.J.; Feinman, R.D. Thermodynamics of weight loss diets. *Nutr. Metab.* **2004**, *1*, 15. [CrossRef] [PubMed]
37. Kong, Z.; Fan, X.; Sun, S.; Song, L.; Shi, Q.; Nie, J. Comparison of high-intensity interval training and moderate-to-vigorous continuous training for cardiometabolic health and exercise enjoyment in obese young women: A randomized controlled trial. *PLoS ONE* **2016**, *11*, e0158589. [CrossRef]
38. Kong, Z.; Sun, S.; Liu, M.; Shi, Q. Short-Term High-Intensity Interval Training on Body Composition and Blood Glucose in Overweight and Obese Young Women. *J. Diabetes Res.* **2016**, *2016*, 4073618. [CrossRef]
39. Klement, R.J.; Frobel, T.; Albers, T.; Fikenzer, S.; Prinzhausen, J.; Kämmerer, U. A pilot case study on the impact of a self-prescribed welketogenic diet on biochemical parameters and running performance in healthy and physically active individuals. *Nutr. Med.* **2013**, *1*, 10.
40. Kodama, S.; Saito, K.; Tanaka, S.; Maki, M.; Yachi, Y.; Asumi, M.; Sugawara, A.; Totsuka, K.; Shimano, H.; Ohashi, Y. Cardiorespiratory fitness as a quantitative predictor of all-cause mortality and cardiovascular events in healthy men and women: A meta-analysis. *JAMA* **2009**, *301*, 2024–2035. [CrossRef]
41. Almallah, M.H.; Sakr, S.; Alqunaibet, A. Cardiorespiratory Fitness and Cardiovascular Disease Prevention: An Update. *Curr. Atheroscler. Rep.* **2018**, *20*, 1. [CrossRef]
42. Brinkworth, G.D.; Noakes, M.; Clifton, P.M.; Buckley, J.D. Effects of a low carbohydrate weight loss diet on exercise capacity and tolerance in obese subjects. *Obesity* **2009**, *17*, 1916–1923. [CrossRef]

2

Sugar-Sweetened Beverages and Cardiometabolic Health: An Update of the Evidence

Vasanti S. Malik [1,2,*] and Frank B. Hu [2,3,4]

1 Department of Nutritional Sciences, Faculty of Medicine, University of Toronto, 1 King's College Circle, Toronto, ON M5S 1A8, Canada
2 Department of Nutrition, Harvard T.H. Chan School of Public Health, 665 Huntington Avenue, Boston, MA 02115, USA
3 Department of Epidemiology, Harvard T.H. School of Public Health, Boston, MA 02115, USA
4 Channing Division of Network Medicine, Brigham and Women's Hospital and Harvard Medical School, Boston, MA 02115, USA
* Correspondence: vasanti.malik@utoronto.ca

Abstract: Sugar-sweetened beverages (SSBs) have little nutritional value and a robust body of evidence has linked the intake of SSBs to weight gain and risk of type 2 diabetes (T2D), cardiovascular disease (CVD), and some cancers. Metabolic Syndrome (MetSyn) is a clustering of risk factors that precedes the development of T2D and CVD; however, evidence linking SSBs to MetSyn is not clear. To make informed recommendations about SSBs, new evidence needs to be considered against existing literature. This review provides an update on the evidence linking SSBs and cardiometabolic outcomes including MetSyn. Findings from prospective cohort studies support a strong positive association between SSBs and weight gain and risk of T2D and coronary heart disease (CHD), independent of adiposity. Associations with MetSyn are less consistent, and there appears to be a sex difference with stroke with greater risk in women. Findings from short-term trials on metabolic risk factors provide mechanistic support for associations with T2D and CHD. Conclusive evidence from cohort studies and trials on risk factors support an etiologic role of SSB in relation to weight gain and risk of T2D and CHD. Continued efforts to reduce intake of SSB should be encouraged to improve the cardiometabolic health of individuals and populations.

Keywords: sugar-sweetened beverages; metabolic syndrome; weight gain; type 2 diabetes; cardiovascular disease; cardiometabolic risk

---

1. Introduction

Metabolic syndrome (MetSyn) is known as a clustering of interrelated risk factors for type 2 diabetes (T2D) and cardiovascular disease (CVD) that occur together more often than by chance alone. Although there is some confusion regarding the clinical definition of MetSyn and whether it is a unique syndrome or a mixture of unrelated phenotypes, the most widespread consensus for a diagnosis is the presence of at least three of five risk factors including hyperglycemia, raised blood pressure, elevated triglyceride levels, low high-density lipoprotein cholesterol levels, and central adiposity [1]. Given the complexity of the definition, the prevalence of MetSyn is difficult to estimate; however, data on individual risk factors suggest that MetSyn is rising across the globe in parallel with obesity trends. It was estimated that 23% of adults in the United States (US) (~50 million) have MetSyn [2,3]. This figure was relatively constant over recent years despite population-level increases in hyperglycemia and waist circumference because of decreases in hypertriglyceridemia and elevated blood pressure corresponding to medication use [4]. However, the burden of MetSyn remains high in the US and is rising in low- and middle-income countries (LMICs) [3]. This is of great concern, since individuals with MetSyn are at twice the risk of developing CVD and have a five-fold higher risk of developing T2D over the next 5–10 years [1]. Preventing or reversing MetSyn could, therefore, be an effective way to stem the rising tide of T2D and CVD.

Sugar-sweetened beverages (SSBs) are the largest source of added sugar in the diet. They include carbonated and non-carbonated soft drinks, fruit drinks, and sports drinks that contain added caloric sweeteners, and they are low in nutritional quality. To date, a large body of evidence supports a strong link between intake of SSBs and weight gain [5] and risk of T2D [6], which is the basis of many dietary guidelines and policies targeting SSBs [7]. Emerging evidence suggests that SSBs are also an important risk factor for cardiovascular diseases and related risk factors [8–12]. However, evidence linking SSBs to MetSyn is not clear. For clinicians and policy-makers to make informed recommendations about SSBs and cardiometabolic health, new evidence needs to be considered alongside existing literature. In this review, we provide an overview of global SSB intake trends and an updated summary on the evidence from prospective cohort studies and trials linking SSBs to weight gain and related cardiometabolic conditions including MetSyn. Findings from cross-sectional or case-control studies were not considered since these designs are more prone to confounding and other biases. Biological mechanisms, alternative beverage options, and policy strategies to limit SSB consumption are also discussed.

2. SSB Intake Trends

Consumption of SSBs has decreased modestly in the US since around 2002 [13]; however, intake levels are still high and, in some groups, nearly exceed the Dietary Guidelines for Americans' [14] and World Health Organization's (WHO) [7] recommendation for no more than 10% of daily calories from all added sugar. National Health and Nutrition Examination Survey (NHANES) data show that US adults consumed an average of 145 kcal/day from SSB, corresponding to 6.5% of total calories, between 2011 and 2014 with higher intake levels reported among younger age groups and among non-Hispanic black and Hispanic men and women [15].

In contrast to the US and other high-income countries where consumption of SSBs is either declining or plateauing, intake of SSBs is increasing in many LMICs as a consequence of widespread urbanization and beverage marketing. A report based on survey data from adults in 187 countries found that SSB consumption was higher in upper–middle-income countries and lower–middle-income countries compared to high-income or low-income countries [16]. Of the 21 world regions evaluated, SSB consumption was highest in the Caribbean and lowest in East Asia [16]. Another study among adolescents in 53 LMICs found that soda intake was most frequent in Central and South America, and least frequent in Southeast Asia. Across all populations surveyed, 54% consumed soda at least once a day, and one in five adolescents in Central and South America consumed soda three or more times per day [17]. These trends are supported by another study that reported that per capita sales of SSB (in daily calories per person) increased in most LMICs, while sales declined in some high-income regions, indicative of consumption patterns [18]. Chile was identified as having the highest per capita sales of SSB in 2014, followed by Mexico, the US, Argentina, and Saudi Arabia [18]. The fastest growth in sales of SSB between 2009 and 2014 was seen in Chile, along with China, Thailand, and Brazil [18] (Figure 1). For some regions, disparities in SSB intake tend to track with disparities in obesity and T2D prevalence. For example, in the US, lower socioeconomic status (SES) groups tend to have higher SSB intake levels, and these groups also tend to have a higher risk for developing obesity and T2D.

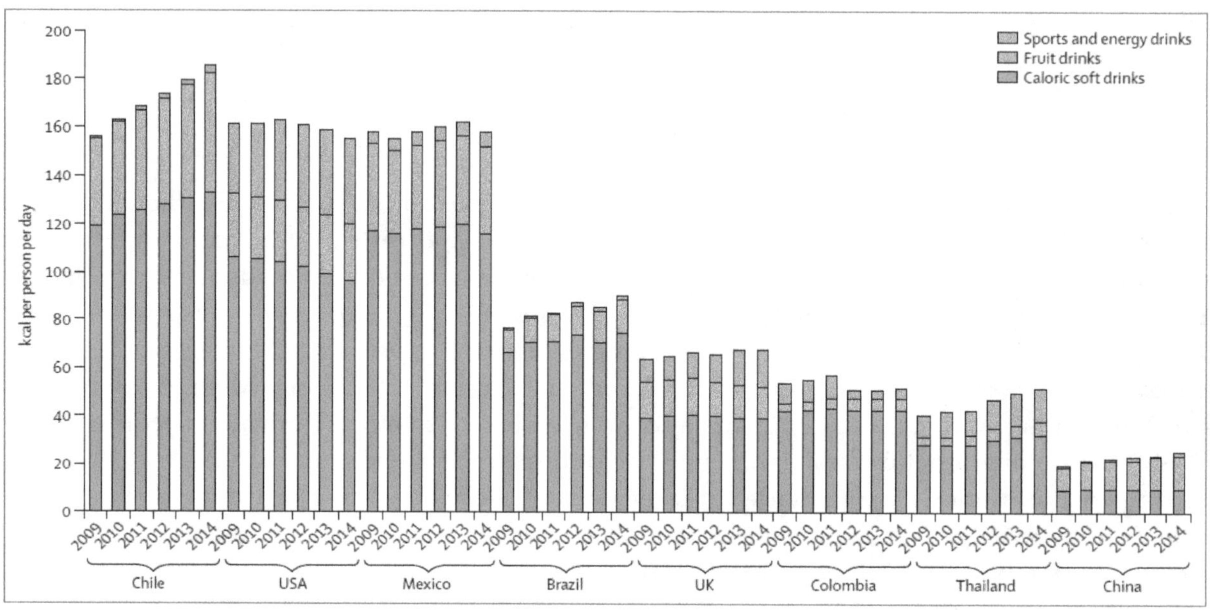

Figure 1. Sales of sugar-sweetened beverages (SSBs) in kcal per person per day by beverage type in 2009–2014 in selected countries. Data from Euromonitor Passport International, which were obtained from nutrition fact panels and websites of sugar-sweetened beverage companies; kcal = kilocalories [18].

3. Weight Gain and Obesity

Many observational studies have evaluated the relationship between consumption of SSBs and weight gain or obesity. The majority [5,19–23] of systematic reviews and meta-analyses on this topic found positive associations between SSBs and weight gain or risk of overweight or obesity. However, others reported null associations [24]. Our previous meta-analysis, the most comprehensive to date, found that a one-serving-per-day increase in SSB was associated with an additional weight gain of 0.12 kg over one year [5]. In this analysis, we included estimates that were not adjusted for total energy intake since the association between SSBs and weight gain is likely mediated through calories. In addition, all of the studies included in the meta-analysis had repeated measurements of diet and weight, and evaluated weight change in relation to change in SSB intake. This type of analysis strategy has some of the features of a quasi-experimental design, although it lacks the element of randomization. An advantage of this design is the generalizability to a real-world setting, because participants are able to change their diet and lifestyle without investigator-driven intervention. Although the results of the meta-analysis seem modest, adult weight gain in the general population is a gradual process, occurring over decades and averaging about one pound (0.45 kg) per year [25]; thus, small gains in weight from SSBs could be substantial over many years.

The association between SSBs and obesity is strengthened by our previous analysis of gene–SSB interactions [26]. Based on data from three large cohorts, we found that individuals who consumed one or more servings of SSB per day had genetic effects on body mass index (BMI) and obesity risk that were twice as large as those who consumed SSBs less than once per month. These data suggest that regular consumers of SSB may be more susceptible to genetic effects on obesity, or that persons with a greater genetic predisposition to obesity may be more susceptible to the deleterious effects of SSBs on BMI.

Compared to observational studies, most trials have evaluated short-term effects on weight change rather than long-term patterns. In our previous meta-analysis of five trials, we found that adding SSBs to the diet significantly increased body weight [5]. Another meta-analysis of seven randomized controlled trials (RCTs) also found a significant increase in body weight when SSBs were added to the diet [24]. However, in their meta-analysis of eight trials attempting to reduce SSB intake, no overall effect on BMI was observed, but a significant benefit on weight loss/less weight gain was observed among individuals who were overweight at baseline [24]. Of note, this meta-analysis included two of the largest and most rigorously conducted RCTs in children and adolescents [27,28] to date.

Another meta-analysis evaluating the effects of dietary sugars on body weight found that, in trials of adults with ad libitum diets, reducing intake of free sugar or SSB was associated with a decrease in body weight, while increasing intake was associated with a comparable weight increase [23]. Because isoenergetic exchange of dietary sugars with other carbohydrates showed no change in body weight, it seems likely that the change in body weight that occurs with modifying intakes of SSBs is mediated via changes in calories [23]. The majority of studies on SSBs and body weight focused on prevention of weight gain rather than weight loss, which is an important distinguishing factor. From a public health point of view, identifying determinants of weight gain is more impactful than short-term weight loss in reducing obesity prevalence [29]. This is because, once an individual develops obesity, it is difficult to achieve and maintain weight loss. For this reason, fewer studies have evaluated the impact of SSB restriction on weight loss.

4. Metabolic Syndrome and Risk Factors

Few prospective studies have examined intake of SSBs in relation to the development of MetSyn, most likely due to challenges in outcome assessment. However, these along with studies of individual risk factors generally show adverse associations that are consistent with studies linking SSBs to weight gain and risk of T2D. Our previous meta-analysis of three cohort studies found a higher risk of about 20% (relative risk (RR), 1.20; 95% confidence interval (CI), 1.02–1.42) comparing highest to lowest categories of SSB intake [6]. However, a recent meta-analysis of three cohort studies by Narain et al. found a marginal positive association between intake of SSB and risk of MetSyn [30]. The discrepancy may be due to inclusion of different studies. The more recent meta-analysis included a new study among children and adolescents [31], which was combined with studies in adults and excluded a study from the Multi-Ethnic Study of Atherosclerosis (MESA) cohort [32], which we included. We also included the cohort-wide estimate from the Framingham Heart study that combined diet and regular soft drinks, while Narain et al. used an estimate from a sub-group with regular soft drink consumption but limited power [33]. Recent studies not included in these meta-analyses have also found positive associations. A study in the Prevención con Dieta Mediterránea (PREDIMED) trial found a positive association between SSBs and fruit juice with MetSyn among participants at high risk for CVD, but cautioned that associations should be interpreted conservatively due to low intake levels [34]. In a cohort of healthy Korean adults, a positive association between SSB and MetSyn was observed in women but not men [35]. According to the authors, the sex difference could be due to the action of sex hormones. Some studies of MetSyn found marginal associations with SSBs; however, because they adjusted for total energy intake, the results may have been underestimated [32,36].

Studies examining individual risk factors rather than MetSyn tend to be more consistent. In the Coronary Artery Risk Development in Young Adults (CARDIA) study, higher SSB consumption was associated with a number of cardiometabolic outcomes: high waist circumference (RR: 1.09; 95% CI 1.04, 1.14), high low-density lipoprotein (LDL) cholesterol (RR: 1.18; 95% CI 1.02, 1.35), high triglycerides (RR: 1.06; 95% CI 1.01, 1.13), and hypertension (RR: 1.06; 95% CI 1.01, 1.12) [37]. Although central adiposity is a risk factor for CVD independent of body weight, few cohort studies have examined this relationship with SSBs, likely due to challenges in measurement. In the Mexican Teacher's cohort, compared to no change, increasing soda consumption by one serving per day was associated with a ~1-cm increase in waist circumference (0.9 cm; 95% CI = 0.5, 1.4) over two years [38]. Similar findings were observed in a Spanish cohort [39]. Both of these studies used waist circumference as a proxy for central adiposity. However, waist circumference does not distinguish between different types of abdominal fat accumulation, e.g., visceral vs. subcutaneous adipose tissues, which may be differently associated with cardiometabolic risk. In the Framingham Third Generation cohort, Ma and colleagues found that SSB intake was associated with a long-term adverse change in visceral adiposity as measured by abdominal computed tomography scan (i.e., increased visceral adipose tissue (VAT) volume and decrease in VAT attenuation), independent of weight gain [40].

In a systematic review including five prospective cohort studies examining SSB intake in relation to vascular risk factors, positive associations were observed for blood pressure, triglycerides, LDL cholesterol, and blood glucose, and an inverse association was observed for high-density lipoprotein (HDL) cholesterol [12]. These findings were supported by cross-sectional analyses in the Health Professionals Follow-up Study (HPFS) and Nurses' Health Study (NHS) cohorts that found associations between SSB and higher plasma triglycerides, along with inflammatory cytokines and other cardiometabolic risk factors [9,41]. Accumulating evidence also suggests a role of SSBs in the development of hypertension [42–44]. A meta-analysis of six cohort studies found that a one serving/day increase in SSB intake was associated with ~8% higher risk of hypertension (RR: 1.08, 95% CI: 1.06, 1.11) [42]. Similar results were reported in two previous meta-analyses [43,44]. Regular consumption of SSBs was also associated with hyperuricemia and with gout [45,46].

Findings from short-term trials and experimental studies also provide important evidence linking SSBs with cardiometabolic risk factors, and they provide mechanistic support for the epidemiologic evidence linking intake of SSBs to higher risk of T2D and coronary heart disease (CHD). Many of these studies explored the effects of sugars used to flavor SSBs such as high-fructose corn syrup (HFCS) (~42–55% fructose, glucose and water) or sucrose (50% fructose and glucose) in liquid form. A meta-analysis of 39 RCTs found that higher compared to lower intakes of dietary sugars or SSB significantly raised triglyceride concentrations (mean difference (MD): 0.11 mmol/L; 95% CI: 0.07, 0.15), total cholesterol (MD: 0.16 mmol/L; 95% CI: 0.10, 0.24), LDL cholesterol (MD: 0.12 mmol/L; 95% CI: 0.05, 0.19), and HDL cholesterol (MD: 0.02 mmol/L; 95% CI: 0.00, 0.03) [47]. The most pronounced effects were noted in studies that ensured energy balance and when no difference in weight change was reported, suggesting that the effects of SSBs on lipids are independent of body weight [47]. This meta-analysis also found a significant blood-pressure-raising effect of sugars, particularly in studies ≥8 weeks in duration (MD 6.9 mm Hg (95% CI: 3.4, 10.3) for systolic blood pressure, and 5.6 mm Hg (95% CI: 2.5, 8.8) for diastolic blood pressure) [47].

In a two-week parallel-arm trial, Stanhope and colleagues showed that consuming beverages containing 10%, 17.5%, or 25% of energy requirements from HFCS produced a significant linear dose–response increase in postprandial triglycerides, fasting LDL cholesterol, and 24-h mean uric acid concentrations [48]. In another study, uric acid was found to increase after six months of consuming 1 L/day of sucrose-sweetened cola compared to isocaloric consumption of milk, water, or diet beverages [49]. The change in uric acid correlated with changes in liver fat ($p = 0.005$), triglycerides ($p = 0.02$), and insulin ($p = 0.002$) [49] In a 10-week trial among overweight healthy participants, consuming a sucrose-rich diet compared to a diet rich in artificial sweeteners, significant increases in postprandial glycemia, insulinemia, and lipidemia were observed [50]. A randomized crossover trial among normal-weight healthy men found that, after three weeks, SSBs consumed in small to moderate quantities resulted in impaired glucose and lipid metabolism and promoted inflammation [51]. Other trials have found inconsistent results on markers of inflammation, which may be due to differences in study duration. [52,53].

5. Diabetes and CVD

Although experimental evidence from RCTs is lacking due to high cost and other feasibility considerations, findings from prospective cohort studies have shown strong and consistent associations in well-powered studies. A meta-analysis of 17 prospective cohort studies evaluating SSB consumption and risk of T2D found that a one-serving-per-day increment in SSB was associated with an 18% higher risk of T2D (95% CI: 9% to 28%) among studies that did not adjust for adiposity [54] (Figure 2). Among studies that adjusted for adiposity, the estimate was attenuated to 13% (6% to 21%), suggesting a partial mediating role of adiposity in this association. Positive yet weaker associations were also noted for juice and artificially sweetened beverages (ASB). This study also estimated the population attributable fraction for T2D from consumption of SSB in the US and United Kingdom (UK). Based on their estimates, 8.7% (95% CI, 3.9% to 12.9%) of T2D cases in the US and 3.6% (95% CI, 1.7% to 5.6%) in the UK would be attributable to the consumption of SSBs [54]. These results, which are consistent with previous meta-analyses [6,55,56], confirm that the consumption of SSBs is associated with increased risk of T2D independently of adiposity and suggests that the consumption of SSBs over many years could be related to a substantial number of new cases. Recent studies in the Mexican Teacher's cohort [57] and Northern Manhattan study [58], a multi ethnic urban cohort in New York City, provide additional support linking intake of SSBs to risk of T2D, and have expanded the generalizability of the findings across different populations.

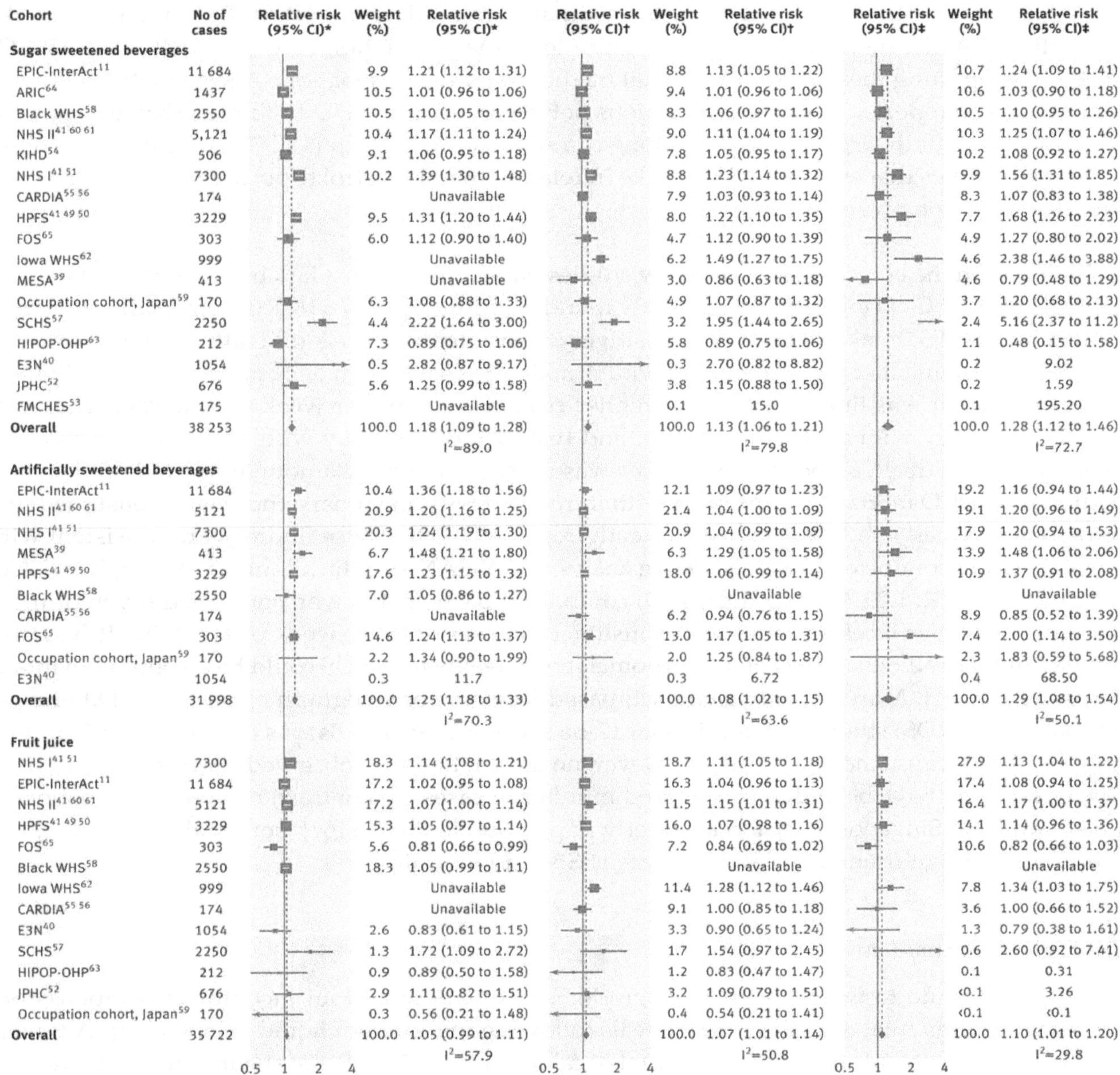

Cohort	No of cases	Weight (%)	Relative risk (95% CI)*	Weight (%)	Relative risk (95% CI)†	Weight (%)	Relative risk (95% CI)‡
Sugar sweetened beverages							
EPIC-InterAct[11]	11 684	9.9	1.21 (1.12 to 1.31)	8.8	1.13 (1.05 to 1.22)	10.7	1.24 (1.09 to 1.41)
ARIC[64]	1437	10.5	1.01 (0.96 to 1.06)	9.4	1.01 (0.96 to 1.06)	10.6	1.03 (0.90 to 1.18)
Black WHS[58]	2550	10.5	1.10 (1.05 to 1.16)	8.3	1.06 (0.97 to 1.16)	10.5	1.10 (0.95 to 1.26)
NHS II[41 60 61]	5,121	10.4	1.17 (1.11 to 1.24)	9.0	1.11 (1.04 to 1.19)	10.3	1.25 (1.07 to 1.46)
KIHD[54]	506	9.1	1.06 (0.95 to 1.18)	7.8	1.05 (0.95 to 1.17)	10.2	1.08 (0.92 to 1.27)
NHS I[41 51]	7300	10.2	1.39 (1.30 to 1.48)	8.8	1.23 (1.14 to 1.32)	9.9	1.56 (1.31 to 1.85)
CARDIA[55 56]	174		Unavailable	7.9	1.03 (0.93 to 1.14)	8.3	1.07 (0.83 to 1.38)
HPFS[41 49 50]	3229	9.5	1.31 (1.20 to 1.44)	8.0	1.22 (1.10 to 1.35)	7.7	1.68 (1.26 to 2.23)
FOS[65]	303	6.0	1.12 (0.90 to 1.40)	4.7	1.12 (0.90 to 1.39)	4.9	1.27 (0.80 to 2.02)
Iowa WHS[62]	999		Unavailable	6.2	1.49 (1.27 to 1.75)	4.6	2.38 (1.46 to 3.88)
MESA[39]	413		Unavailable	3.0	0.86 (0.63 to 1.18)	4.6	0.79 (0.48 to 1.29)
Occupation cohort, Japan[59]	170	6.3	1.08 (0.88 to 1.33)	4.9	1.07 (0.87 to 1.32)	3.7	1.20 (0.68 to 2.13)
SCHS[57]	2250	4.4	2.22 (1.64 to 3.00)	3.2	1.95 (1.44 to 2.65)	2.4	5.16 (2.37 to 11.2)
HIPOP-OHP[63]	212	7.3	0.89 (0.75 to 1.06)	5.8	0.89 (0.75 to 1.06)	1.1	0.48 (0.15 to 1.58)
E3N[40]	1054	0.5	2.82 (0.87 to 9.17)	0.3	2.70 (0.82 to 8.82)	0.2	9.02
JPHC[52]	676	5.6	1.25 (0.99 to 1.58)	3.8	1.15 (0.88 to 1.50)	0.2	1.59
FMCHES[53]	175		Unavailable	0.1	15.0	0.1	195.20
Overall	38 253	100.0	1.18 (1.09 to 1.28) I^2=89.0	100.0	1.13 (1.06 to 1.21) I^2=79.8	100.0	1.28 (1.12 to 1.46) I^2=72.7
Artificially sweetened beverages							
EPIC-InterAct[11]	11 684	10.4	1.36 (1.18 to 1.56)	12.1	1.09 (0.97 to 1.23)	19.2	1.16 (0.94 to 1.44)
NHS II[41 60 61]	5121	20.9	1.20 (1.16 to 1.25)	21.4	1.04 (1.00 to 1.09)	19.1	1.20 (0.96 to 1.49)
NHS I[41 51]	7300	20.3	1.24 (1.19 to 1.30)	20.9	1.04 (0.99 to 1.09)	17.9	1.20 (0.94 to 1.53)
MESA[39]	413	6.7	1.48 (1.21 to 1.80)	6.3	1.29 (1.05 to 1.58)	13.9	1.48 (1.06 to 2.06)
HPFS[41 49 50]	3229	17.6	1.23 (1.15 to 1.32)	18.0	1.06 (0.99 to 1.14)	10.9	1.37 (0.91 to 2.08)
Black WHS[58]	2550	7.0	1.05 (0.86 to 1.27)		Unavailable		Unavailable
CARDIA[55 56]	174		Unavailable	6.2	0.94 (0.76 to 1.15)	8.9	0.85 (0.52 to 1.39)
FOS[65]	303	14.6	1.24 (1.13 to 1.37)	13.0	1.17 (1.05 to 1.31)	7.4	2.00 (1.14 to 3.50)
Occupation cohort, Japan[59]	170	2.2	1.34 (0.90 to 1.99)	2.0	1.25 (0.84 to 1.87)	2.3	1.83 (0.59 to 5.68)
E3N[40]	1054	0.3	11.7	0.3	6.72	0.4	68.50
Overall	31 998	100.0	1.25 (1.18 to 1.33) I^2=70.3	100.0	1.08 (1.02 to 1.15) I^2=63.6	100.0	1.29 (1.08 to 1.54) I^2=50.1
Fruit juice							
NHS I[41 51]	7300	18.3	1.14 (1.08 to 1.21)	18.7	1.11 (1.05 to 1.18)	27.9	1.13 (1.04 to 1.22)
EPIC-InterAct[11]	11 684	17.2	1.02 (0.95 to 1.08)	16.3	1.04 (0.96 to 1.13)	17.4	1.08 (0.94 to 1.25)
NHS II[41 60 61]	5121	17.2	1.07 (1.00 to 1.14)	11.5	1.15 (1.01 to 1.31)	16.4	1.17 (1.00 to 1.37)
HPFS[41 49 50]	3229	15.3	1.05 (0.97 to 1.14)	16.0	1.07 (0.98 to 1.16)	14.1	1.14 (0.96 to 1.36)
FOS[65]	303	5.6	0.81 (0.66 to 0.99)	7.2	0.84 (0.69 to 1.02)	10.6	0.82 (0.66 to 1.03)
Black WHS[58]	2550	18.3	1.05 (0.99 to 1.11)		Unavailable		Unavailable
Iowa WHS[62]	999		Unavailable	11.4	1.28 (1.12 to 1.46)	7.8	1.34 (1.03 to 1.75)
CARDIA[55 56]	174		Unavailable	9.1	1.00 (0.85 to 1.18)	3.6	1.00 (0.66 to 1.52)
E3N[40]	1054	2.6	0.83 (0.61 to 1.15)	3.3	0.90 (0.65 to 1.24)	1.3	0.79 (0.38 to 1.61)
SCHS[57]	2250	1.3	1.72 (1.09 to 2.72)	1.7	1.54 (0.97 to 2.45)	0.6	2.60 (0.92 to 7.41)
HIPOP-OHP[63]	212	0.9	0.89 (0.50 to 1.58)	1.2	0.83 (0.47 to 1.47)	0.1	0.31
JPHC[52]	676	2.9	1.11 (0.82 to 1.51)	3.2	1.09 (0.79 to 1.51)	<0.1	3.26
Occupation cohort, Japan[59]	170	0.3	0.56 (0.21 to 1.48)	0.4	0.54 (0.21 to 1.41)	<0.1	<0.1
Overall	35 722	100.0	1.05 (0.99 to 1.11) I^2=57.9	100.0	1.07 (1.01 to 1.14) I^2=50.8	100.0	1.10 (1.01 to 1.20) I^2=29.8

Figure 2. Prospective associations for an incremental increase in beverage consumption with incident type 2 diabetes (T2D): random effects meta-analysis. * Unadjusted for adiposity; † adjusted for adiposity; ‡ adjusted for adiposity and within person variation [54].

Emerging evidence linking intake of SSBs to CVD is strengthened by consistent associations of SSBs with cardiometabolic risk factors, in addition to weight gain and risk of T2D. A meta-analysis of nine prospective cohort studies found that a one-serving-per-day increase in SSB was associated with a 13% higher risk of stroke (RR: 1.13, 95% CI: 1.02, 1.24) based on one study, and 22% higher risk of myocardial infarction (MI) (RR: 1.22, 95% CI: 1.14, 1.30) based on two studies [10]. In the categorical analysis comparing high vs. low SSB intake, there was a 19% higher risk of MI (RR: 1.19, 95% CI: 1.09, 1.31) based on three studies, but no significant association was observed for stroke (three studies) [10]. For the association with stroke, moderate heterogeneity was evident. After stratification by sex and stroke type, the pooled results suggested that women who consume SSBs have a higher risk of ischemic stroke (RR: 1.33, 95% CI: 1.07, 1.66), while no differences were noted for men or for men and women with hemorrhagic stroke [10]. These findings are consistent with a previous meta-analysis of four prospective cohort studies, which found a 17% higher risk of CHD (95% CI: 7% to 28%) comparing extreme SSB intake categories and a 16% higher risk of CHD per one-serving-per-day increment (10% to 23%) [11]. Similar to studies of T2D, when estimates that did not adjust for BMI or energy intake were included in the meta-analysis, the magnitude of the association increased (RR: 1.26, 95% CI: 1.16, 1.37), suggesting these factors as partial mediators of the association. A systematic review by Keller et al. also reported positive associations between SSB and CHD but noted that associations were only apparent in large studies with long durations of follow-up [12]. This review also found that, among studies that evaluated SSB intake in relation to risk of stroke, positive associations were observed only among women.

Building on the clinical evidence, a few studies have also shown a link between SSB intake and risk of all-cause or CVD mortality. We recently found that, among over 118,000 women and men from the NHS and HPFS, intake of SSBs was positively associated with risk of death from any cause in a dose-dependent manner [59]. Compared with drinking SSBs less than once per month, drinking one to four per month was linked with a 1% higher risk, two to six per week with a 6% higher risk, one to two per day with a 14% higher risk, and two or more per day with a 21% higher risk [59]. The higher risk of death associated with SSBs was more pronounced among women than men and was driven by CVD mortality. Compared with infrequent SSB consumers, those who consumed two or more per day had a 31% higher risk of death from CVD [59]. These findings are consistent with a previous study conducted in a prospective analysis of NHANES, which found a 29% higher risk of CVD mortality (RR: 1.29, 95% CI: 1.04, 1.60) comparing participants who consumed seven or more servings of SSBs per week to those who consumed one serving per week or less [60]. It was also estimated in NHANES that 7.4% of all cardiometabolic deaths in the US could be attributed to intake of SSBs in 2012 [61]. More recently, in the US-based Reasons for Geographic and Racial Differences in Stroke (REGARDS) study, each additional 12-oz serving/day of SSBs was associated with an 11% higher risk of all-cause mortality [62]. However, no association was observed for risk of death from CHD, which may have been due to a limited number of cases. In contrast, results from a cohort of Chinese adults in Singapore [63] and an elderly population in the US [64], both with very low intake levels, found no significant association between SSBs and mortality.

6. Biological Mechanisms

SSBs contribute to weight gain through decreased satiety and an incomplete compensatory reduction in energy intake at subsequent meals following ingestion of liquid calories [20]. A typical 12-oz (360 mL) serving of soda contains ~140–150 calories and ~35–37.5 g of sugar. If these calories are added to the diet without compensating for the additional calories, one can of soda per day could in theory lead to a weight gain of five pounds in one year [65]. Short-term feeding trials that show greater energy intake [66] and weight gain [50,66–69] from consuming SSBs compared to ASBs indirectly illustrate this point. While few studies have evaluated this mechanism, some evidence supporting incomplete compensation for liquid calories has been provided by studies showing greater energy intake and weight gain after isocaloric consumption of beverages compared to solid food [70–72]. These studies suggest that calories from sugar in liquid beverages may not suppress intake of solid foods to the level needed to maintain energy balance; however, the mechanisms responsible for this response are largely unknown.

SSBs contribute to the development of T2D and cardiometabolic risk in part through their ability to induce weight gain, but also independently through metabolic effects of constituent sugars (Figure 3). Consumption of SSBs has been shown to induce rapid spikes in blood glucose and insulin levels [73,74]. As such, these beverages have moderate-to-high glycemic index (GI) values [75], which, in combination with the large quantities consumed, contribute to a high dietary glycemic load (GL). High-GL diets can promote insulin resistance [76], exacerbate inflammatory biomarkers [77], and are associated with higher risk of T2D [78,79] and CHD [80]. Consuming fructose from SSBs as a component of sucrose or HFCS may further impact cardiometabolic risk. Fructose alone is poorly absorbed but is enhanced by glucose in the gut, thus accounting for the rapid and complete absorption of both fructose and glucose when ingested as sucrose or HFCS. Fructose, when consumed in moderate amounts, is metabolized in the liver where it is converted to glucose, lactate, and fatty acids to serve as metabolic substrates for other cells in the body [81]. When consumed in excess, this can lead to increased hepatic de novo lipogenesis, atherogenic dyslipidemia, and insulin resistance. The increase in hepatic lipid promotes production and secretion of very-low-density lipoproteins (VLDLs) leading to increased concentrations of postprandial triglycerides. Consumption of fructose-containing sugars is associated with production of small dense LDL cholesterol, which may be due to increased levels of VLDL-induced lipoprotein remodeling [48,82]. Fructose was also shown to promote the accumulation of VAT and the deposition of ectopic fat [83–86], processes indicative of cardiometabolic risk. Accumulating evidence suggests that the metabolic effects of fructose may be modified by physical activity level with more adverse effects observed under conditions of high fructose intake and low levels of physical activity [87]. According to this model, the adverse metabolic effects of fructose would occur when fructose intake chronically exceeds the capacity of the liver to release lactate and glucose for muscle, i.e., when there is a mismatch between fructose intake and energy output in the muscle. Fructose is the only sugar known to increase production of uric acid [87]. The production of uric acid in the liver has been shown to reduce endothelial nitric oxide, which may be implicated in the association between SSBs and CHD [88]. Hyperuricemia often precedes development of obesity and T2D, and clinical evidence suggests that hyperuricemia may mediate the association between SSB consumption and hypertension through the development of renal disease, endothelial dysfunction, and activation of the renin–angiotensin system [88]. In addition, hyperuricemia is associated with the development of gout [45,46], and gout and hyperuricemia are associated with hypertension, T2D, MetSyn, kidney disease, and CVD [88,89].

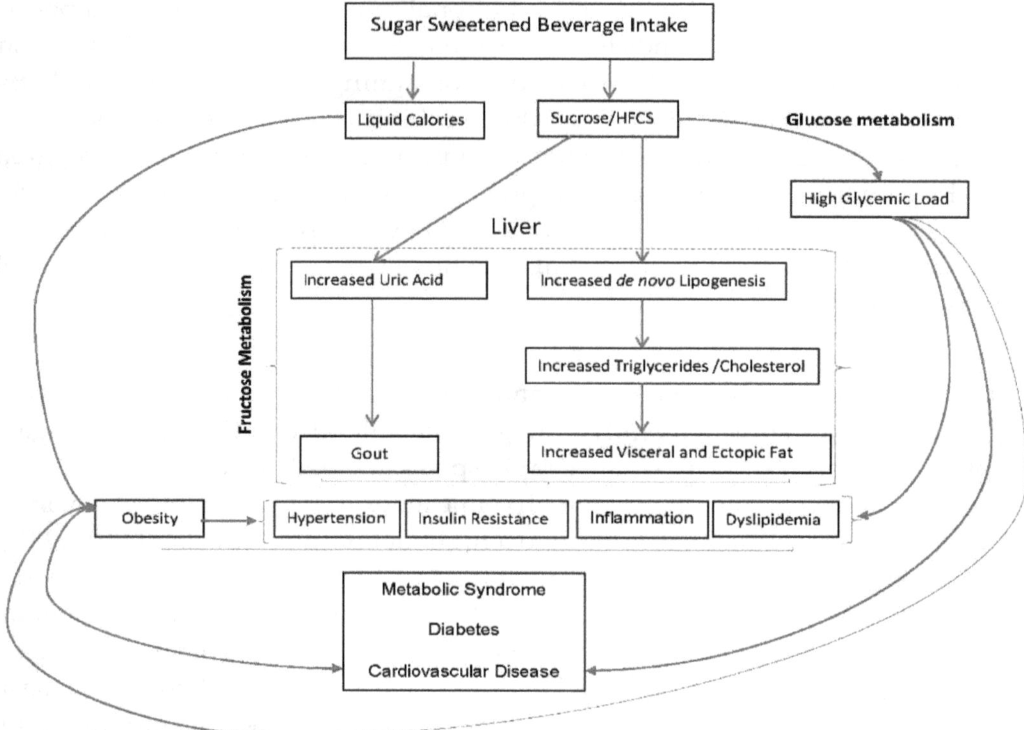

Figure 3. Biological mechanisms linking intake of sugar-sweetened beverages (SSB) to the development of obesity, metabolic syndrome (Met Syn), diabetes, and cardiovascular disease (CVD). Incomplete compensation for liquid calories leads to obesity, which is a risk factor for cardiometabolic outcomes. Increased diabetes, MetSyn, and CVD risk also occur independent of weight through development of risk factors precipitated by adverse glycemic effects and increased fructose metabolism in the liver. Excess fructose ingestion promotes hepatic uric acid production, de novo lipogenesis, and accumulation of visceral and ectopic fat, and also leads to gout. HFCS = high-fructose corn syrup.

7. Alternative Beverages

Several beverages have been suggested as alternatives to SSBs including water, 100% fruit juice, coffee, tea, and ASBs. Unlike SSBs, water does not contain liquid calories and, for most people with access to safe drinking water, it is the optimal calorie-free beverage. We found that replacement of one serving per day of SSBs with one serving of water was associated with less weight gain [90] and a lower risk of T2D [91]. With more consumers opting for water, several types of sparkling and flavored waters have emerged on the market, which may make switching to water more feasible for habitual SSB consumers.

Although 100% fruit juice might be perceived as a healthy choice since juice contains some vitamins and nutrients, they also contain a relatively high number of calories from natural sugars. Previous cohort studies have found positive associations between consumption of fruit juice and weight gain [92] and T2D [93], while the opposite has been shown for whole fruit [25,94]. Sugars in juice are absorbed more quickly than those in fruit and vegetables, which are absorbed more slowly due in part to their fiber content [95,96]. The rapid absorption of liquid fructose (from juice) compared to solid forms is more likely to result in higher concentrations of fructose in the liver and increase the rate of hepatic extraction of fructose, de novo lipogenesis, and production of lipids [97,98]. A recent study in the REGARDS cohort found that fruit juice intake was associated with a higher risk of all-cause mortality [62]. However, other studies have shown benefits of juice on cardiometabolic markers [92,99]. This suggests a need for further research that can evaluate different types of juice, since the nutrient profile and sugar content across various juices may differ. Nonetheless, based on the current evidence, it is recommended that daily intake of fruit juice be limited to 8 oz for adults.

Numerous studies have shown that regular consumption of coffee (decaffeinated or regular) and tea can have favorable effects on T2D and CVD risk [100,101], possibly due to their high polyphenol content. These beverages can thus be considered healthful alternatives to SSBs for individuals without contraindications, provided that caloric sweeteners and creamers are used sparingly, and that intake does not exceed the guidelines for caffeine. We found that substituting one serving per day of SSBs with one cup of coffee was associated with a 17% lower risk of T2D [102].

ASBs provide few to no calories but retain a sweet flavor, making them an attractive alternative to SSBs. Paradoxically, some cohort studies have reported positive associations between ASB consumption and weight gain and risk of T2D and CVD [32,36]. These findings may be due in part to residual confounding by unmeasured or poorly measured lifestyle factors or reverse causation, since individuals with obesity or metabolic risk may switch to ASBs for health reasons, which can result in spurious associations between ASBs and cardiometabolic outcomes. Studies with repeated measurements of diet, which are less prone to reverse causation, have shown only marginal nonsignificant associations with ASBs [8,9,25,59,102]. Cohort-based substitution analysis has also shown inverse associations with weight gain, T2D and mortality with replacement of SSBs with ASBs [59,90,91]. In addition, short-term trials that assessed ASBs as a replacement for SSBs reported modest benefits on body weight and metabolic risk factors [5,103]. On the other hand, some mechanisms have been proposed linking ASBs to adverse cardiometabolic health such as the intense sweetness of artificial sweeteners conditioning toward a preference for sweets or stimulating a cephalic insulin response, and more recently through alterations in gut microflora linked to insulin resistance [104]. However, these mechanisms are not well understood, and different types of artificial sweeteners may have different metabolic effects.

Consumption of ASBs in place of SSBs could be a helpful strategy to reduce cardiometabolic risk among heavy SSB consumers with the ultimate goal of switching to water or other healthful beverages. Further studies are needed to evaluate potential metabolic consequences of consuming ASBs over the life course and better understand underlying biological mechanisms. Understanding potential health impacts of ASB consumption is especially important in the context of sugar reduction policies such as taxation and labeling, which may lead to product reformulation and more ASBs in the food supply.

8. Policy Considerations

In response to the strong evidence linking consumption of SSBs to weight gain and risk of T2D and CVD, national and international organizations are already calling for reductions in intake of these beverages to help curb obesity and improve cardiometabolic health [105]. Both the WHO and 2015–2020 US Dietary Guidelines recommend an upper limit of 10% of total energy from added sugar, and numerous associations specifically recommend limiting intake of SSBs. In addition to widespread public health recommendations, public policies are needed to change consumption pattern at the population level (Box 1). The most common actions implemented to reduce SSB consumption include taxation, reduction of availability in schools, restrictions on marketing to children, public awareness campaigns, and front-of-package labelling [18,106]. Several cities in the US and globally have implemented excise taxes on SSBs as a strategy to reduce intake levels and generate revenue to support various public efforts. The most rigorously evaluated SSB tax to date is in Mexico, where a nationwide excise tax of 10% (one peso per liter) was implemented in 2014. Two years after the tax was implemented, a net decrease of 7.6% in sales of sugary drinks was observed, while sales of untaxed beverages such as water increased by 2.1% [107]. It was estimated that, between 2013 to 2022, the tax alone will prevent nearly 200,000 cases of obesity and save $980 million in direct healthcare costs, with the majority of benefits in young adults [108]. In Berkeley, California, the first US city to levy a penny-per-ounce excise tax on SSBs, sales of SSBs fell 9.6%, while sales of untaxed beverages, such as water and milk, increased 3.5%, comparing pre-tax to one-year-post-implementation trends [109]. Whether these early benefits of the tax will continue over the long term and translate into improvements in health will be important factors to monitor over time. In the US, the recently revised nutrition facts label will now require manufacturers (compliance by 1 January2020 to 1 July

2021, depending on annual food sales) to disclose the added sugar content of products, and will be accompanied by a percent daily value, with a goal of helping consumers make healthier choices. To achieve meaningful changes in beverage consumption patterns, a combination of multiple strategies will be needed, together with consumer education, and will serve as important steps in changing social norms surrounding beverage habits. Implementing and evaluating these policy actions in relation to behavior changes in the short term and clinical outcomes in the long term should remain a priority for scientists and policy-makers.

Box 1. Policy strategies to reduce consumption of sugar-sweetened beverages (SSBs).

- Governments should impose financial incentives such as taxation of SSBs of at least a 10% price increase, and implement limits for use of Supplemental Nutrition Assistance Program (SNAP) benefits for SSBs or subsidizing SNAP purchases of healthier foods, to encourage healthier beverages choices.
- Regulations are needed to reduce exposure to marketing of unhealthy foods and beverages in the media and at sports events or other activities, particularly in relation to children.
- Front-of-package labelling or other nutrition labeling strategies should be implemented to help guide consumers to make healthy food and beverage choices. These changes should be accompanied by concurrent public health awareness campaigns.
- Policies should be adopted to reduce the availability of SSBs in the workplace, healthcare facilities, government institutions, and other public spaces, and ensure access to safe water and healthy alternatives. Policies that make healthful beverages the default choice should also be adopted.
- Educational campaigns about the health risks associated with overconsumption of SSBs should be aimed at healthcare professionals and clinical populations.
- National and international campaigns targeting obesity and chronic disease prevention should include the health risks associated with overconsumption of SSBs.
- National and international dietary recommendations should include specific guidelines for healthy beverage consumption.

9. Conclusions

Intake of SSBs remains high in the US and is rising in many parts of the world. Based on findings from prospective cohort studies and short-term experimental trials of cardiometabolic risk factors, there is strong evidence for an etiological relationship between intake of SSBs and weight gain and risk of T2D and CHD. The evidence for a link with stroke is less clear and warrants further research, including the potential sex difference. Few studies have investigated intake of SSBs in relation to MetSyn, and this may be due to challenges in assessment and controversy about its clinical utility. However, findings on individual risk factors suggest a link. Since development of MetSyn often precedes onset of T2D and CHD, preventing or reversing MetSyn could be an effective way to curtail rising T2D and CHD rates.

SSBs are thought to promote weight gain through incomplete compensation for liquid calories at subsequent meals. These beverages may increase T2D and CHD in part through weight gain and independently through metabolic effects of constituent sugars. A mechanistic area that warrants future research is exploring the health effects of sugar consumed in solid form compared to SSB, and further elucidating compensatory effects of liquid vs. solid sugars. With the strength of evidence sufficient to call for reductions in intake of SSB for optimal cardiometabolic health, important research gaps exist regarding suitable alternative beverages, including the long-term health effects of consuming ASBs. Continued evaluation of SSB policies that are already in place is needed, as are more and higher-quality RCTs to identify effective strategies to reduce intake of SSBs at the individual and population level. SSBs present a clear target for health policy; however, chronic disease prevention should focus on improving overall diet quality by consuming more healthful foods and limiting unhealthy ones. Given the high levels of intake across the globe, reducing consumption of SSBs is an important step in improving diet quality that could have a measurable impact on weight control and improving cardiometabolic health.

Author Contributions: Original draft preparation, V.S.M.; critical review and editing, F.B.H. Both authors approved the submitted version and take responsibility for the accuracy and integrity of the work.

Acknowledgments: This research was supported by NIH grants P30 DK46200 and HL607.

References

1. Alberti, K.G.; Eckel, R.H.; Grundy, S.M.; Zimmet, P.Z.; Cleeman, J.I.; Donato, K.A.; Fruchart, J.C.; James, W.P.; Loria, C.M.; Smith, S.C., Jr.; et al. Harmonizing the metabolic syndrome: A joint interim statement of the International Diabetes Federation Task Force on Epidemiology and Prevention; National Heart, Lung, and Blood Institute; American Heart Association; World Heart Federation; International Atherosclerosis Society; and International Association for the Study of Obesity. *Circulation* **2009**, *120*, 1640–1645. [PubMed]
2. Beltran-Sanchez, H.; Harhay, M.O.; Harhay, M.M.; McElligott, S. Prevalence and trends of metabolic syndrome in the adult U.S. population, 1999–2010. *J. Am. Coll. Cardiol.* **2013**, *62*, 697–703. [CrossRef] [PubMed]
3. Saklayen, M.G. The Global Epidemic of the Metabolic Syndrome. *Curr. Hypertens. Rep.* **2018**, *20*, 12. [CrossRef] [PubMed]
4. Palmer, M.K.; Toth, P.P. Trends in Lipids, Obesity, Metabolic Syndrome, and Diabetes Mellitus in the United States: An NHANES Analysis (2003–2004 to 2013–2014). *Obesity* **2019**, *27*, 309–314. [CrossRef] [PubMed]
5. Malik, V.S.; Pan, A.; Willett, W.C.; Hu, F.B. Sugar-sweetened beverages and weight gain in children and adults: A systematic review and meta-analysis. *Am. J. Clin. Nutr.* **2013**, *98*, 1084–1102. [CrossRef] [PubMed]
6. Malik, V.S.; Popkin, B.M.; Bray, G.A.; Despres, J.P.; Willett, W.C.; Hu, F.B. Sugar-sweetened beverages and risk of metabolic syndrome and type 2 diabetes: A meta-analysis. *Diabetes Care* **2010**, *33*, 2477–2483. [CrossRef] [PubMed]
7. *Guideline: Sugar Intake for Adults and Children*; World Health Organization: Geneva, Switzerland, 2015.
8. Fung, T.T.; Malik, V.; Rexrode, K.M.; Manson, J.E.; Willett, W.C.; Hu, F.B. Sweetened beverage consumption and risk of coronary heart disease in women. *Am. J. Clin. Nutr.* **2009**, *89*, 1037–1042. [CrossRef]
9. De Koning, L.; Malik, V.S.; Kellogg, M.D.; Rimm, E.B.; Willett, W.C.; Hu, F.B. Sweetened beverage consumption, incident coronary heart disease, and biomarkers of risk in men. *Circulation* **2012**, *125*, 1735–1741. [CrossRef]
10. Narain, A.; Kwok, C.S.; Mamas, M.A. Soft drinks and sweetened beverages and the risk of cardiovascular disease and mortality: A systematic review and meta-analysis. *Int. J. Clin. Pract.* **2016**, *70*, 791–805. [CrossRef]
11. Huang, C.; Huang, J.; Tian, Y.; Yang, X.; Gu, D. Sugar sweetened beverages consumption and risk of coronary heart disease: A meta-analysis of prospective studies. *Atherosclerosis* **2014**, *234*, 11–16. [CrossRef]
12. Keller, A.; Heitmann, B.L.; Olsen, N. Sugar-sweetened beverages, vascular risk factors and events: A systematic literature review. *Public Health Nutr.* **2015**, *18*, 1145–1154. [CrossRef] [PubMed]
13. Welsh, J.A.; Sharma, A.J.; Grellinger, L.; Vos, M.B. Consumption of added sugars is decreasing in the United States. *Am. J. Clin. Nutr.* **2011**, *94*, 726–734. [CrossRef] [PubMed]
14. Dietary Guidelines for Americans 2015–2020. Available online: http://health.gov/dietaryguidelines/2015/guidelines/ (accessed on 7 August 2019).
15. Rosinger, A.; Herrick, K.; Gahche, J.; Park, S. Sugar-sweetened Beverage Consumption Among U.S. Adults, 2011–2014. *NCHS Data Brief* **2017**, *270*, 1–8.
16. Singh, G.M.; Micha, R.; Khatibzadeh, S.; Shi, P.; Lim, S.; Andrews, K.G.; Engell, R.E.; Ezzati, M.; Mozaffarian, D.; Global Burden of Diseases Nutrition and Chronic Diseases Expert Group (NutriCoDE). Global, Regional, and National Consumption of Sugar-Sweetened Beverages, Fruit Juices, and Milk: A Systematic Assessment of Beverage Intake in 187 Countries. *PLoS ONE* **2015**, *10*, e0124845. [CrossRef] [PubMed]
17. Yang, L.; Bovet, P.; Liu, Y.; Zhao, M.; Ma, C.; Liang, Y.; Xi, B. Consumption of Carbonated Soft Drinks Among Young Adolescents Aged 12 to 15 Years in 53 Low- and Middle-Income Countries. *Am. J. Public Health* **2017**, *107*, 1095–1100. [CrossRef] [PubMed]

18. Popkin, B.M.; Hawkes, C. Sweetening of the global diet, particularly beverages: Patterns, trends, and policy responses. *Lancet Diabetes Endocrinol.* **2016**, *4*, 174–186. [CrossRef]
19. Hu, F.B.; Malik, V.S. Sugar-sweetened beverages and risk of obesity and type 2 diabetes: Epidemiologic evidence. *Physiol. Behav.* **2010**, *100*, 47–54. [CrossRef]
20. Malik, V.S.; Popkin, B.M.; Bray, G.A.; Despres, J.P.; Hu, F.B. Sugar-sweetened beverages, obesity, type 2 diabetes mellitus, and cardiovascular disease risk. *Circulation* **2010**, *121*, 1356–1364. [CrossRef]
21. Malik, V.S.; Schulze, M.B.; Hu, F.B. Intake of sugar-sweetened beverages and weight gain: A systematic review. *Am. J. Clin. Nutr.* **2006**, *84*, 274–288. [CrossRef]
22. Vartanian, L.R.; Schwartz, M.B.; Brownell, K.D. Effects of soft drink consumption on nutrition and health: A systematic review and meta-analysis. *Am. J. Public Health* **2007**, *97*, 667–675. [CrossRef]
23. Te Morenga, L.; Mallard, S.; Mann, J. Dietary sugars and body weight: Systematic review and meta-analyses of randomised controlled trials and cohort studies. *BMJ* **2013**, *346*, e7492. [CrossRef] [PubMed]
24. Kaiser, K.A.; Shikany, J.M.; Keating, K.D.; Allison, D.B. Will reducing sugar-sweetened beverage consumption reduce obesity? Evidence supporting conjecture is strong, but evidence when testing effect is weak. *Obes. Rev.* **2013**, *14*, 620–633. [CrossRef] [PubMed]
25. Mozaffarian, D.; Hao, T.; Rimm, E.B.; Willett, W.C.; Hu, F.B. Changes in diet and lifestyle and long-term weight gain in women and men. *N. Engl. J. Med.* **2011**, *364*, 2392–2404. [CrossRef] [PubMed]
26. Qi, Q.; Chu, A.Y.; Kang, J.H.; Jensen, M.K.; Curhan, G.C.; Pasquale, L.R.; Ridker, P.M.; Hunter, D.J.; Willett, W.C.; Rimm, E.B.; et al. Sugar-sweetened beverages and genetic risk of obesity. *N. Engl. J. Med.* **2012**, *367*, 1387–1396. [CrossRef] [PubMed]
27. Ebbeling, C.B.; Feldman, H.A.; Chomitz, V.R.; Antonelli, T.A.; Gortmaker, S.L.; Osganian, S.K.; Ludwig, D. A randomized trial of sugar-sweetened beverages and adolescent body weight. *N. Engl. J. Med.* **2012**, *367*, 1407–1416. [CrossRef] [PubMed]
28. De Ruyter, J.C.; Olthof, M.R.; Seidell, J.C.; Katan, M.B. A trial of sugar-free or sugar-sweetened beverages and body weight in children. *N. Engl. J. Med.* **2012**, *367*, 1397–1406. [CrossRef] [PubMed]
29. Hu, F.B. Resolved: There is sufficient scientific evidence that decreasing sugar-sweetened beverage consumption will reduce the prevalence of obesity and obesity-related diseases. *Obes. Rev.* **2013**, *14*, 606–619. [CrossRef]
30. Narain, A.; Kwok, C.S.; Mamas, M.A. Soft drink intake and the risk of metabolic syndrome: A systematic review and meta-analysis. *Int. J. Clin. Pract.* **2017**, *71*, e12927. [CrossRef]
31. Mirmiran, P.; Yuzbashian, E.; Asghari, G.; Hosseinpour-Niazi, S.; Azizi, F. Consumption of sugar sweetened beverage is associated with incidence of metabolic syndrome in Tehranian children and adolescents. *Nutr. Metab.* **2015**, *12*, 25. [CrossRef]
32. Nettleton, J.A.; Lutsey, P.L.; Wang, Y.; Lima, J.A.; Michos, E.D.; Jacobs, D.R., Jr. Diet soda intake and risk of incident metabolic syndrome and type 2 diabetes in the Multi-Ethnic Study of Atherosclerosis (MESA). *Diabetes Care* **2009**, *32*, 688–694. [CrossRef]
33. Dhingra, R.; Sullivan, L.; Jacques, P.F.; Wang, T.J.; Fox, C.S.; Meigs, J.B.; D'Agostino, R.B.; Gaziano, J.M.; Vasan, R.S. Soft drink consumption and risk of developing cardiometabolic risk factors and the metabolic syndrome in middle-aged adults in the community. *Circulation* **2007**, *116*, 480–488. [CrossRef] [PubMed]
34. Ferreira-Pego, C.; Babio, N.; Bes-Rastrollo, M.; Corella, D.; Estruch, R.; Ros, E.; Fitó, M.; Serra-Majem, L.; Arós, F.; Fiol, M.; et al. Frequent Consumption of Sugar- and Artificially Sweetened Beverages and Natural and Bottled Fruit Juices Is Associated with an Increased Risk of Metabolic Syndrome in a Mediterranean Population at High Cardiovascular Disease Risk. *J. Nutr.* **2016**, *146*, 1528–1536. [PubMed]
35. Kang, Y.; Kim, J. Soft drink consumption is associated with increased incidence of the metabolic syndrome only in women. *Br. J. Nutr.* **2017**, *117*, 315–324. [CrossRef] [PubMed]
36. Lutsey, P.L.; Steffen, L.M.; Stevens, J. Dietary intake and the development of the metabolic syndrome: The Atherosclerosis Risk in Communities study. *Circulation* **2008**, *117*, 754–761. [CrossRef] [PubMed]
37. Duffey, K.J.; Gordon-Larsen, P.; Steffen, L.M.; Jacobs, D.R., Jr.; Popkin, B.M. Drinking caloric beverages increases the risk of adverse cardiometabolic outcomes in the Coronary Artery Risk Development in Young Adults (CARDIA) Study. *Am. J. Clin. Nutr.* **2010**, *92*, 954–959. [CrossRef] [PubMed]
38. Stern, D.; Middaugh, N.; Rice, M.S.; Laden, F.; Lopez-Ridaura, R.; Rosner, B.; Willett, W.; Lajous, M. Changes in Sugar-Sweetened Soda Consumption, Weight, and Waist Circumference: 2-Year Cohort of Mexican Women. *Am. J. Public Health* **2017**, *107*, 1801–1808. [CrossRef]

39. Funtikova, A.N.; Subirana, I.; Gomez, S.F.; Fito, M.; Elosua, R.; Benitez-Arciniega, A.A.; Schröder, H. Soft drink consumption is positively associated with increased waist circumference and 10-year incidence of abdominal obesity in Spanish adults. *J. Nutr.* **2015**, *145*, 328–334. [CrossRef]
40. Ma, J.; McKeown, N.M.; Hwang, S.J.; Hoffmann, U.; Jacques, P.F.; Fox, C.S. Sugar-Sweetened Beverage Consumption Is Associated With Change of Visceral Adipose Tissue Over 6 Years of Follow-Up. *Circulation* **2016**, *133*, 370–377. [CrossRef]
41. Yu, Z.; Ley, S.H.; Sun, Q.; Hu, F.B.; Malik, V.S. Cross-sectional association between sugar-sweetened beverage intake and cardiometabolic biomarkers in US women. *Br. J. Nutr.* **2018**, *119*, 570–580. [CrossRef]
42. Kim, Y.; Je, Y. Prospective association of sugar-sweetened and artificially sweetened beverage intake with risk of hypertension. *Arch. Cardiovasc. Dis.* **2016**, *109*, 242–253. [CrossRef]
43. Jayalath, V.H.; de Souza, R.J.; Ha, V.; Mirrahimi, A.; Blanco-Mejia, S.; Di Buono, M.; Jenkins, A.L.; Leiter, L.A.; Wolever, T.; Beyene, J.; et al. Sugar-sweetened beverage consumption and incident hypertension: A systematic review and meta-analysis of prospective cohorts. *Am. J. Clin. Nutr.* **2015**, *102*, 914–921. [CrossRef] [PubMed]
44. Xi, B.; Huang, Y.; Reilly, K.H.; Li, S.; Zheng, R.; Barrio-Lopez, M.T.; Martinez-Gonzalez, M.A.; Zhou, D. Sugar-sweetened beverages and risk of hypertension and CVD: A dose-response meta-analysis. *Br. J. Nutr.* **2015**, *113*, 709–717. [CrossRef] [PubMed]
45. Choi, H.K.; Curhan, G. Soft drinks, fructose consumption, and the risk of gout in men: Prospective cohort study. *BMJ* **2008**, *336*, 309–312. [CrossRef] [PubMed]
46. Choi, H.K.; Willett, W.; Curhan, G. Fructose-rich beverages and risk of gout in women. *JAMA* **2010**, *304*, 2270–2278. [CrossRef] [PubMed]
47. Te Morenga, L.A.; Howatson, A.J.; Jones, R.M.; Mann, J. Dietary sugars and cardiometabolic risk: Systematic review and meta-analyses of randomized controlled trials of the effects on blood pressure and lipids. *Am. J. Clin. Nutr.* **2014**, *100*, 65–79. [CrossRef] [PubMed]
48. Stanhope, K.L.; Medici, V.; Bremer, A.A.; Lee, V.; Lam, H.D.; Nunez, M.V.; Chen, G.X.; Keim, N.L.; Havel, P.J. A dose-response study of consuming high-fructose corn syrup-sweetened beverages on lipid/lipoprotein risk factors for cardiovascular disease in young adults. *Am. J. Clin. Nutr.* **2015**, *101*, 1144–1154. [CrossRef]
49. Bruun, J.M.; Maersk, M.; Belza, A.; Astrup, A.; Richelsen, B. Consumption of sucrose-sweetened soft drinks increases plasma levels of uric acid in overweight and obese subjects: A 6-month randomised controlled trial. *Eur. J. Clin. Nutr.* **2015**, *69*, 949–953. [CrossRef]
50. Raben, A.; Moller, B.K.; Flint, A.; Vasilaris, T.H.; Christina Moller, A.; Juul Holst, J.; Astrup, A. Increased postprandial glycaemia, insulinemia, and lipidemia after 10 weeks' sucrose-rich diet compared to an artificially sweetened diet: A Randomised controlled trial. *Food Nutr. Res.* **2011**, *55*, 5961. [CrossRef]
51. Aeberli, I.; Gerber, P.A.; Hochuli, M.; Kohler, S.; Haile, S.R.; Gouni-Berthold, I.; Berthold, H.K.; Spinas, G.A.; Berneis, K. Low to moderate sugar-sweetened beverage consumption impairs glucose and lipid metabolism and promotes inflammation in healthy young men: A randomized controlled trial. *Am. J. Clin. Nutr.* **2011**, *94*, 479–485. [CrossRef]
52. Sorensen, L.B.; Raben, A.; Stender, S.; Astrup, A. Effect of sucrose on inflammatory markers in overweight humans. *Am. J. Clin. Nutr.* **2005**, *82*, 421–427. [CrossRef]
53. Kuzma, J.N.; Cromer, G.; Hagman, D.K.; Breymeyer, K.L.; Roth, C.L.; Foster-Schubert, K.E.; Holte, S.E.; Weigle, D.S.; Kratz, M. No differential effect of beverages sweetened with fructose, high-fructose corn syrup, or glucose on systemic or adipose tissue inflammation in normal-weight to obese adults: A randomized controlled trial. *Am. J. Clin. Nutr.* **2016**, *104*, 306–314. [CrossRef] [PubMed]
54. Imamura, F.; O'Connor, L.; Ye, Z.; Mursu, J.; Hayashino, Y.; Bhupathiraju, S.N.; Forouhi, N.G. Consumption of sugar sweetened beverages, artificially sweetened beverages, and fruit juice and incidence of type 2 diabetes: Systematic review, meta-analysis, and estimation of population attributable fraction. *Br. J. Sports Med.* **2016**, *50*, 496–504. [CrossRef] [PubMed]
55. Fagherazzi, G.; Vilier, A.; Saes Sartorelli, D.; Lajous, M.; Balkau, B.; Clavel-Chapelon, F. Consumption of artificially and sugar-sweetened beverages and incident type 2 diabetes in the Etude Epidemiologique aupres des femmes de la Mutuelle Generale de l'Education Nationale-European Prospective Investigation into Cancer and Nutrition cohort. *Am. J. Clin. Nutr.* **2013**, *97*, 517–523. [PubMed]
56. Consumption of sweet beverages and type 2 diabetes incidence in European adults: Results from EPIC-InterAct. *Diabetologia* **2013**, *56*, 1520–1530. [CrossRef] [PubMed]
57. Stern, D.; Mazariegos, M.; Ortiz-Panozo, E.; Campos, H.; Malik, V.S.; Lajous, M.; López-Ridaura, R. Sugar-Sweetened Soda Consumption Increases Diabetes Risk Among Mexican Women. *J. Nutr.* **2019**, *149*, 795–803. [CrossRef] [PubMed]

58. Gardener, H.; Moon, Y.P.; Rundek, T.; Elkind, M.S.V.; Sacco, R.L. Diet Soda and Sugar-Sweetened Soda Consumption in Relation to Incident Diabetes in the Northern Manhattan Study. *Curr. Dev. Nutr.* **2018**, *2*, nzy008. [CrossRef] [PubMed]
59. Malik, V.S.; Li, Y.; Pan, A.; De Koning, L.; Schernhammer, E.; Willett, W.C.; Hu, F.B. Long-Term Consumption of Sugar-Sweetened and Artificially Sweetened Beverages and Risk of Mortality in US Adults. *Circulation* **2019**, *139*, 2113–2125. [CrossRef] [PubMed]
60. Yang, Q.; Zhang, Z.; Gregg, E.W.; Flanders, W.D.; Merritt, R.; Hu, F.B. Added Sugar Intake and Cardiovascular Diseases Mortality Among US Adults. *JAMA Intern Med.* **2014**, *174*, 516–524. [CrossRef] [PubMed]
61. Micha, R.; Penalvo, J.L.; Cudhea, F.; Imamura, F.; Rehm, C.D.; Mozaffarian, D. Association Between Dietary Factors and Mortality From Heart Disease, Stroke, and Type 2 Diabetes in the United States. *JAMA* **2017**, *317*, 912–924. [CrossRef] [PubMed]
62. Collin, L.J.; Judd, S.; Safford, M.; Vaccarino, V.; Welsh, J.A. Association of Sugary Beverage Consumption With Mortality Risk in US Adults: A Secondary Analysis of Data from the REGARDS Study. *JAMA Netw. Open* **2019**, *2*, e193121. [CrossRef] [PubMed]
63. Odegaard, A.O.; Koh, W.P.; Yuan, J.M.; Pereira, M.A. Beverage habits and mortality in Chinese adults. *J. Nutr.* **2015**, *145*, 595–604. [CrossRef] [PubMed]
64. Paganini-Hill, A.; Kawas, C.H.; Corrada, M.M. Non-alcoholic beverage and caffeine consumption and mortality: The Leisure World Cohort Study. *Prev. Med.* **2007**, *44*, 305–310. [CrossRef] [PubMed]
65. Malik, V.S.; Hu, F.B. Sweeteners and Risk of Obesity and Type 2 Diabetes: The Role of Sugar-Sweetened Beverages. *Curr. Diab. Rep.* **2012**, *12*, 195–203. [CrossRef] [PubMed]
66. DellaValle, D.M.; Roe, L.S.; Rolls, B.J. Does the consumption of caloric and non-caloric beverages with a meal affect energy intake? *Appetite* **2005**, *44*, 187–193. [CrossRef] [PubMed]
67. Raben, A.; Vasilaras, T.H.; Moller, A.C.; Astrup, A. Sucrose compared with artificial sweeteners: Different effects on ad libitum food intake and body weight after 10 wk of supplementation in overweight subjects. *Am. J. Clin. Nutr.* **2002**, *76*, 721–729. [CrossRef] [PubMed]
68. Tordoff, M.G.; Alleva, A.M. Effect of drinking soda sweetened with aspartame or high-fructose corn syrup on food intake and body weight. *Am. J. Clin. Nutr.* **1990**, *51*, 963–969. [CrossRef] [PubMed]
69. Reid, M.; Hammersley, R.; Hill, A.J.; Skidmore, P. Long-term dietary compensation for added sugar: Effects of supplementary sucrose drinks over a 4-week period. *Br. J. Nutr.* **2007**, *97*, 193–203. [CrossRef]
70. DiMeglio, D.P.; Mattes, R.D. Liquid versus solid carbohydrate: Effects on food intake and body weight. *Int. J. Obes. Relat. Metab. Disord.* **2000**, *24*, 794–800. [CrossRef]
71. Pan, A.; Hu, F.B. Effects of carbohydrates on satiety: Differences between liquid and solid food. *Curr. Opin. Clin. Nutr. Metab. Care* **2011**, *14*, 385–390. [CrossRef]
72. Mourao, D.M.; Bressan, J.; Campbell, W.W.; Mattes, R.D. Effects of food form on appetite and energy intake in lean and obese young adults. *Int. J. Obes.* **2007**, *31*, 1688–1695. [CrossRef]
73. Tey, S.L.; Salleh, N.B.; Henry, J.; Forde, C.G. Effects of aspartame-, monk fruit-, stevia- and sucrose-sweetened beverages on postprandial glucose, insulin and energy intake. *Int. J. Obes.* **2017**, *41*, 450–457. [CrossRef] [PubMed]
74. Solomi, L.; Rees, G.A.; Redfern, K.M. The acute effects of the non-nutritive sweeteners aspartame and acesulfame-K in UK diet cola on glycaemic response. *Int. J. Food Sci. Nutr.* **2019**, 1–7. [CrossRef] [PubMed]
75. Atkinson, F.S.; Foster-Powell, K.; Brand-Miller, J.C. International tables of glycemic index and glycemic load values: 2008. *Diabetes Care* **2008**, *31*, 2281–2283. [CrossRef] [PubMed]
76. Ludwig, D.S. The glycemic index: Physiological mechanisms relating to obesity, diabetes, and cardiovascular disease. *JAMA* **2002**, *287*, 2414–2423. [CrossRef] [PubMed]
77. Liu, S.; Manson, J.E.; Buring, J.E.; Stampfer, M.J.; Willett, W.C.; Ridker, P.M. Relation between a diet with a high glycemic load and plasma concentrations of high-sensitivity C-reactive protein in middle-aged women. *Am. J. Clin. Nutr.* **2002**, *75*, 492–498. [CrossRef] [PubMed]
78. Bhupathiraju, S.N.; Tobias, D.K.; Malik, V.S.; Pan, A.; Hruby, A.; Manson, J.E.; Willett, W.C.; Hu, F.B. Glycemic index, glycemic load, and risk of type 2 diabetes: Results from 3 large US cohorts and an updated meta-analysis. *Am. J. Clin. Nutr.* **2014**, *100*, 218–232. [CrossRef] [PubMed]

79. Livesey, G.; Taylor, R.; Livesey, H.F.; Buyken, A.E.; Jenkins, D.J.A.; Augustin, L.S.A.; Sievenpiper, J.L.; Barclay, A.W.; Liu, S.; Wolever, T.M.S.; et al. Dietary Glycemic Index and Load and the Risk of Type 2 Diabetes: A Systematic Review and Updated Meta-Analyses of Prospective Cohort Studies. *Nutrients* **2019**, *11*, 1280. [CrossRef]
80. Livesey, G.; Livesey, H. Coronary Heart Disease and Dietary Carbohydrate, Glycemic Index, and Glycemic Load: Dose-Response Meta-analyses of Prospective Cohort Studies. *Mayo Clin. Proc. Innov. Qual. Outcomes* **2019**, *3*, 52–69. [CrossRef]
81. Sun, S.Z.; Empie, M.W. Fructose metabolism in humans—What isotopic tracer studies tell us. *Nutr. Metab. (London)* **2012**, *9*, 89. [CrossRef]
82. Goran, M.I.; Tappy, L.; Lê, K.A. *Dietary Sugars and Health*; CRC Press, Taylor & Francis Group: Boca Raton, FL, USA, 2015.
83. Teff, K.L.; Grudziak, J.; Townsend, R.R.; Dunn, T.N.; Grant, R.W.; Adams, S.H.; Keim, N.L.; Cummings, B.P.; Stanhope, K.L.; Havel, P.J. Endocrine and metabolic effects of consuming fructose- and glucose-sweetened beverages with meals in obese men and women: Influence of insulin resistance on plasma triglyceride responses. *J. Clin. Endocrinol. Metab.* **2009**, *94*, 1562–1569. [CrossRef]
84. Stanhope, K.L.; Schwarz, J.M.; Keim, N.L.; Griffen, S.C.; Bremer, A.A.; Graham, J.L.; Hatcher, B.; Cox, C.L.; Dyachenko, A.; Zhang, W.; et al. Consuming fructose-sweetened, not glucose-sweetened, beverages increases visceral adiposity and lipids and decreases insulin sensitivity in overweight/obese humans. *J. Clin. Investig.* **2009**, *119*, 1322–1334. [CrossRef] [PubMed]
85. Stanhope, K.L.; Griffen, S.C.; Bair, B.R.; Swarbrick, M.M.; Keim, N.L.; Havel, P.J. Twenty-four-hour endocrine and metabolic profiles following consumption of high-fructose corn syrup-, sucrose-, fructose-, and glucose-sweetened beverages with meals. *Am. J. Clin. Nutr.* **2008**, *87*, 1194–1203. [CrossRef] [PubMed]
86. Stanhope, K.L.; Havel, P.J. Endocrine and metabolic effects of consuming beverages sweetened with fructose, glucose, sucrose, or high-fructose corn syrup. *Am. J. Clin. Nutr.* **2008**, *88*, 1733S–1737S. [CrossRef] [PubMed]
87. Tappy, L.; Rosset, R. Health outcomes of a high fructose intake: The importance of physical activity. *J. Physiol.* **2019**, *597*, 3561–3571. [CrossRef] [PubMed]
88. Richette, P.; Bardin, T. Gout. *Lancet* **2009**. [CrossRef]
89. Nakagawa, T.; Tuttle, K.R.; Short, R.A.; Johnson, R.J. Hypothesis: Fructose-induced hyperuricemia as a causal mechanism for the epidemic of the metabolic syndrome. *Nat. Clin. Pract. Nephrol.* **2005**, *1*, 80–86. [CrossRef] [PubMed]
90. Pan, A.; Malik, V.S.; Hao, T.; Willett, W.C.; Mozaffarian, D.; Hu, F.B. Changes in water and beverage intake and long-term weight changes: Results from three prospective cohort studies. *Int. J. Obes.* **2013**, *37*, 1378. [CrossRef] [PubMed]
91. Pan, A.; Malik, V.S.; Schulze, M.B.; Manson, J.E.; Willett, W.C.; Hu, F.B. Plain-water intake and risk of type 2 diabetes in young and middle-aged women. *Am. J. Clin. Nutr.* **2012**, *95*, 1454–1460. [CrossRef] [PubMed]
92. Schulze, M.B.; Manson, J.E.; Ludwig, D.S.; Colditz, G.A.; Stampfer, M.J.; Willett, W.C.; Hu, F.B. Sugar-sweetened beverages, weight gain, and incidence of type 2 diabetes in young and middle-aged women. *JAMA* **2004**, *292*, 927–934. [CrossRef]
93. Bazzano, L.A.; Li, T.Y.; Joshipura, K.J.; Hu, F.B. Intake of fruit, vegetables, and fruit juices and risk of diabetes in women. *Diabetes Care* **2008**, *31*, 1311–1317. [CrossRef]
94. Muraki, I.; Imamura, F.; Manson, J.E.; Hu, F.B.; Willett, W.C.; van Dam, R.M.; Sun, Q. Fruit consumption and risk of type 2 diabetes: Results from three prospective longitudinal cohort studies. *BMJ* **2013**, *347*, f5001. [CrossRef] [PubMed]
95. Ravn-Haren, G.; Dragsted, L.O.; Buch-Andersen, T.; Jensen, E.N.; Jensen, R.I.; Nemeth-Balogh, M.; Paulovicsová, B.; Bergström, A.; Wilcks, A.; Licht, T.R.; et al. Intake of whole apples or clear apple juice has contrasting effects on plasma lipids in healthy volunteers. *Eur. J. Nutr.* **2013**, *52*, 1875–1889. [CrossRef] [PubMed]
96. Pepin, A.; Stanhope, K.L.; Imbeault, P. Are Fruit Juices Healthier Than Sugar-Sweetened Beverages? A Review. *Nutrients* **2019**, *11*, 1006. [CrossRef] [PubMed]
97. Sundborn, G.; Thornley, S.; Merriman, T.R.; Lang, B.; King, C.; Lanaspa, M.A.; Johnson, R.J. Are Liquid Sugars Different from Solid Sugar in Their Ability to Cause Metabolic Syndrome? *Obesity* **2019**, *27*, 879–887. [CrossRef] [PubMed]

98. Lanaspa, M.A.; Sanchez-Lozada, L.G.; Choi, Y.J.; Cicerchi, C.; Kanbay, M.; Roncal-Jimenez, C.A.; Schreiner, G. Uric acid induces hepatic steatosis by generation of mitochondrial oxidative stress: Potential role in fructose-dependent and -independent fatty liver. *J. Biol. Chem.* **2012**, *287*, 40732–40744. [CrossRef] [PubMed]
99. Ghanim, H.; Mohanty, P.; Pathak, R.; Chaudhuri, A.; Sia, C.L.; Dandona, P. Orange juice or fructose intake does not induce oxidative and inflammatory response. *Diabetes Care* **2007**, *30*, 1406–1411. [CrossRef] [PubMed]
100. Van Dam, R.M. Coffee consumption and risk of type 2 diabetes, cardiovascular diseases, and cancer. *Appl. Physiol. Nutr. Metab.* **2008**, *33*, 1269–1283. [CrossRef]
101. Bhupathiraju, S.N.; Pan, A.; Malik, V.S.; Manson, J.E.; Willett, W.C.; van Dam, R.M.; Hu, F.B. Caffeinated and caffeine-free beverages and risk of type 2 diabetes. *Am. J. Clin. Nutr.* **2013**, *97*, 155–166. [CrossRef]
102. De Koning, L.; Malik, V.S.; Rimm, E.B.; Willett, W.C.; Hu, F.B. Sugar-sweetened and artificially sweetened beverage consumption and risk of type 2 diabetes in men. *Am. J. Clin. Nutr.* **2011**, *93*, 1321–1327. [CrossRef]
103. Malik, V.S. Non-sugar sweeteners and health. *BMJ* **2019**, *364*, k5005. [CrossRef]
104. Swithers, S.E. Not so Sweet Revenge: Unanticipated Consequences of High-Intensity Sweeteners. *Behav. Anal.* **2015**, *38*, 1–17. [CrossRef] [PubMed]
105. Yale Rudd Center for Food Policy and Obesity. SUgar-Sweetened Beverage Taxes and Sugar Intake: Policy Statements, Endorsements, and Recommendations. Available online: http://www.yaleruddcenter.org/resources/upload/docs/what/policy/SSBtaxes/SSBTaxStatements.pdf (accessed on 10 January 2013).
106. Muth, N.D.; Dietz, W.H.; Magge, S.N.; Johnson, R.K.; American Academy Of Pediatrics; Section On Obesity; Committee On Nutrition; American Heart Association. Public Policies to Reduce Sugary Drink Consumption in Children and Adolescents. *Pediatrics* **2019**, *143*, e20190282. [CrossRef] [PubMed]
107. Colchero, M.A.; Rivera-Dommarco, J.; Popkin, B.M.; Ng, S.W. In Mexico, Evidence Of Sustained Consumer Response Two Years After Implementing A Sugar-Sweetened Beverage Tax. *Health Aff.* **2017**, *36*, 564–571. [CrossRef] [PubMed]
108. Sanchez-Romero, L.M.; Penko, J.; Coxson, P.G.; Fernandez, A.; Mason, A.; Moran, A.E.; Ávila-Burgos, L.; Odden, M.; Barquera, S.; Bibbins-Domingo, K. Projected Impact of Mexico's Sugar-Sweetened Beverage Tax Policy on Diabetes and Cardiovascular Disease: A Modeling Study. *PLoS Med.* **2016**, *13*, e1002158. [CrossRef] [PubMed]
109. Silver, L.D.; Ng, S.W.; Ryan-Ibarra, S.; Taillie, L.S.; Induni, M.; Miles, D.R.; Poti, J.M.; Popkin, B.M. Changes in prices, sales, consumer spending, and beverage consumption one year after a tax on sugar-sweetened beverages in Berkeley, California, US: A before-and-after study. *PLoS Med.* **2017**, *14*, e1002283. [CrossRef] [PubMed]

3

The Effects of Alcohol Consumption on Cardiometabolic Health Outcomes Following Weight Loss in Premenopausal Women with Obesity

John W. Apolzan *, Robbie A. Beyl, Corby K. Martin, Frank L. Greenway and Ursula White *

Pennington Biomedical Research Center, Louisiana State University System, Baton Rouge, LA 70808, USA; Robbie.Beyl@pbrc.edu (R.A.B.); Corby.Martin@pbrc.edu (C.K.M.); Frank.Greenway@pbrc.edu (F.L.G.)

* Correspondence: John.Apolzan@pbrc.edu (J.W.A.); Ursula.White@pbrc.edu (U.W.)

Abstract: Alcohol (i.e., ethanol) is consumed regularly by much of the adult population; yet, the health effects associated with its use are not well-characterized. Clinical interventions to investigate the effects of moderate alcohol consumption on metabolic outcomes, including adiposity and cardiovascular risk factors, are limited and have yielded conflicting data. In addition, no study has reported the effects of routine alcohol intake during weight loss in a controlled feeding trial. We present the first randomized controlled pilot trial to investigate the effects of moderate alcohol consumption on metabolic outcomes during weight loss in women with obesity. Both groups consumed 30% energy restricted diets and were randomized to either an ethanol-free control (CTL) group or a group (EtOH) that consumed 35 g ethanol daily for eight weeks. Our findings demonstrate that, despite similar weight loss, the decrease in mean arterial pressure was attenuated in the EtOH group, relative to the CTL group ($p = 0.02$). In addition, decreases in other outcomes, including visceral adipose tissue ($p = 0.23$), circulating lipids (triglycerides ($p = 0.11$) and cholesterol ($p = 0.11$)), and uric acid ($p = 0.07$) tended to be attenuated with alcohol consumption. These pilot data provide potential evidence that moderate alcohol consumption may mitigate the beneficial effects of weight loss and support the need for larger Randomized Controlled Trials (RCTs) to better investigate the metabolic effects of moderate alcohol intake in humans.

Keywords: ethanol; alcohol; weight loss; body weight; obesity; triglycerides; visceral fat; cholesterol; uric acid; blood pressure

---

1. Introduction

Alcohol (i.e., ethanol) is one of the most widely used recreational substances by humans and is consumed regularly by much of the population. Recent data reported that as many as ~58% of adults consumed alcohol within the previous month [1]. Other evidence from the National Health and Nutrition Examination Survey (NHANES) suggests that alcohol constitutes an estimated 5% of total daily energy intake in U.S. adults [2]. Despite the widespread consumption of alcohol, the health effects associated with its use have not been firmly established.

While the link between excessive alcohol intake and poor health outcomes, including liver cirrhosis, obesity-related cardiometabolic disorders, and mortality, is well-documented in humans, the consequences of moderate alcohol consumption remain obscure. Experimental intervention studies to examine the effects on body weight gain and obesity have been scarce and largely inconsistent, reporting either a positive association [3,4] or no effect [3–7] with alcohol intake. Routine alcohol consumption has also been associated with adipose tissue (AT) distribution, with limited cross-sectional studies describing a positive correlation with increased visceral adipose tissue (VAT) accumulation [8–11]. Yet, other studies suggest either an inverse or no association [7,12]. Interestingly, moderate alcohol consumption has been suggested to have both beneficial and unfavorable effects on cardiovascular morbidities and insulin sensitivity [13].

Many of the discrepancies in prior studies are due to the inclusion of various alcohol types (i.e., wine, beer, and spirits), which prevents the characterization of ethanol-specific effects, as wine and beer contain antioxidants and other micronutrients. The interpretation of existing data is also complicated by different intervention time periods, potential sex differences, the use of self-reported dietary data and other potential confounders. Many of these analyses have been primarily epidemiological and cross-sectional in nature; hence, there is a paucity of data from longitudinal assessments in humans to examine the metabolic response to routine moderate alcohol consumption in randomized controlled trials (RCTs). In addition, although ethanol consumption has been shown to be a risk factor for health consequences associated with weight gain, no study has examined the physiological effects of alcohol intake during a weight loss intervention, despite the favorable effects of energy restriction.

We report, herein, the first pilot RCT to investigate the effects of moderate alcohol consumption on metabolic outcomes during weight loss in women with obesity who consumed 30% energy restricted diets and were randomized to either an ethanol-free control (CTL) group or a group that consumed 35 g ethanol daily (EtOH) for eight weeks. We hypothesized that alcohol consumption would mitigate the favorable metabolic health effects resulting from weight loss.

2. Materials and Methods

2.1. Participant Characteristics

The study reported herein was conducted according to the guidelines in the Declaration of Helsinki. All participants were given verbal and written explanations about the study, provided signed informed consent, and received a monetary stipend. The study was approved by the Association for the Accreditation of Human Research Protection Programs (AAHRPP) accredited Pennington Biomedical Institutional Review Board. The study was registered at ClinicalTrials.gov (NCT 03521817).

Participants were healthy, pre-menopausal females who were 21–40 years of age with a BMI between 27–50 kg/m^2. Twelve participants were enrolled in the study. The inclusion criteria are as follows: (1) being willing to practice appropriate birth control, (2) being willing to eat at Pennington Biomedical Research Center (PBRC) at least 3 times per week, (3) beingwilling to consume alcohol (EtOH group), (4) being willing to abstain from alcohol (CTL group), and (5) being a daily or almost daily drinker, defined as typically consuming at least 8 drinks per week, but no more than 4 per day. Exclusion criteria included but are not limited to: (1) non-drinkers of alcohol, (2) habitual binge drinkers, defined by the consumption of ≥ 4 standard drinks per day or ≥ 28 drinks per week, (3) self-reported alcoholics or a history of alcoholism, (4) any attendance or inpatient stay for alcohol or drug treatment, (5) display any characteristic of current or future substance abuse disorders, (6) presence of any psychiatric, behavioral, or medical disorder that, in the opinion of the PIs, Co-Is, or MI, may interfere with study participation, the ability to adhere to the protocol, or has the potential for increased substance abuse, (7) prescription medications that interact with alcohol intake, (8) abnormal screening laboratory safety tests, (9) smokers, (10) diagnosis of Type 1 or 2 diabetes mellitus, cancer, or major organ disease, (11) serious digestive disorders, (12) conditions that affect metabolism or body weight (i.e., uncontrolled thyroid conditions, bariatric surgery, pregnancy, breastfeeding), (13) hysterectomy and/or hysterectomy with bilateral salphingo-oopherectomy, (14) hormonal pharmaceutical contraceptives including oral contraception (birth control pills), injectables (Depo-Provera), or the patch (Xulane), (15) Polycystic Ovary Syndrome (PCOS), and (16) use of medications that affect body weight or metabolism (i.e., atypical antipsychotics, weight loss medications).

2.2. *Study Design*

This study was a single blind between-subject randomized controlled study design. The investigators were blinded to the treatment group, but due to the nature of the study, participants were not blinded. All women underwent a 30% energy restriction for 8-weeks and were randomized to either an ethanol-consuming group or a non-ethanol control group at the start of the study. Participants initially visited the center for a screening visit (SV). If they volunteered and met the inclusion/exclusion criteria, they attended a pre-randomization visit. Following the pre-randomization visit, an alcohol tolerance test occurred (with study dose). Pending acceptance and adherence to the alcohol tolerance test, participants returned to the center for Clinic Visit (CV) 1 and randomization. The intervention lasted 8 weeks. Participants were required to come to the center a minimum of 3 times per week. Finally, participants came in for the final CV. Thus, participation lasted approximately 10–12 weeks in total.

2.2.1. Screening Visit 1

SV was conducted the morning after a ~10-h overnight fast. Demographics, vital signs, and medical history were assessed. A physical exam was administered. Anthropometric characteristics (i.e., height, metabolic weight, body mass index (BMI), blood pressure, and waist and hip circumference) were measured. A blood sample was collected and analyzed for laboratory safety tests. Menstrual cycle status was determined.

A semi-standardized Lifestyle Interview was administered by trained behavioral staff (Master's Level Psychologists) and overseen by a clinical psychologist (CKM). The interview was used to identify barriers to participation in the study, including scheduling challenges, ability to attend appointments, etc. The Substance Abuse Subtle Screening Inventory (SASSI) [14,15] and Michigan Alcoholism Screening Test (MAST) [16,17] questionnaires were administered. All participants were also screened and excluded based on the presences of psychological conditions that could interfere with the ability to adhere to protocol or indicate that participating in the research could be unsafe, for example, due to a history of substance dependence. Specifically, the Structured Clinical Interview for DSM-5 Clinical Version (SCID-5-CV [18]) was administered to identify mood disorders, psychotic disorders, substance abuse, etc. Furthermore, the Structured Clinical Interview for DSM-5 Personality Disorders (SCID-5 PD [19]) was administered to identify DSM-5 Personality Disorders.

This, and other information, was used to provide an overall eligibility assessment for each candidate. A multidisciplinary team consisting of behavioral experts, dietitians, clinical staff, a Medical Investigator (FLG), and study staff discussed and approved candidates for official admission to the study.

2.2.2. Pre-Randomization Visit

Before enrollment in the study, all women were required to undergo an overnight alcohol tolerance test at the required ethanol dose. This was the dose of alcohol that was to be consumed for the duration of the study in the EtOH group. Furthermore, women were provided with a step log (pedometer provided; New Lifestyles YAMX Digi-Walker) and asked to return it at CV1. Pending adherence to the overnight alcohol test, a one-week ethanol-free washout following the overnight tolerance test, and the return of the pedometer with step count, participants underwent CV1.

The purpose of the ethanol-free washout following the overnight tolerance test was two-fold. First, participants demonstrated the ability to forgo alcohol for 1 week. Secondly it provided a stable baseline period for all subjects prior to study enrollment at CV1.

2.2.3. Clinic Visit (CV) 1

At CV1 and 2, women reported to PBRC after an overnight fast during the luteal phase of the menstrual cycle. Anthropometric characteristics (height; metabolic weight; mean arterial pressure (1/3 [systolic BP – diastolic BP] + diastolic BP)) were measured.

Subcutaneous abdominal AT (SAT) and visceral AT (VAT) volumes were defined and quantified with magnetic resonance imaging (MRI) using a 3.0 T scanner (GE, Discovery 750 w) by obtaining ~581 images from the dome of the liver to the pubic symphysis. Images were analyzed by a single trained analyst. Estimates of VAT and SAT volumes were converted to mass using an assumed density of 0.92 kg/L. Blood draws were performed, and serum and plasma were archived.

2.3. *Randomization*

Eligible participants were then randomized (1:1) to consume 35 g/day of ethanol (EtOH group; $n = 7$) or to control (CTL; $n = 5$) via block randomization (using SAS 9.4) for 8 weeks. After randomization, participants began the dietary intervention.

2.4. *8-Week Dietary Intervention*

Participants were provided all meals. Meals were prepared by the PBRC metabolic kitchen (5-day meal rotation). Participants were given both verbal and written instructions as to the consumption of the food. On weekdays, a minimum of one meal (i.e., breakfast, lunch, or dinner) was consumed at PBRC at least 3 times per week, (excluding holidays), whereas the other weekday meals were packaged for takeout. In addition, alcohol, weekend, and holiday meals were packaged for takeout. Participants' energy requirements were determined from their estimated resting metabolic rate (RMR), calculated via the Mifflin-St. Jeor formula [20] with an activity factor of 1.5. The energy requirements were then multiplied by 0.70 so that all participants will restrict energy needs by 30% compared to weight maintenance. Each group (control and ethanol) had the same 30% reduction in calories and will consume the same percentage of each additional macronutrient (20% protein, 50% carbohydrate, and 30% fat).

The ethanol group consumed a 30% energy restriction diet that also included ~2.5 standard drinks, or 35 g of ethanol, administered as 80-proof distilled spirits (e.g., 80 proof gin, rum, vodka, whiskey, or tequila). In the United States, one "standard" drink contains roughly 14 g of pure alcohol. The remaining calories (Mifflin-St. Jeor formula, with an activity factor of 1.5 multiplied by 0.70 minus the ~240 kcals from ethanol) was consumed as 20% protein, 50% carbohydrate, and 30% fat. The control group l consumed these ~240 kcal as included in the aforementioned macronutrient percentages (20% protein, 50% carbohydrate, and 30% fat) as a beverage to match the ethanol group.

The alcohol was purchased, logged, handled, and dispensed by the study pharmacist. Measured doses of alcohol were prepared by the study pharmacist. Sealed, individual bottles (~7) of alcohol were dispensed to the participant once per week (on the Monday; excluding holidays) through the outpatient clinic. Each bottle contained a pre-measured dose of alcohol, and participants drank the pre-measured dose of alcohol each day of the week.

Participants were asked to have an in-clinic check in once per week when coming for their in-house meal (generally Monday am). At this check a metabolic weight was obtained, adverse events and changes in medication were assessed. The ethanol group was also administered the modified weekly version of the alcohol-related questionnaires (SASSI and MAST).

2.5. *Instructions for Alcohol Consumption*

Participants were given general information about alcohol and informed of the effects of its use on the body. The participants were warned of the risks associated with performing daily activities and operating vehicles or other machinery after alcohol ingestion. Alcohol was instructed to be consumed when participants were in for the evening and driving was concluded for the day. Subjects were provided information about the warning signs of alcohol dependency.

2.6. *Dietary and Alcohol Compliance*

Subjects were instructed to report if any additional food, beverages, and alcoholic drinks were consumed. Subjects who were under-compliant (<85%) or over-compliant (>100%) were counseled by study staff on the importance of compliance.

2.7. *Participant Follow-up*

At the end of the intervention, participants were contacted (phone) by trained study staff at 2 weeks and 4 weeks after completion of the study in order to assess if the women have acquired any alcohol abuse and/or dependency issues.

2.8. *Blood Parameters*

A chemistry panel was performed at SV1, CV1, and CV2. This included glucose, cholesterol (HDL and LDL), triglyceride, and uric acid. Furthermore, insulin, free fatty acids (FFA), and glycerol (GLY) were measured with standardized procedures.

2.9. *Statistical Analysis*

Analyses were carried out using SAS, Version 9.4 (SAS Institute, Cary, NC) with a significance level of $\alpha = 0.05$. All data reported are mean ± SEM. Two-way ANOVAs were used to test if changes in covariates (Week 8 — Baseline) differed between treatment groups (primary outcome). Treatment effects, which represent the change induced in the EtOH group relative to the change in the CTL group, are denoted with symbol Δ. Normality of the residuals from the mixed model were checked and observations with a residual value of ± 3 were investigated. One participant in the CTL group was dropped from the study due to time commitments, and another in the CTL group was excluded from the analysis, as she was non-compliant with the study design.

3. Results

The analyses included 10 women who completed the study (CTL group—$n = 3$; EtOH group—$n = 7$) who were of Caucasian ($n = 6$), African American ($n = 3$), or Other decent ($n = 1$). One person (Other) was of Hispanic, Latino, or Spanish Origin. At SV1, they were 33 ± 3 years with a mean body weight of 97.8 ± 4.4 kg and BMI of 35.4 ± 1.6 kg/m^2. The control group had 4917 ± 1706 step/day and the EtOH group had 6902 ± 1117 steps/day at baseline ($p = 0.36$). The clinical and metabolic characteristics of participants in the CTL and EtOH groups are included in Table 1.

There was no significant difference in the change in body weight between the CTL and the EtOH groups ($\Delta = -1.2 \pm 1.4$ kg; $p = 0.43$). There was no significant difference in the change in SAT (1A; $\Delta = 0.05 \pm 0.3$ kg; $p = 0.87$) or VAT (1B; $\Delta = -0.18 \pm 0.14$ kg; $p = 0.23$) mass between the CTL and the EtOH groups. Furthermore, there was no significant difference in the change in triglycerides (2A; $\Delta = -42.9 \pm 24.3$ mg/dL; $p = 0.11$) or cholesterol (2B; $\Delta = -21.1 \pm 11.8$ mg/dL; $p = 0.11$) between the CTL and the EtOH groups. The decrease in mean arterial pressure was significantly attenuated by alcohol consumption in the EtOH group as compared to the CTL group ($\Delta = -8.0 \pm 2.8$ mmHg; $p = 0.02$). There was no significant difference in the change in mean steps between the CTL and the EtOH groups ($\Delta = 743 \pm 1547$ steps/d CTL, $\Delta = -113 \pm 1013$ steps/d EtOH, $\Delta = 855.8 \pm 1849.3$ steps/d; $p = 0.66$).

Table 1. Baseline, treatment, and changes in the clinical and metabolic characteristics of participants in the ethanol-free control (CTL) and the group that consumed 35 g ethanol daily for eight weeks (EtOH).

	CTL Δ W0 vs. W8	EtOH Δ W0 vs. W8	Δ CTL vs. Δ EtOH	Effect Size Δ CTL vs. Δ EtOH	*p*-Value Δ CTL vs. Δ EtOH
BMI (kg/m^2)	−2.2 ± 0.4 [a]	−2.0 ± 0.3 [a]	−0.2 ± 0.5	−0.2	0.76
Body weight (kg)	−6.6 ± 1.2 [a]	−5.4 ± 0.8 [a]	−1.2 ± 1.4	−0.6	0.43
SAT (kg)	−1.1 ± 0.3 [a]	−1.2 ± 0.2 [a]	0.05 ± 0.3	0.1	0.87
VAT (kg)	−0.2 ± 0.1	−0.1 ± 0.1	−0.2 ± 0.1	−0.9	0.23
Triglycerides (mg/dL)	−26.3 ± 20.3	16.6 ± 13.3	−42.9 ± 24.3	−1.2	0.11
FFA (mmol/L)	0.1 ± 0.1	0.2 ± 0.1 [a]	−0.1 ± 0.1	−0.3	0.62
Glycerol (mmol/L)	−0.01 ± 0.02	0.02 ± 0.02	−0.03 ± 0.03	−0.8	0.33
Cholesterol (mg/dL)	−26.7 ± 9.9 [a]	-5.6 ± 6.5	−21.1 ± 11.8	−1.2	0.11
HDL (mg/dL)	−5.7 ± 3.7	-4.3 ± 2.4	−1.4 ± 4.4	−0.2	0.76
LDL (mg/dL)	−15.7 ± 8.3	-4.6 ± 5.4	−11.1 ± 9.9	−0.8	0.29
Mean Arterial Pressure (mmHg)	−8.3 ± 2.3 [a]	−0.4 ± 1.5	−8.0 ± 2.8	−2.0	0.02
Glucose (mg/dL)	−3.0 ± 4.5	3.3 ± 3.0	−6.3 ± 5.4	−0.8	0.28
Insulin (mU/L)	−6.8 ± 3.3	−5.2 ± 2.1 [a]	−1.6 ± 3.9	−0.3	0.70
HOMA-IR	−1.7 ± 0.85	−1.1 ± 0.6	−0.6 ± 1.0	−0.4	0.58
Uric Acid (mg/dL)	−0.5 ± 0.3	0.3 ± 0.2	−0.8 ± 0.4	−1.4	0.07

Values presented as mean ± SEM; [a] $p < 0.05$ for within-group change in measured outcome

4. Discussion

The authors believe this to be the first study to test the effects of EtOH consumption on the cardiometabolic effects of weight loss in premenopausal women with obesity during controlled feeding. The results from this pilot study suggest that the ingestion of EtOH may have negative effects on the metabolic benefits of weight loss. Our findings demonstrate that the decrease in mean arterial pressure was attenuated in the EtOH group, relative to the CTL group. In addition, decreases in other outcomes, including VAT and circulating lipids (triglycerides and cholesterol), tended to be attenuated with alcohol consumption. With the increasing focus on personalized medicine, alcohol consumption may play a significant role as a modifiable risk factor affecting the metabolic health outcomes associated with weight loss. Future work may consider adding physical activity to determine if it can improve metabolic health outcomes with alcohol consumption.

Limited randomized trials have examined the effects of EtOH on circulating lipid levels. A previous controlled feeding study recruited weight-stable premenopausal women who were ~80–130% of desirable weight and were provided 30 g of alcohol per day for 60 days [21]. Alcohol consumption did not affect total cholesterol or triglyceride levels, but HDL increased, and LDL decreased [21]. Another crossover-controlled feeding study examined postmenopausal women who were 90–140% of ideal in weight maintenance [22]. This study performed a dose response with three treatment groups including control, 15 g alcohol, and 30 g alcohol. The 15 and 30 g alcohol groups had decreased triglycerides compared to the control group. The 30 g alcohol group decreased total cholesterol compared to the control group, and the 15 g alcohol group was not different than either group. The 30 g alcohol group increased HDL compared to control and 15 g alcohol drink group, whereas LDL was decreased in the 15 and 30 g alcohol groups compared to the control group [22]. Similarly, a study in women with obesity was randomized to either ~2.5 drinks of white wine or grape juice [23]. Post study, the white wine group had decreased triglycerides and LDL cholesterol and increased HDL cholesterol. Herein, we found that HDL levels were fairly consistent between groups, but triglycerides tended to have a greater reduction in the EtOH vs. the control group. Overall, lipid metabolism is likely affected by moderate ethanol intake. In energy balance (weight maintenance) alcohol may have positive health effects on lipid metabolism, whereas alcohol may attenuate the positive effects of weight loss on lipid metabolism in women.

Interestingly, early data from Eric Jequier's group demonstrated that the addition of alcohol to the diet decreased lipid (fat) oxidation, suggesting that ethanol consumption may favor lipid storage [24] in a cross-sectional study with low to modest habitual alcohol intake. This coincides with our results suggesting that VAT loss tended to be attenuated in the EtOH vs. control groups. However, the effects of ethanol on adipose tissue (AT) distribution are controversial. Several studies have reported that routine alcohol intake is positively correlated with increased visceral adipose tissue (VAT) accumulation [8–11]. Other studies suggest either an inverse or no association with central adiposity [7,12]. A previous study examined the effects of drinking red wine (~17 g ethanol) over two years and found no differences between the ethanol groups and control group in visceral adiposity [25]. The results reported herein found that VAT loss tended to be attenuated with EtOH consumption. A strong positive association between visceral adiposity and blood pressure exists [26]. Interestingly, to date, alcohol intake has been shown to have somewhat mixed effects on blood pressure response [27–29], however, and not surprisingly the current study found a strong attenuation in mean arterial blood pressure loss with EtOH.

It is possible that alcohol consumption may have diuretic action and influence dehydration; however, the extent of these effects is not fully understood. A previous RCT study showed that spirits (consumed at an amount similar to our study) caused only a small and transient diuretic effect at 4 h, and that there were no differences in 24 hr urine output or urine osmolarity when compared to subjects that consumed water [30]. Another study reported that more urine was excreted after 4 h when beer (4% alcohol), compared to the non-alcoholic beverage, was consumed during euhydration ($p < 0.001$), while there was no significant difference between groups during hypohydration ($p = 0.06$) [31]. Yet, a subsequent RCT using the beverage hydration index found that cumulative urine output at 4 h after ingestion of lager beer (4% alcohol) was not different from the response to water ingestion [32]. Taken together, these data suggest that the moderate consumption of alcohol may play a limited role in hydration. Of note, in our study, the alcoholic drinks were consumed with non-caloric mixers, which contain water.

Furthermore, various hormones, including vasopressin, can impact hydration and influence metabolic outcomes such as blood pressure, and studies have shown that alcohol consumption can alter vasopressin [33]. Our data demonstrate that alcohol consumption attenuated the lowering of mean blood pressure during weight loss, relative to the control group; however, neither vasopressin, nor other similar hormones, were measured in our study. Though hormonal regulation is plausible, the precise mechanisms underlying these findings need to be elucidated in future studies, as it is likely that there are several independent mechanisms acting to increase blood pressure with alcohol consumption [34].

In previous studies, moderate alcohol consumption has been associated with benefits to glycemia particularly in nondiabetic subjects [35–38]. Postmenopausal women with 90–140% of the ideal weight (27.4 kg/m^2) were enrolled in a randomized crossover trial with 0, 15, or 30 g of alcohol [39]. The study found that fasting insulin decreased in the 30 g of alcohol vs. control conditions. Insulin sensitivity improved with the consumption of 30 g of alcohol vs. control conditions in non-diabetic premenopausal women [39]. Similarly, in a study where women with overweight were randomized to either white wine or white grape juice for six weeks, fasting insulin was lower in the white wine vs. grape juice groups [23]. Alcohol seems to confer benefits to insulin sensitivity during weight maintenance. However, in a nonrandomized study that provided 30 g of alcohol to insulin resistant individuals, no benefits to insulin sensitivity were seen [40]. In the current study, our results suggest no difference between groups. This may be due to the difference in baseline body weight of the participants among studies, or the fact that, in energy balance (weight maintenance), alcohol may have positive health effects on insulin sensitivity, whereas alcohol may attenuate the positive effects of weight loss on insulin sensitivity in women.

Well-powered longitudinal assessments from a randomized, controlled trial (RCT) with clinically relevant end points are necessary in order to examine the influence of chronic alcohol consumption on cardiometabolic health, central adiposity, and the mechanisms underlying ethanol-associated changes in metabolism. Post-hoc power analyses indicated that if 38 total participants were enrolled ($n = 19$/group), this study would have been powered to see differences in all of the main variables that did not reach significance: visceral adipose tissue, circulating lipids (triglycerides and cholesterol), and uric acid. NHANES data underestimates the overall energy intake due to self-report methodology and further underestimates the percentage daily alcohol energy intake in alcohol consumers. In persons that consume alcohol, energy intake from ethanol is estimated to be ~10% [41]. Therefore, if the average daily total energy intake is ~2400 kcal in women with obesity, most alcohol users are likely consuming ~240 kcal/d (10% of total energy) from alcohol. Hence, our dose of ethanol is externally valid.

This study has numerous strengths. These include that it was a randomized controlled trial (RCT), and a controlled feeding trial. It is important to note that all food (and beverage) intake was provided for all subjects, and the intervention did not affect physical activity. For eight weeks, participants were only provided with, and expected, food and beverage from the Pennington Biomedical metabolic research kitchen. The study did not involve behavior change (i.e., behavioral weight loss), nor was it recommended. As expected, physical activity did not change during the course of the intervention. While a pilot study, multiple effect sizes were robust. Some weaknesses include the lack of physical activity data throughout the study, no measurement of hydration status, low sample size, and the lack of a true control group. Furthermore, only premenopausal women were included—given that there are sex differences in adipose tissue distribution [42] (a primary endpoint) and likely the mechanisms that influence this and other metabolic outcomes—in order to reduce potential confounders.

5. Conclusions

These pilot data provide potential evidence that moderate alcohol consumption may counteract the beneficial effects of weight loss and support the need for larger RCTs to better investigate the metabolic effects of moderate alcohol intake during weight loss in humans. Personalized medicine remains a focus of the National Institutes of Health (NIH). While preliminary, this pilot study suggests that a dietary pattern which incorporates moderate alcohol consumption may attenuate some of the beneficial effects of weight loss, but well-powered follow-up studies are needed.

Author Contributions: Conceptualization, J.W.A. and U.W.; methodology, J.W.A., U.W., C.K.M., and F.L.G.; formal analysis, J.W.A., U.W., and R.A.B.; investigation, J.W.A., U.W., and R.A.B.; resources, J.W.A. and U.W.; data curation, J.W.A., U.W., and R.A.B.; writing—original draft preparation, J.W.A. and U.W.; writing—review and editing, J.W.A, U.W., R.A.B., C.K.M., and F.L.G.; supervision, J.W.A., U.W., C.K.M., and F.L.G.; project administration, J.W.A. and U.W.; funding acquisition, J.W.A. and U.W. All authors have read and agreed to the published version of the manuscript.

Acknowledgments: The authors would like to thank the participants for their time and effort. We would like to thank our consultant Louis Cataldie. Furthermore, we would like to thank the PBRC Cores including the outpatient unit (Erin LeJeune), pharmacy (Claire Hazlett), recruiting (Alison Carville and Grace Bella), advertising (Lauren Giffin), and imaging (Owen T. Carmichael and Kori Murray), and clinical chemistry (Stephen Lee and Stacey Roussel).

References

1. 2018 National Survey on Drug Use and Health (NSDUH). Available online: https://www.samhsa.gov/data/sites/default/files/cbhsq-reports/NSDUHDetailedTabs2018R2/NSDUHDetTabsSect2pe2018.htm#tab2-1b (accessed on 12 February 2019).
2. Eicher-Miller, H.A.; Boushey, C.J. How Often and How Much? Differences in Dietary Intake by Frequency and Energy Contribution Vary among U.S. Adults in NHANES 2007-2012. *Nutrients* **2017**, *9*, 86. [CrossRef]
3. Crouse, J.R.; Grundy, S.M. Effects of alcohol on plasma lipoproteins and cholesterol and triglyceride metabolism in man. *J. Lipid Res.* **1984**, *25*, 486–496.
4. Romeo, J.; Gonzalez-Gross, M.; Warnberg, J.; Diaz, L.E.; Marcos, A. Does beer have an impact on weight gain? Effects of moderate beer consumption on body composition. *Nutr. Hosp.* **2007**, *22*, 223–228.

5. Cordain, L.; Bryan, E.D.; Melby, C.L.; Smith, M.J. Influence of moderate daily wine consumption on body weight regulation and metabolism in healthy free-living males. *J. Am. Coll. Nutr.* **1997**, *16*, 134–139. [CrossRef]

6. Cordain, L.; Melby, C.L.; Hamamoto, A.E.; O'Neill, D.S.; Cornier, M.A.; Barakat, H.A.; Israel, R.G.; Hill, J.O. Influence of moderate chronic wine consumption on insulin sensitivity and other correlates of syndrome X in moderately obese women. *Metab. Clin. Exp.* **2000**, *49*, 1473–1478. [CrossRef]

7. Beulens, J.W.; van Beers, R.M.; Stolk, R.P.; Schaafsma, G.; Hendriks, H.F. The effect of moderate alcohol consumption on fat distribution and adipocytokines. *Obesity (Silver Spring)* **2006**, *14*, 60–66. [CrossRef]

8. Cigolini, M.; Targher, G.; Bergamo Andreis, I.A.; Tonoli, M.; Filippi, F.; Muggeo, M.; De Sandre, G. Moderate alcohol consumption and its relation to visceral fat and plasma androgens in healthy women. *Int. J. Obes. Relat. Metab. Disord. J. Int. Assoc. Study Obes.* **1996**, *20*, 206–212.

9. Molenaar, E.A.; Massaro, J.M.; Jacques, P.F.; Pou, K.M.; Ellison, R.C.; Hoffmann, U.; Pencina, K.; Shadwick, S.D.; Vasan, R.S.; O'Donnell, C.J.; et al. Association of lifestyle factors with abdominal subcutaneous and visceral adiposity: The Framingham Heart Study. *Diabetes Care* **2009**, *32*, 505–510. [CrossRef] [PubMed]

10. Kim, K.H.; Oh, S.W.; Kwon, H.; Park, J.H.; Choi, H.; Cho, B. Alcohol consumption and its relation to visceral and subcutaneous adipose tissues in healthy male Koreans. *Ann. Nutr. Metab.* **2012**, *60*, 52–61. [CrossRef] [PubMed]

11. Komiya, H.; Mori, Y.; Yokose, T.; Tajima, N. Smoking as a risk factor for visceral fat accumulation in Japanese men. *Tohoku J. Exp. Med.* **2006**, *208*, 123–132. [CrossRef] [PubMed]

12. Greenfield, J.R.; Samaras, K.; Jenkins, A.B.; Kelly, P.J.; Spector, T.D.; Campbell, L.V. Moderate alcohol consumption, dietary fat composition, and abdominal obesity in women: Evidence for gene-environment interaction. *J. Clin. Endocrinol. Metab* **2003**, *88*, 5381–5386. [CrossRef] [PubMed]

13. Mukamal, K.J.; Clowry, C.M.; Murray, M.M.; Hendriks, H.F.; Rimm, E.B.; Sink, K.M.; Adebamowo, C.A.; Dragsted, L.O.; Lapinski, P.S.; Lazo, M.; et al. Moderate Alcohol Consumption and Chronic Disease: The Case for a Long-Term Trial. *Alcohol. Clin. Exp. Res.* **2016**, *40*, 2283–2291. [CrossRef] [PubMed]

14. Lazowski, L.E.; Geary, B.B. Validation of the Adult Substance Abuse Subtle Screening Inventory-4 (SASSI-4). *Eur. J. Psychol. Assess.* **2019**, 86–97. [CrossRef]

15. Lazowski, L.E.; Geary, B.B.; Baker, S.L. *The Adult Substance Abuse Subtle Screening Inventory-4 (SASSI-4) User Guide & Manual*; The Sassi Institute: Springville, IN, USA, 2016.

16. Selzer, M.L. The Michigan alcoholism screening test: The quest for a new diagnostic instrument. *Am. J. Psychiatry* **1971**, *127*, 1653–1658. [CrossRef]

17. Selzer, M.L.; Vinokur, A.; van Rooijen, L. A self-administered Short Michigan Alcoholism Screening Test (SMAST). *J. Stud. Alcohol.* **1975**, *36*, 117–126. [CrossRef]

18. First, M.B.; Williams, J.B.; Karg, R.S.; Spitzer, R.L. *Structured Clinical Interview for DSM-5 Disorders—Clinical Version (SCID-5-CV)*; American Psychiatric Association: Arlington, VA, USA, 2016.

19. First, M.B.; Williams, J.B.; Karg, R.S.; Spitzer, R.L. *Structured Clinical Interview for DSM-5 Personality Disorders (SCID-5-PD)*; American Psychiatric Association: Arlington, VA, USA, 2016.

20. Mifflin, M.D.; St Jeor, S.T.; Hill, L.A.; Scott, B.J.; Daugherty, S.A.; Koh, Y.O. A new predictive equation for resting energy expenditure in healthy individuals. *Am. J. Clin. Nutr.* **1990**, *51*, 241–247. [CrossRef]

21. Clevidence, B.A.; Reichman, M.E.; Judd, J.T.; Muesing, R.A.; Schatzkin, A.; Schaefer, E.J.; Li, Z.; Jenner, J.; Brown, C.C.; Sunkin, M.; et al. Effects of alcohol consumption on lipoproteins of premenopausal women. A controlled diet study. *Arterioscler. Thromb. Vasc. Biol.* **1995**, *15*, 179–184. [CrossRef]

22. Baer, D.J.; Judd, J.T.; Clevidence, B.A.; Muesing, R.A.; Campbell, W.S.; Brown, E.D.; Taylor, P.R. Moderate alcohol consumption lowers risk factors for cardiovascular disease in postmenopausal women fed a controlled diet. *Am. J. Clin. Nutr.* **2002**, *75*, 593–599. [CrossRef]

23. Joosten, M.M.; Beulens, J.W.; Kersten, S.; Hendriks, H.F. Moderate alcohol consumption increases insulin sensitivity and ADIPOQ expression in postmenopausal women: A randomised, crossover trial. *Diabetologia* **2008**, *51*, 1375–1381. [CrossRef]

24. Suter, P.M.; Schutz, Y.; Jequier, E. The effect of ethanol on fat storage in healthy subjects. *N. Engl. J. Med.* **1992**, *326*, 983–987. [CrossRef]

25. Golan, R.; Shelef, I.; Shemesh, E.; Henkin, Y.; Schwarzfuchs, D.; Gepner, Y.; Harman-Boehm, I.; Witkow, S.; Friger, M.; Chassidim, Y.; et al. Effects of initiating moderate wine intake on abdominal adipose tissue in adults with type 2 diabetes: A 2-year randomized controlled trial. *Public Health Nutr.* **2017**, *20*, 549–555. [CrossRef] [PubMed]
26. Chandra, A.; Neeland, I.J.; Berry, J.D.; Ayers, C.R.; Rohatgi, A.; Das, S.R.; Khera, A.; McGuire, D.K.; de Lemos, J.A.; Turer, A.T. The relationship of body mass and fat distribution with incident hypertension: Observations from the Dallas Heart Study. *J. Am. Coll. Cardiol.* **2014**, *64*, 997–1002. [CrossRef] [PubMed]
27. Roerecke, M.; Kaczorowski, J.; Tobe, S.W.; Gmel, G.; Hasan, O.S.M.; Rehm, J. The effect of a reduction in alcohol consumption on blood pressure: A systematic review and meta-analysis. *Lancet Public Health* **2017**, *2*, e108–e120. [CrossRef]
28. Sesso, H.D.; Cook, N.R.; Buring, J.E.; Manson, J.E.; Gaziano, J.M. Alcohol consumption and the risk of hypertension in women and men. *Hypertension* **2008**, *51*, 1080–1087. [CrossRef] [PubMed]
29. Gillman, M.W.; Cook, N.R.; Evans, D.A.; Rosner, B.; Hennekens, C.H. Relationship of alcohol intake with blood pressure in young adults. *Hypertension* **1995**, *25*, 1106–1110. [CrossRef] [PubMed]
30. Polhuis, K.; Wijnen, A.H.C.; Sierksma, A.; Calame, W.; Tieland, M. The Diuretic Action of Weak and Strong Alcoholic Beverages in Elderly Men: A Randomized Diet-Controlled Crossover Trial. *Nutrients* **2017**, *9*, 660. [CrossRef]
31. Hobson, R.M.; Maughan, R.J. Hydration status and the diuretic action of a small dose of alcohol. *Alcohol Alcohol.* **2010**, *45*, 366–373. [CrossRef]
32. Maughan, R.J.; Watson, P.; Cordery, P.A.; Walsh, N.P.; Oliver, S.J.; Dolci, A.; Rodriguez-Sanchez, N.; Galloway, S.D. A randomized trial to assess the potential of different beverages to affect hydration status: Development of a beverage hydration index. *Am. J. Clin. Nutr.* **2016**, *103*, 717–723. [CrossRef]
33. Taivainen, H.; Laitinen, K.; Tahtela, R.; Kilanmaa, K.; Valimaki, M.J. Role of plasma vasopressin in changes of water balance accompanying acute alcohol intoxication. *Alcohol. Clin. Exp. Res.* **1995**, *19*, 759–762. [CrossRef]
34. Husain, K.; Ansari, R.A.; Ferder, L. Alcohol-induced hypertension: Mechanism and prevention. *World J. Cardiol.* **2014**, *6*, 245–252. [CrossRef]
35. Bonnet, F.; Disse, E.; Laville, M.; Mari, A.; Hojlund, K.; Anderwald, C.H.; Piatti, P.; Balkau, B.; Group, R.S. Moderate alcohol consumption is associated with improved insulin sensitivity, reduced basal insulin secretion rate and lower fasting glucagon concentration in healthy women. *Diabetologia* **2012**, *55*, 3228–3237. [CrossRef] [PubMed]
36. Kiechl, S.; Willeit, J.; Poewe, W.; Egger, G.; Oberhollenzer, F.; Muggeo, M.; Bonora, E. Insulin sensitivity and regular alcohol consumption: Large, prospective, cross sectional population study (Bruneck study). *BMJ* **1996**, *313*, 1040–1044. [CrossRef] [PubMed]
37. Kroenke, C.H.; Chu, N.F.; Rifai, N.; Spiegelman, D.; Hankinson, S.E.; Manson, J.E.; Rimm, E.B. A cross-sectional study of alcohol consumption patterns and biologic markers of glycemic control among 459 women. *Diabetes Care* **2003**, *26*, 1971–1978. [CrossRef] [PubMed]
38. Schrieks, I.C.; Heil, A.L.; Hendriks, H.F.; Mukamal, K.J.; Beulens, J.W. The effect of alcohol consumption on insulin sensitivity and glycemic status: A systematic review and meta-analysis of intervention studies. *Diabetes Care* **2015**, *38*, 723–732. [CrossRef] [PubMed]
39. Davies, M.J.; Baer, D.J.; Judd, J.T.; Brown, E.D.; Campbell, W.S.; Taylor, P.R. Effects of moderate alcohol intake on fasting insulin and glucose concentrations and insulin sensitivity in postmenopausal women: A randomized controlled trial. *JAMA* **2002**, *287*, 2559–2562. [CrossRef]
40. Kim, S.H.; Abbasi, F.; Lamendola, C.; Reaven, G.M. Effect of moderate alcoholic beverage consumption on insulin sensitivity in insulin-resistant, nondiabetic individuals. *Metabolism* **2009**, *58*, 387–392. [CrossRef]
41. Jequier, E. Alcohol intake and body weight: A paradox. *Am. J. Clin. Nutr.* **1999**, *69*, 173–174.
42. Karastergiou, K.; Smith, S.R.; Greenberg, A.S.; Fried, S.K. Sex differences in human adipose tissues—the biology of pear shape. *Biol. Sex Differ.* **2012**, *3*, 13. [CrossRef]

4

The Role of Omega-3 Fatty Acids in the Setting of Coronary Artery Disease and COPD

Alex Pizzini [1,†], Lukas Lunger [2,†], Thomas Sonnweber [1], Guenter Weiss [1] and Ivan Tancevski [1,*]

1 Department of Internal Medicine II, Infectious Diseases, Pneumology, Rheumatology, Medical University of Innsbruck, 6020 Innsbruck, Austria; alex.pizzini@i-med.ac.at (A.P.); Thomas.Sonnweber@i-med.ac.at (T.S.); Guenter.Weiss@i-med.ac.at (G.W.)

2 Department of Urology, Klinikum rechts der Isar, Technische Universität München, 81675 Munich, Germany; lukas.lunger@tum.de

* Correspondence: Ivan.Tancevski@i-med.ac.at

† Authors with equal contribution.

Abstract: Chronic obstructive pulmonary disease (COPD) is a growing healthcare concern and will represent the third leading cause of death worldwide within the next decade. COPD is the result of a complex interaction between environmental factors, especially cigarette smoking, air pollution, and genetic preconditions, which result in persistent inflammation of the airways. There is growing evidence that the chronic inflammatory state, measurable by increased levels of circulating cytokines, chemokines, and acute phase proteins, may not be confined to the lungs. Cardiovascular disease (CVD) and especially coronary artery disease (CAD) are common comorbidities of COPD, and low-grade systemic inflammation plays a decisive role in its pathogenesis. Omega-3 polyunsaturated fatty acids (*n*-3 PUFAs) exert multiple functions in humans and are crucially involved in limiting and resolving inflammatory processes. *n*-3 PUFAs have been intensively studied for their ability to improve morbidity and mortality in patients with CVD and CAD. This review aims to summarize the current knowledge on the effects of *n*-3 PUFA on inflammation and its impact on CAD in COPD from a clinical perspective.

Keywords: omega 3; PUFA; *n*-3 PUFA; COPD; inflammation; coronary artery disease; ischemic heart disease; CAD; CHD

---

1. Introduction

Chronic obstructive pulmonary disease (COPD) is one of the leading causes of morbidity and mortality worldwide [1]. Data from the Global Burden of Disease Study estimate that, to date, approximately 328 million people suffer from COPD globally, and suggest that this number may be even higher because of a substantial number of undiagnosed cases and increasing exposure to environmental factors, which promote COPD development and progression. It is estimated that, by the year 2030, COPD will represent the third leading cause of death worldwide [1–5].

COPD is the result of a complex interaction between lifestyle factors, especially cigarette smoking and air pollution, and genetic preconditions, resulting in persistent inflammation of the airways even after smoking cessation, causing sustained peripheral airflow limitation [1,6]. The latter is defined as the ratio between forced expiratory volume in one second (FEV1) versus forced vital capacity (FVC) being less than 0.7, determined via spirometry after bronchodilator therapy [1]. The exact mechanisms behind these processes are not yet understood, but the challenge to oxidative stress and the resulting imbalance of proteases and anti-proteases seem to be causative [6]. Moreover, there is growing evidence that the chronic inflammatory state reflected by increased levels of circulating cytokines, chemokines, and acute phase proteins may not be confined to the lungs [7]. Cardiovascular disease (CVD) and coronary artery disease (CAD) are the typical and most common comorbidities of COPD, and significantly impact on patients' prognosis and quality of life (Figure 1) [8–11].

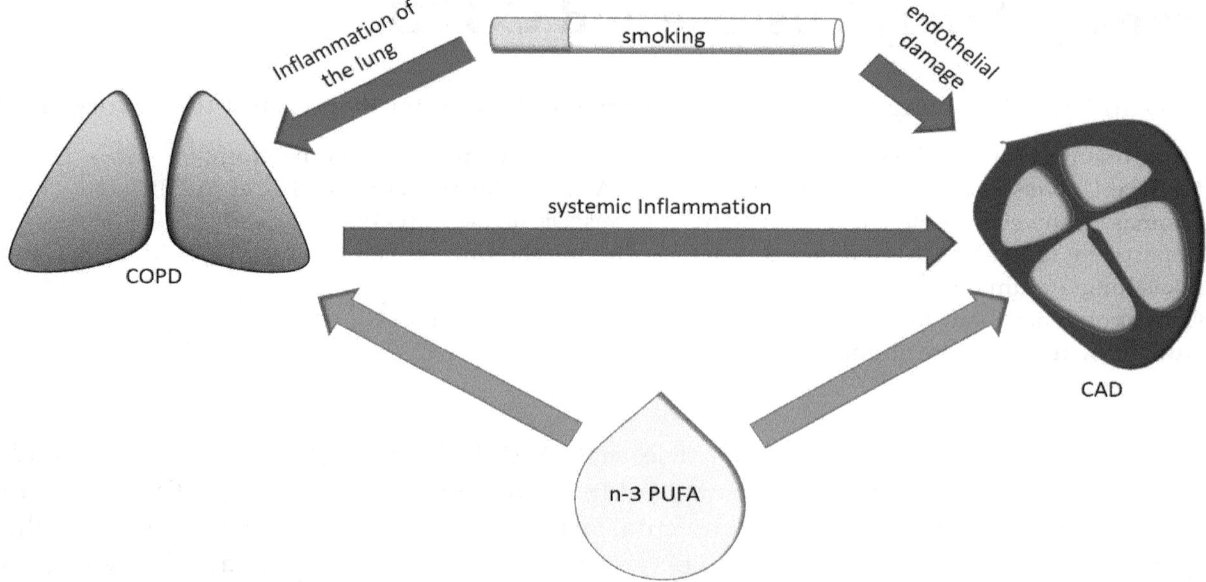

Figure 1. Interplay between smoking, pulmonary and systemic inflammation, coronary artery disease and omega-3 polyunsaturated fatty acids (*n*-3 PUFAs). COPD = chronic obstructive pulmonary disease, CAD = coronary artery disease.

Omega-3 polyunsaturated fatty acids (*n*-3 PUFAs) exert multiple functions in humans and are crucially involved in limiting and resolving inflammatory processes [12,13]. Eicosapentaenoic (EPA) and docosahexaenoic (DHA) acid are the main long-chain PUFA of the *n*-3 PUFA family, and seafood is the richest dietary source of these essential fatty acids, whereas their metabolic precursor, α-linolenic acid (ALA), is contained in substantial amounts only in vegetables [14].

2. Systemic Inflammation in COPD

The principal pathological features of COPD are obstructive bronchiolitis and emphysema, as well as increased mucus secretion. These conditions are the result of a rather complex and chronic inflammatory process, which is initiated mostly by chronic inhalation of irritants, predominantly cigarette smoking, air pollutants, and biomass fuel [6]. In this context, it ought to be mentioned that each puff of a cigarette contains more than 2000 xenobiotic compounds and 1014 free radicals, which injure lung epithelial cells with dose-dependent cytotoxicity [15,16]. These irritants subsequently activate pattern recognition receptors, such as Toll-like receptors (TLR), either directly, or indirectly by causing injury to epithelial cells, which release damage-associated molecular patterns. Interleukin (IL)-1ß has been demonstrated to be crucially involved in this first step, and IL-1 receptor knockout mice exposed to cigarette smoke showed reduced pulmonary inflammation and were significantly protected from development of emphysema compared with littermate controls [17]. On activation, innate immune cells release pro-inflammatory cytokines and chemokines, such as tumor necrosis factor α (TNFα) and IL-8, which leads to further recruitment of neutrophils and inflammatory monocytes to the lung [18]. Activated neutrophils and macrophages, in turn, foster lung destruction through the release of reactive oxygen species and proteolytic enzymes such as neutrophil elastase and matrix metalloproteinases [19,20].

Activation of the adaptive immune system is a second step in the pathogenesis of COPD, and cigarette smoke is crucially involved in activation of dendritic cells in the lower respiratory tract, leading to T cell activation [21]. CD8 cytotoxic T cells are the predominant T cells in the airways of

COPD patients [15], however, CD4+ T helper-1 cells and CD4+ T helper-17 cells are also found in high quantities [6,22,23]. Furthermore, B cells organized into lymphoid follicles are frequently detected in the airways of patients with COPD, as shown in central bronchial biopsy specimens [24].

Several inflammatory cytokines, including TNFα; IL-6; IL-8; IL-18; and acute phase proteins such as C-reactive protein (CRP), serum amyloid A, and fibrinogen, as well as white blood cells (WBC), are detected at increased concentrations in the circulation of patients affected by COPD [25,26]. Similarly, these cytokines are also increased in the sputum and bronchoalveolar lavage fluid of COPD patients [8], suggesting a close relationship between airway and systemic inflammation. The latter has been described as an overspill of inflammatory mediators from the peripheral lung to systemic circulation contributing to the development of comorbidities of COPD [7]. Agusti et al. analyzed six inflammatory biomarkers (WBC, CRP, IL-6, IL-8, fibrinogen, and TNFα) in one of the largest available COPD cohorts, the ECLIPSE cohort [26]. The study included COPD patients, smokers without airflow limitation, and non-smokers. Thirty percent of COPD patients had no signs of systemic inflammation, whereas 16% had persistent systemic inflammation. The study group with persistent inflammation had significantly increased all-cause mortality, as compared with individuals without chronic inflammation (13% vs. 2%). The authors concluded that systemic inflammation is not a constant feature in all COPD patients, because approximately one-third of those analyzed did not have any abnormal biomarker neither at baseline nor at one year after follow-up. In a logistic regression analysis, body mass index (BMI), age, current smoking, and airflow limitation were identified as risk factors for persistent inflammation in COPD patients. Similarly, Garcia-Aymerich et al. were able to identify a COPD phenotype characterized by high proportion of obesity, cardiovascular disease, diabetes, and systemic inflammation in approximately one-third of patients recruited at the first hospital admission because of acute exacerbated COPD (AECOPD) [27]. Yet, the mechanisms linking COPD to the development or progression of COPD associated comorbidities are not fully understood, as these studies only show associations and do not prove causality.

3. Coronary Artery Disease in COPD

CAD prevalence rates in COPD patients range from 7% to 34% [28–30]. COPD and CAD have a close relationship, as they share common risk factors such as advanced age, cigarette smoking, and environmental pollution. There are evident epidemiologic data connecting COPD with CAD. In a cross-sectional study of patients with suspected CAD, patients with COPD had a significantly higher frequency of obstructive coronary lesions as compared with CAD patients without airflow limitation [31]. Additionally, the severity of airflow limitation correlated with coronary lesion size and quantity. No difference was found between COPD and non-COPD CAD patients regarding risk factors, and a univariate analysis revealed COPD as an independent predictor of CAD. Multiple other studies have shown similar results and identified COPD as a powerful and independent risk factor for CVD and CAD. Spirometry tests, especially FEV1, and airflow obstruction defined as FEV1/FVC less than 0.70, for instance, have strong predictive potential for CAD. For every 10% decrease in FEV1, cardiovascular mortality was found to increase by about 28%, and even among individuals with severe airways obstruction, the leading causes of death are predominantly sequels of cardiovascular disease [31–34]. On the other side, studies investigating airflow limitation in patients with CAD are scarce, but the prevalence of obstructive ventilation in CAD patients might be underestimated in the literature [28].

The pathophysiological mechanism linking COPD to its comorbidities is not yet certain, but chronic exposure to low-grade systemic inflammation might play a central role. Inflammation is a key factor in the development and progression of atherosclerotic lesions, and numerous cytokines, mediators, and immune cells have been identified to promote vascular inflammation, cholesterol deposition in the arterial wall, and the formation of atherosclerotic plaques [35,36].

Most large epidemiologic studies identified C-reactive protein (CRP) as a key player and predictor of CAD [35,37], as well as "upstream" inflammatory cytokines like IL-6, IL-18, and TNFα strongly correlated with disease activity and severity in CAD [38,39]. Similar systemic alterations of systemic inflammatory markers are found in those COPD patients that revealed an increased prevalence of cardiovascular disease [26].

However, even though persistent inflammation may constitute the pathophysiological link between COPD and CAD, alternative mechanistic approaches ought to be mentioned.

Pulmonary emphysema, a phenotype of COPD, is a pathologic condition characterized by abnormal and permanent enlargement of the airspaces distal to the terminal bronchioles that leads to destruction of airspace walls and usually to progressive airflow limitation [1]. Studies about the pathogenesis of emphysema revealed an association with endothelial apoptosis [40–42] and endothelial dysfunction [43]. The subsequently altered pulmonary perfusion can lead to impaired left ventricular filling, reduced stroke volume, and lower cardiac output [44]. The endothelial damage, however, is not limited to the lungs and large cross-sectional studies linked the presence of emphysema to subclinical atherosclerosis and peripheral arterial stiffness [45] as a consequence of endothelial and vascular smooth muscle dysfunction [46]. Arterial stiffness is a strong predictor of cardiovascular disease [47,48], and emphysema severity based on quantitative computed tomography scans in turn was revealed as the most powerful predictor of arterial stiffness [49]. Moreover, systemic vascular dysfunction seems to already be present in the earlier stages of COPD, and particularly in patients with emphysema, although presenting with a largely preserved FEV1 [50].

Still, many other potential mechanisms, for instance, physical inactivity secondary to more advanced COPD stages, chronic hypoxia, genetic predisposition, as well as direct endothelial damage caused by cigarette smoking, may help to further explain the frequent association between COPD and CAD [51].

4. Anti-Inflammatory Proprieties of *n*-3 PUFA and the Benefits in Cardiovascular Disease

n-3 PUFA exert multiple functions in humans and are crucially involved in limiting and resolving inflammatory processes. A recent American Heart Association science advisory recommends consuming nonfried seafood, especially species higher in long chain *n*-3 PUFA, one to two times per week for cardiovascular benefits [52]. However, data about the specific *n*-3 PUFA supplementation for influencing the risk of CVD are still ambiguous, underlined by recent findings from randomized controlled trials and meta-analyses, which led to a class III recommendation by the American Heart Association for dietary supplementation with *n*-3 PUFAs in populations at high risk of CVD [53]. This is further supported by a Cochrane Systematic Review providing information that EPA and DHA slightly reduce serum triglycerides and raise high density lipoprotein cholesterol (HDL-C), however, little or no effect on all-cause deaths and cardiovascular events and probably little or no difference in terms of cardiovascular death, coronary deaths or events, stroke, or heart irregularities was described. [54]. The hypothesized protective mechanisms are not solely related to reduced overall inflammation, but also include effects on lipid metabolism and thrombogenesis, as well as anti-arrhythmic proprieties, reducing the rate of sudden cardiac death in secondary prevention [53,55,56].

Increased bioavailability of *n*-3 PUFAs, by means of EPA and DHA, change the balance between *n*-3 and *n*-6 PUFA with arachidonic acid (AA) as the major precursor of the latter, favoring the synthesis of anti-inflammatory eicosanoids [57]. The incorporation of EPA and DHA into human inflammatory cells occurs in a dose-response fashion, and because less substrate is available for synthesis of AA-derived eicosanoids, *n*-3 PUFA supplementation to human diet has been shown to result in decreased production of prostaglandin E2 (PGE2), thromboxane A2, Leukotriene B4 (LTB4), 5-hydroxyeicosatetraenoic acid, and leukotriene E4 by inflammatory cells [57]. Plenty of evidence supporting this hypothesis is available from rheumatoid arthritis disease, a disease primarily characterized by inflammation [58]. There are many studies about patients with rheumatoid arthritis, where fish oil supplements decreased LTB4 production by neutrophils and monocytes, 5-hydroxyeicosatetraenoic acid production by neutrophils, and PGE2 production by mononuclear cells [58]. A recently published prospective trial concluded that the intake of fish oil resulted in a shift of *n*-6/*n*-3 PUFA ratio and in a higher incorporation of *n*-3 PUFA precursors for the anti-inflammatory lipid mediators in plasma phospholipids. This further induced a significant improvement in the clinical status by improving joint inflammation, as well as reducing inflammatory parameters (CRP, erythrocyte sedimentation rate) [59]. However, the altered ratio between *n*-6/*n*-3 PUFA occurred solely through an increase of *n*-3 PUFA, while *n*-6 PUFA remained unchanged. In the literature, similar concerns with the *n*-6/*n*-3 PUFA ratio were identified and discussed. Depending on how the proportion of *n*-6 PUFA changes, the proportion of *n*-3 PUFA could decrease, remain unchanged, or increase and still lead to a lower *n*-6/*n*-3 PUFA ratio, although the active biochemical effects of a decrease, no change, or an increase in the proportion of *n*-3 PUFA are distinctly different. Moreover, the single aspect of an *n*-3/*n*-6 PUFA ratio neglects the source of *n*-3 PUFA, and it is well established that the biological effects of α-linolenic acid (ALA), EPA, and DHA are diverse [60]. In terms of cardiovascular diseases, one would hypothesize that higher levels of *n*-6 PUFA and lower levels of *n*-3 PUFA could increase cardiovascular risk. This has not been demonstrated, as both *n*-6 and *n*-3 fatty acids are associated with reduced cardiovascular risk in several studies [61]. Similarly, two prospective trials concluded that the ratio of *n*-6/*n*-3 polyunsaturated fatty acids is of no value in modifying cardiovascular disease risk [62–64].

The anti-inflammatory mechanism of *n*-3 PUFA also expands on leukocyte recruitment by affecting the expression of adhesion molecules on endothelial cells [65]. This step is crucial, as monocytes in particular migrate into the vessel wall, differentiate into macrophages, and may become foam cells, contributing to the initiation and progression of inflammatory atherosclerotic lesions [66,67]. Moreover, resolution of inflammation is an actively programmed biochemical progress, regulated by specialized pro-resolving mediators (SPM) derived from *n*-3 and *n*-6 PUFA (Figure 2) [68]. While *n*-3 PUFAs are synthesized to resolvins, protectins, and maresins, *n*-6 PUFAs are synthesized to lipoxins [69]. SPMs are predominantly involved in the regulation of neutrophil activity, as well as cyto- and chemokine release, and induce the resolution of an inflammatory tissue state towards tissue homeostasis [70].

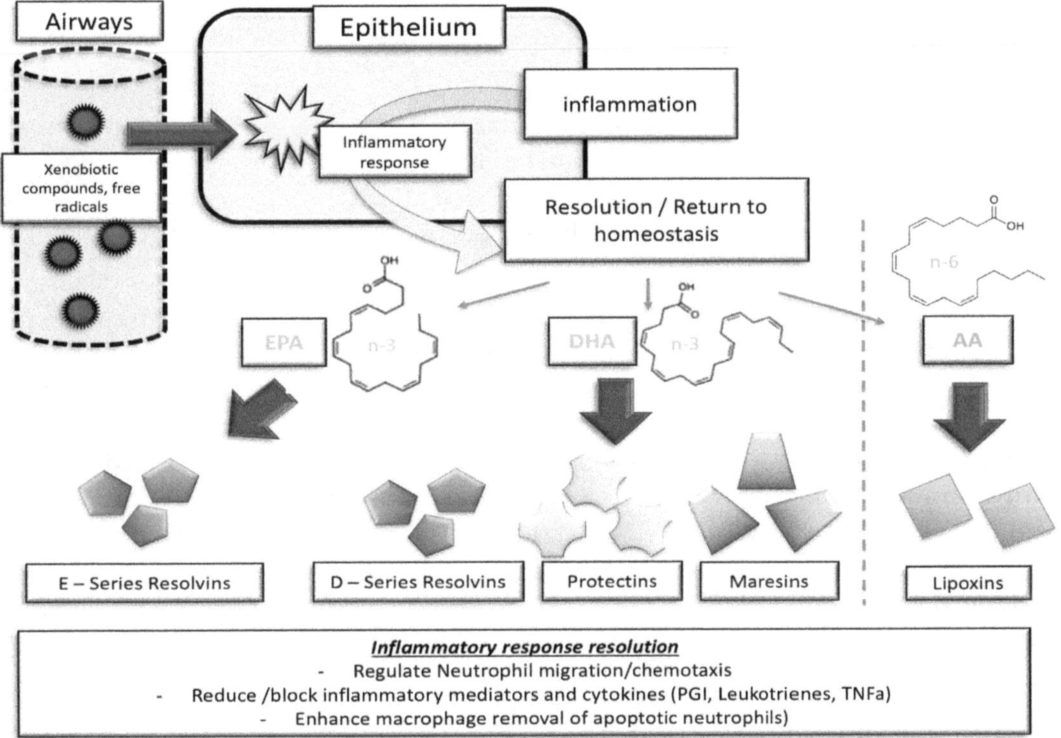

Figure 2. Inflammatory response and inflammatory resolution: the role of molecular mediators derived from *n*-3 PUFA and *n*-6 PUFA. EPA = eicosapentaenoic acid, DHA = docosahexaenoic acid, AA = arachidonic acid, PGI = prostaglandins, TNFα = tumor necrosis factor α.

Figure 2 illustrates the complexity of SPM involvement in inflammation resolution. Resolvin E1, derived from EPA, is involved in the limitation of neutrophil migration, the enhancement of neutrophil and eosinophil clearance, and the reduction of IL-23 and 12 release. Also, resolvin E1 inhibits platelet and vascular smooth muscle activation [71].

Similarly, resolvin D1, derived from DHA, limits neutrophil transmigration, and promotes the clearance of apoptotic cells and allergens. Moreover, resolvin D1 stimulates the production of IgM and IgG. Resolvin D2, on top of limiting neutrophil activity and enhancing macrophage activity, reduces the possibility of leukocyte–endothelial interaction by stimulating NO production [71].

Protectin D1 effectively inhibits T cell migration and apoptosis, and reduces the production and release of TNFα and Interferon gamma, besides limiting neutrophil activity and promoting macrophage activation [70].

Maresin 1, on the other hand, predominately affects pulmonary tissue by reducing the overall amount of neutrophils in the lung, limiting edema, tissue hypoxia, and pro-inflammatory cytokines [70]. Also, IL-5 and IL-13 secretion is reduced, thereby affecting innate lymphoid cells. Another beneficial effect of this SPM is the stimulation of regulatory T cells, stimulating innate lymphoid cells type 2 mediated effects [70]. Finally, *n*-3 PUFAs also directly impact arterial stiffness by decreasing the pulse wave velocity and improving arterial compliance [72], as was shown in a meta-analysis by Pase et al. Similarly, the effects were further confirmed by more recent randomized controlled trials in patients with metabolic syndrome and patients at elevated cardiovascular risk [73,74].

5. *n*-3 PUFA in COPD Patients, Smokers, and Subjects at Risk

The beneficial effects of an inflammation-modulating diet using *n*-3 PUFA in patients with acute lung injury or acute respiratory distress syndrome have been reported previously [75,76]. Therefore, it was hypothesized that *n*-3 PUFA might also have beneficial effects in patients with COPD and the effect might extend to linked comorbidities potentially related to systemic inflammation, including CAD.

Investigations on *n*-3 PUFA and the impact on airflow limitation and smoking were published in the past (a schematic overview of the discussed studies is given in Table 1). One of the first available studies was conducted by Sharp et al. in 1994 [77]. A large cross-sectional cohort study (Honolulu Heart Program) revealed a protective function of elevated fish consumption (major source of *n*-3 PUFA) in smokers by decelerating the FEV1 decline. However, the effect was limited to subjects with a maximum inhalation of 30 cigarettes per day, indicating a dose-dependent limitation. Interestingly, an analysis of the same cohort also showed a decrease in the risk of CAD morbidity and mortality in smokers with increased fish intake (defined as >2 times/week), suggesting a relationship between airflow limitation, CAD, and *n*-3 PUFA [78]. No information is available on whether patients matching the current definition of COPD were included in this analysis.

Table 1. Summary of the reviewed studies related to omega-3 polyunsaturated fatty acid (*n*-3 PUFA) in chronic obstructive pulmonary disease (COPD) patients, smokers and subjects at risk. ALA = alpha linoleic acid, CAD = coronary artery diseases, CRP = C-reactive protein, CVD = cardiovascular disease, FFQ = food frequency questionnaire, DHA = docosahexaenoic acid, EPA = eicosapentaenoic acid, FEV1 = forced expiratory volume in one second, FVC = forced vital capacity, HF = heart failure, IL = interleukin, RCT = randomized controlled trial, STA = stearinic acid, TNFα = tumor necrosis factor alpha.

Author/Year/Type	Cohort Size/Description	*n*-3 PUFA Source	Outcome	COPD	Limitations	Association with CAD (Same Study or Same Cohort)
Sharp et al., 1994, observational	*n* = 6346, Honolulu Heart Program—mean age 54 years	Fish consumption/week—FFQ	Slower decline of FEV1 in smokers.	Obstructive lung disease was solely based on FEV1<65%. Symptoms are not reported.	No details provided about COPD patients. PUFA source reported as fish consumption per week.	Decrease in the risk of coronary heart disease morbidity and mortality in smokers with elevated fish intake.
Shahar et al., 1994, observational	*n* = 8960, Atherosclerosis Risk in Communities Study (ARIC); age: 45–64 years	*n*-3 PUFA (EPA and DHA)—FFQ	Strong inverse relation between COPD and intake of *n*-3 PUFA. Besides COPD, better lung function also in smokers and former smokers.	COPD patients included, however, using a different definition.	Outdated definition of COPD.	*n*-3 PUFAs were associated with hypocoagulable hemostasis. Lower levels of plasma PUFA (especially *n*-6 PUFA) among participants who developed coronary heart disease. Increased risk of HF in subjects with higher plasma levels of saturated fatty acids. *n*-3 PUFAs were associated with a decreased risk of HF in women.
Garcia-Larsen et al., 2015, cross-sectional	*n* = 1232, age 22–28 y	*n*-3 PUFA—FFQ	Positive association between *n*-3 PUFA consumption and ventilatory function (FEV1% and FVC%).	-	Results were not significant after adjustment for multiple comparisons.	-
Leng et al., 2017, observational	*n* = 1829, Lovelace Smokers cohort and *n* = 508 the Veterans Smokers cohort, age 40–74 years	*n*-3 PUFA, EPA, DPA, DHA—FFQ	EPA, DPA, and DHA were associated with better FEV1; DPA was associated with a lower age-related FEV1 decline.	25% COPD patients.	Both cohorts showed a mean FEV1/FVC ratio of >0.7. Included COPD patients mild-to-moderate stages.	-
Wood et al., 2010, observational	*n* = 195, Hunter community study, age 55–85 years	*n*-3 PUFA—FFQ	Increased proportion of dietary fat was associated with increased IL-6 levels, which were significant predictors of FEV1% and FVC in men. No association between *n*3-PUFA and %FEV1.	No information given (no absolute limitation of FEV1% and FEV1/FVC > 0.7).	No information is given about the relation between *n*-3 PUFA and IL-6.	IL-6 is an important marker of cardiovascular and coronary artery disease. No data about CAD or CVD reported.
Scaglia et al., 2016, cross-sectional	*n* = 100 (1:1 smokers vs. never-smokers), 18–75 years	Red blood cell membrane determination of ALA, EPA, DPA, and DHA	Significantly lower levels of DHA in smokers compared with non-smokers.	-	Spirometry not included; no information about lung diseases.	-

Table 1. *Cont.*

Author/Year/Type	Cohort Size/Description	*n*-3 PUFA Source	Outcome	COPD	Limitations	Association with CAD (Same Study or Same Cohort)
Matsuyama et al., 2005, prospective interventional, 2 years duration	$n = 64$, mean age 66 years.	Supplementation *n*-3 PUFA vs. *n*-6 PUFA	Decrease of Borg dyspnea scale and a decrease of arterial oxygen saturation after 6 min walking test in *n*-3 PUFA group. Leukotriene B4 levels in serum and sputum and tumor necrosis factor alpha and interleukin-8 levels in sputum decreased significantly in the *n*-3 group. No change in FEV1.	Limited to COPD only with FEV1% < 60% and BMI <25 kg/m^2, no active smokers.	Sample size	Impact on inflammatory parameters related to CAD and CVD, however, no data about CAD and CVD in this population are reported.
De Batlle, 2012, cross-sectional	$n = 250$, PAC-COPD study group, mean age 68 years	*n*-3 PUFA: DHA, EPA, ALA—FFQ	ALA was associated with lower TNFα concentrations in serum. AA (*n*-6 PUFA) was related to higher IL-6 and CRP serum concentrations.	COPD patients recruited during their first hospital admission. Mostly moderate to severe COPD.	No repeated measurements, inflammatory sputum parameters not assessed.	Association between ALA and cardiovascular disease, however, no information about CVD or CAD in this population are reported.
Broekhuizen et al., 2005, prospective interventional double-blind RCT over 8 weeks (PUFA vs. Placebo)	$n = 80$, mean age 63 years	9 g PUFA (STA, ALA, EPA, DHA) or placebo daily	Increase in peak exercise capacity and duration of constant work rate. No changes in terms of CRP, IL-6 and TNFa	Mostly severe to very severe COPD patients with mean FEV1% 35–38%.	Limited observation period of 8 weeks.	Association between the analyzed inflammatory parameters and CAD and CVD, however, no information about CVD or CAD in this population are reported.
Calder et al., 2018, prospective interventional RCT over 12 weeks	$n = 45$, mean age 69 years	2.0 g DHA + EPA, 10 g whey protein concentrate and 10 µg 25-hydroxy-vitamin D3 twice daily for 12 weeks vs. a milk-based comparator	Intervention group gained more fat mass. Reductions in systolic blood pressure, triglycerides and exercise-induced fatigue and dyspnoea, and increases in high-density lipoprotein cholesterol.	Moderate-to-severe COPD and involuntary weight loss or low body mass index (16–18 kg/m^2).	Sample size	Inclusion of metabolic parameters and inflammatory parameters clearly associated with CVD and CAD.

Shahar et al. analyzed the dietary impact of *n*-3 PUFA (assessment of EPA and DHA intake via questionnaire) on 8960 current or former smokers from the "Atherosclerosis Risk in Communities—ARIC" study cohort and studied its relation with COPD [79]. COPD was assessed by a questionnaire on respiratory symptoms and by spirometry. The definition of COPD, however, was slightly different when compared with the current GOLD definition [1]. The authors describe a strong inverse relation between COPD severity and intake of *n*-3 PUFA. Moreover, higher intake of *n*-3 PUFA and fish consumption also predicted better lung function in smokers and former smokers. Many other investigations, including the same cohort, were subsequently published; *n*-3 PUFAs were associated with a modification of hemostatic factors—key components of CAD and acute myocardial infarction—resulting in a hypocoagulable profile [80]. Data from the same cohort also revealed lower levels of plasma PUFA (especially *n*-6 PUFA) among participants who developed CAD [81]. Yamagishi et al. found an increased risk of heart failure in subjects with higher plasma levels of saturated fatty acids, and *n*-3 PUFAs were associated with a decreased risk of heart failure in women in the ARIC cohort [82].

A positive association between *n*-3 PUFA (assessment of *n*-3 PUFA via questionnaire) consumption and ventilatory function (FEV1% and FVC%) was found in 1232 adults aged between 22 and 28 years [83]. The analyzed cohort had no signs of obstructive ventilatory dysfunction, and statistical significance was lost after adjusting for multiple comparisons, suggesting only a weak effect of *n*-3 PUFA. The idea of analyzing a cohort of young adults was related to the fact that reduced maximal attained lung function (as measured by spirometry) may identify individuals who are at increased risk for the subsequent development of COPD [1,84].

Leng et al. conducted a nutritional epidemiological study in two separate cohorts (Hispanic and non-Hispanic white smokers; assessment of EPA, DHA, and docosapentaenoic acid (DPA) intake via questionnaire) to identify nutrients associated with FEV1 and its decline [85]. Of the analyzed *n*-3 PUFAs, EPA, DHA, and DPA intake were positively associated with better FEV1 volumes, and DPA was associated with a reduced age-related FEV1 decline. No increased FEV1 decline of currently smoking participants was observed in one of the two cohorts (Lovelace Smoker's cohort) if high amounts of DPA were consumed. The study only included approximately 25% COPD patients, and both cohorts showed a mean FEV1/FVC ratio of >0.7, limiting the disease to mild-to-moderate stages. No data about CVD prevalence in the two analyzed cohorts are provided.

Conflicting evidence came from another population-based cohort study showing that an increased proportion of dietary fat consumption was associated with increased IL-6 levels, which were significant predictors of FEV1 and FVC [86]. Plasma IL-6 is a clinically relevant marker of inflammation and has been linked to cardiovascular outcomes in some epidemiological studies [87]. *n*-3 PUFA (assessment via questionnaire) intake was not found to be associated with %FEV1 in the linear regression model, and no information is given about the relation between *n*-3 PUFA and IL-6. Overall, the patients included in the study had no absolute limitation of FEV1 (approximately 80% predicted) and obstructive ventilation, a typical feature of COPD, was not found (FEV1/FVC > 0.7.) Moreover, the assessed smoking status revealed non-smokers in 73% of female patients and 39% of male patients and, therefore, the odds of COPD patients being included in the study are low.

In 2016, Scaglia et al. analyzed dietary habits related to PUFA consumption (red blood cell membrane determination of alpha linoleic acid (ALA), EPA, DPA, and DHA) in smokers and lifetime non-smokers [88]. They found significant differences in the dietary consumption of *n*-3 PUFA between the two groups and showed lower levels of DHA and EPA in smokers. They hypothesized that PUFA might interfere with smoking habits, suggesting dietary supplementation as a potential therapeutic option for smoking cessation. Still, this observation was not confirmed in follow up studies thus far and urges further elucidation.

The anti-inflammatory proprieties of *n*-3 PUFA in COPD patients have been studied [89] in sixty-four patients receiving either an *n*-3 PUFA (ALA) or an *n*-6 PUFA (linoleic acid) supplementation diet for two years. Apart from clinical improvements (decrease of dyspnea according to Borg scale and decrease of arterial oxygen saturation after a 6 min walking test), leukotriene B4 levels in serum and sputum, as well as TNFα and IL-8 levels in sputum, decreased significantly in patients consuming an *n*-3 PUFA rich diet, while there was no significant change in individuals receiving dietary supplementation of *n*-6 PUFA.

A cross-sectional study including 250 COPD patients analyzed inflammatory parameters related to dietary intake of *n*-3 (EPA, DHA, ALA) and *n*-6 PUFA [90]. Higher intake of alpha linoleic acid (ALA) was associated with lower TNFα concentrations in serum, while no differences were seen with other assessed inflammatory parameters (IL-6, IL-8, and CRP). A higher ALA intake was related to higher IL-6 and CRP serum concentrations.

The effects of PUFA supplementation (blend of PUFA, 9 g, mainly *n*-3 PUFA, namely ALA, EPA, and DHA) on the outcome of pulmonary rehabilitation were studied in 80 COPD patients randomized to an intervention or a placebo group [91]. The peak exercise capacity increased in both groups. However, a significantly higher increase was observed in the intervention group after eight weeks of training. Also, the duration of the constant work rate increased far more in patients receiving PUFA. However, the measured systemic inflammatory parameters, namely CRP, IL-6, and TNFα, did not change after rehabilitation or after PUFA intervention, contrasting the results of others [89,90], who observed modulation of systemic inflammation after *n*-3 PUFA supplementation. Thus, systemic inflammation is not a common feature of all COPD patients. Therefore, a more detailed analysis of the subgroup of "inflamed COPD" patients would be desirable. Still, it is unanswered as to how the biochemical phenotype of an "inflamed COPD" patient is defined.

The beneficial effects of *n*-3 PUFA in COPD associated cachexia were studied in a randomized controlled trial including 45 patients [92]. Patients in the intervention group received 2.0 g DHA + EPA as well as 10 g whey protein concentrate and 10 μg 25-hydroxy-vitamin D3 twice daily for 12 weeks versus a milk-based comparator. Both groups gained weight, but the intervention group gained more fat mass. Moreover, a significant reduction in systolic blood pressure and increases in high-density lipoprotein cholesterol were observed in the intervention group compared with controls, parameters that can be regarded as risk factors for CAD [93]. No significant changes in the measured inflammatory parameters (CRP, IL-6, IL-8, and TNF) were observed.

In summary, several limitations of the described studies must be discussed. First, the most important limitation is that most of the studies are cross-sectional observational cohort studies. Second, *n*-3 PUFA sources are indirectly measured using food frequency questionnaires. Dietary habits reported from questionnaires are surrogate parameters of the real dietary consumption of *n*-3 PUFA; this may lead to inaccurate *n*-3 PUFA consumption estimations, although studies suggest a plausible correlation between the two factors [94,95]. Third, the causality and the direction of a causal relation cannot be explained when considering a cross-sectional study design. Finally, COPD patients and smokers may have changed their lifestyles and dietary habits, reducing fish consumption. Therefore, further prospective studies are warranted to investigate the impact of *n*-3 PUFA consumption on systemic inflammatory parameters in such patients.

6. *n*-3 PUFA, CAD, and COPD

Evidence on the beneficial effects of *n*-3 PUFA on CAD and CVD in COPD patients is scarce. Many large randomized controlled trials have been conducted to study the benefits of *n*-3 PUFA in CAD and CVD [53,54], however, although most of the included patients were smokers, the prevalence and severity of COPD were rarely reported.

We reviewed all included studies from the Cochrane systematic database review, "Polyunsaturated fatty acids for the primary and secondary prevention of cardiovascular disease", and the American Heart Association Science Advisory, "Omega-3 Polyunsaturated Fatty Acid (Fish Oil) Supplementation and the Prevention of Clinical Cardiovascular Disease", in regard to included COPD patients [53,54]. Of the included 65 studies, only 4 reported on COPD patients in their cohort.

Nodari et al. analyzed the benefits of *n*-3 PUFA (850 to 882 mg of EPA and DHA) in the prevention of atrial fibrillation (AF) recurrence rates after electrical cardioversion in a prospective randomized controlled trial, including 199 patients [96]. After one year of follow-up, the probability of maintained sinus rhythm was significantly higher in the n-3 PUFAs-treated patients as compared with the placebo group. A small subgroup of approximately 10% COPD patients (n = 12 placebo vs. n = 13 intervention) was included in the study, however, no separate details on the subgroup were discussed.

Rauch et al. analyzed the effect of n-3 PUFA (460 mg EPA, 380 mg DHA) if given on top of modern guideline-adjusted therapy in survivors of acute myocardial infarction [97]. The study was designed as a randomized, placebo-controlled trial with a duration of one year, and included 3851 patients, of whom approximately 6% were highlighted as COPD patients (n = 122 placebo vs. n = 108 intervention group). Overall, guideline-adjusted treatment of acute myocardial infarction already resulted in a low rate of sudden cardiac death and other clinical events within one year of follow-up, and the application of n-3 PUFA could not further improve the outcome. No details are provided regarding such effects in the COPD subgroup.

The GISSI-HF investigators published a randomized, double-blind, placebo-controlled trial analyzing the effect of n-3 PUFA (850–882 mg EPA and DHA) in patients with chronic heart failure [98]. In total, 6975 patients with chronic heart failure of New York Heart Association class II–IV were randomly assigned to n-3 PUFA intervention or placebo. A subpopulation of 205 COPD patients was included in the study (n = 793 placebo vs. n = 740 intervention). Primary endpoints were time to death from any cause or death/admission to hospital for a cardiovascular reason. A slight, yet significant reduction of death from any cause or death/admission to hospital for cardiovascular reasons was found in the PUFA group. No specific details are provided for the COPD subpopulation.

Finally, Mozaffarin et al. analyzed the effect of n-3 PUFA (EPA 465 mg and DHA 375 mg) in the prevention of AF in 1516 patients who underwent cardiac surgery [99]. Patients were randomized to receive fish oil or placebo until hospital discharge or postoperative day 10. A small subgroup of approximately 11% of COPD patients (placebo n = 90 vs. intervention n = 80) was included in the study. The authors concluded that perioperative supplementation with n-3 PUFA did not reduce the risk of postoperative AF and, similarly to the aforementioned studies, no details are provided about the COPD subgroup.

In summary, these studies showed a weak benefit of n-3 PUFA supplementation in the setting of atrial fibrillation recurrence rate after electrical cardioversion and a slight reduction of death and hospital admission in patients with left heart failure, both diseases closely associated with CAD. No benefits were seen in survivors of acute myocardial infarction or patients with atrial fibrillation after cardiac surgery. The weak benefits seem to also apply to COPD patients, which were included in 5–20% of the discussed studies. However, as already mentioned earlier, the high number of undiagnosed COPD cases and low awareness of investigators towards this chronic disease in patients with cardiac pathologies led to neglect of this important aspect even in large and prospective trials. In our opinion, it seems plausible that other studies also included COPD patients at a rate of at least 5–10%. Thus, the results from the Cochrane systematic database review and the American Heart Association Science Advisory might also apply to COPD patients.

7. Conclusions and Future Perspectives

COPD represents a growing healthcare concern worldwide. Pathophysiological aspects of COPD imply a local inflammatory reaction, initiated by inhalation of noxious substances, which, in some cases, led to the emergence of inflammatory mediators in the systemic circulation. Epidemiologic and mechanistic studies indicate that COPD is frequently associated with CAD, congestive heart failure, and cardiac arrhythmias, independent of shared risk factors. A possible pathway is highlighted as chronic low-grade systemic inflammation, an aspect that likely also contributes to coronary artery disease. n-3 PUFAs have been intensively studied for their ability to improve morbidity and mortality in patients with CAD. However, little evidence exists toward the beneficial anti-inflammatory aspects of n-3 PUFA in COPD patients, and even less evidence is available in regard to patients with COPD and associated CAD.

Overall, the available literature suggests a weak benefit of n-3 PUFA in COPD patients related to clinical outcomes, and n-3 PUFA mediated borderline amelioration of local and systemic inflammation. To date, the specific interplay between n-3 PUFA, COPD, and CAD has not been investigated in prospective trials.

In-depth keyword guided research on ongoing trials on n-3 PUFA in COPD and CAD revealed a relatively small number of registered trials on http://ClinicalTrials.gov. To date, only one trial investigating the effect of fish oil on endothelial function by FMD (flow-mediated dilation) in COPD has been registered (NCT00835289). Another trial has investigated the effect of both training and nutritional supplementation on body composition, activity, and cardiometabolic risk in COPD (NCT01344135). However, as nutritional supplementation has not occurred in all subjects and as an observational period of eight months may not be enough to reach clinically important cardiovascular and COPD endpoints, prospective, randomized controlled studies are warranted. Future studies ought to measure atherosclerotic disease progression, as well as establish relevant COPD inflammation parameters in order to determine the role of PUFA in inflammation-mediated diseases such as COPD and CAD. Moreover, standardized PUFA administration as well as a sufficient observation period may be crucial to understanding the role of PUFA in these diseases. Successful trials may help introduce a standardized supplementation of PUFA in patients with CAD or COPD or both to reduce disease progression or development.

Author Contributions: Conceptualization, A.P., L.L., and T.S.; writing—original draft preparation, A.P. and L.L.; writing—review and editing, G.W., I.T.; visualization, L.L.; supervision, I.T.

Acknowledgments: Support by the "Verein zur Förderung von Forschung und Weiterbildung in Infektiologie und Immunologie an der Medizinischen Universität Innsbruck" is gratefully acknowledged.

References

1. Vogelmeier, C.F.; Criner, G.J.; Martinez, F.J.; Anzueto, A.; Barnes, P.J.; Bourbeau, J.; Celli, B.R.; Chen, R.; Decramer, M.; Fabbri, L.M.; et al. Global strategy for the diagnosis, management, and prevention of chronic obstructive lung disease 2017 report. GOLD executive summary. *Am. J. Respir. Crit. Care Med.* **2017**, *195*, 557–582. [CrossRef] [PubMed]
2. Lozano, R.; Naghavi, M.; Foreman, K.; Lim, S.; Shibuya, K.; Aboyans, V.; Abraham, J.; Adair, T.; Aggarwal, R.; Ahn, S.Y.; et al. Global and regional mortality from 235 causes of death for 20 age groups in 1990 and 2010: A systematic analysis for the global burden of disease study 2010. *Lancet* **2012**, *380*, 2095–2128. [CrossRef]
3. WHO. Projections of Mortality and Causes of Death, 2015 and 2030. Available online: http://www.who.int/healthinfo/global_burden_disease/projections2015_2030/en/ (accessed on 1 June 2018).
4. WHO. Chronic Obstructive Pulmonary Disease (COPD). Available online: http://www.who.int/respiratory/copd/en/ (accessed on 1 September 2018).
5. Lindberg, A.; Bjerg, A.; Ronmark, E.; Larsson, L.G.; Lundback, B. Prevalence and underdiagnosis of COPD by disease severity and the attributable fraction of smoking report from the obstructive lung disease in Northern Sweden studies. *Respir. Med.* **2006**, *100*, 264–272. [CrossRef] [PubMed]
6. Barnes, P.J.; Burney, P.G.; Silverman, E.K.; Celli, B.R.; Vestbo, J.; Wedzicha, J.A.; Wouters, E.F. Chronic obstructive pulmonary disease. *Nat. Rev. Dis. Primers* **2015**, *1*, 15076. [CrossRef] [PubMed]
7. Barnes, P.J. Chronic obstructive pulmonary disease: Effects beyond the lungs. *PLoS Med.* **2010**, *7*, e1000220. [CrossRef] [PubMed]
8. Barnes, P.J.; Celli, B.R. Systemic manifestations and comorbidities of COPD. *Eur. Respir. J.* **2009**, *33*, 1165–1185. [CrossRef] [PubMed]
9. Soriano, J.B.; Visick, G.T.; Muellerova, H.; Payvandi, N.; Hansell, A.L. Patterns of comorbidities in newly diagnosed COPD and asthma in primary care. *Chest* **2005**, *128*, 2099–2107. [CrossRef] [PubMed]
10. Mannino, D.M.; Thorn, D.; Swensen, A.; Holguin, F. Prevalence and outcomes of diabetes, hypertension and cardiovascular disease in COPD. *Eur. Respir. J.* **2008**, *32*, 962–969. [CrossRef] [PubMed]

11. Miller, J.; Edwards, L.D.; Agusti, A.; Bakke, P.; Calverley, P.M.; Celli, B.; Coxson, H.O.; Crim, C.; Lomas, D.A.; Miller, B.E.; et al. Comorbidity, systemic inflammation and outcomes in the ECLIPSE cohort. *Respir. Med.* **2013**, *107*, 1376–1384. [CrossRef] [PubMed]
12. Serhan, C.N.; Chiang, N.; Van Dyke, T.E. Resolving inflammation: Dual anti-inflammatory and pro-resolution lipid mediators. *Nat. Rev. Immunol.* **2008**, *8*, 349–361. [CrossRef] [PubMed]
13. Calder, P.C. Omega-3 polyunsaturated fatty acids and inflammatory processes: Nutrition or pharmacology? *Br. J. Clin. Pharmacol.* **2013**, *75*, 645–662. [CrossRef] [PubMed]
14. Davis, B.C.; Kris-Etherton, P.M. Achieving optimal essential fatty acid status in vegetarians: Current knowledge and practical implications. *Am. J. Clin. Nutr.* **2003**, *78*, 640S–646S. [CrossRef] [PubMed]
15. Cosio, M.G.; Saetta, M.; Agusti, A. Immunologic aspects of chronic obstructive pulmonary disease. *N. Engl. J. Med.* **2009**, *360*, 2445–2454. [CrossRef] [PubMed]
16. Pryor, W.A.; Prier, D.G.; Church, D.F. Electron-spin resonance study of mainstream and sidestream cigarette smoke: Nature of the free radicals in gas-phase smoke and in cigarette tar. Environ. *Health Perspect.* **1983**, *47*, 345–355. [CrossRef] [PubMed]
17. Churg, A.; Zhou, S.; Wang, X.; Wang, R.; Wright, J.L. The role of interleukin-1beta in murine cigarette smoke-induced emphysema and small airway remodeling. *Am. J. Respir. Cell Mol. Biol.* **2009**, *40*, 482–490. [CrossRef] [PubMed]
18. Brusselle, G.G.; Joos, G.F.; Bracke, K.R. New insights into the immunology of chronic obstructive pulmonary disease. *Lancet* **2011**, *378*, 1015–1026. [CrossRef]
19. Chung, K.F.; Adcock, I.M. Multifaceted mechanisms in COPD: Inflammation, immunity, and tissue repair and destruction. *Eur. Respir. J.* **2008**, *31*, 1334–1356. [CrossRef] [PubMed]
20. Demedts, I.K.; Morel-Montero, A.; Lebecque, S.; Pacheco, Y.; Cataldo, D.; Joos, G.F.; Pauwels, R.A.; Brusselle, G.G. Elevated MMP-12 protein levels in induced sputum from patients with COPD. *Thorax* **2006**, *61*, 196–201. [CrossRef] [PubMed]
21. Freeman, C.M.; Martinez, F.J.; Han, M.K.; Ames, T.M.; Chensue, S.W.; Todt, J.C.; Arenberg, D.A.; Meldrum, C.A.; Getty, C.; McCloskey, L.; et al. Lung dendritic cell expression of maturation molecules increases with worsening chronic obstructive pulmonary disease. *Am. J. Respir. Crit. Care Med.* **2009**, *180*, 1179–1188. [CrossRef] [PubMed]
22. Di Stefano, A.; Caramori, G.; Gnemmi, I.; Contoli, M.; Vicari, C.; Capelli, A.; Magno, F.; D'Anna, S.E.; Zanini, A.; Brun, P.; et al. T helper type 17-related cytokine expression is increased in the bronchial mucosa of stable chronic obstructive pulmonary disease patients. *Clin. Exp. Immunol.* **2009**, *157*, 316–324. [CrossRef] [PubMed]
23. Barnes, P.J. Cellular and molecular mechanisms of chronic obstructive pulmonary disease. *Clin. Chest Med.* **2014**, *35*, 71–86. [CrossRef] [PubMed]
24. Hogg, J.C.; Chu, F.; Utokaparch, S.; Woods, R.; Elliott, W.M.; Buzatu, L.; Cherniack, R.M.; Rogers, R.M.; Sciurba, F.C.; Coxson, H.O.; et al. The nature of small-airway obstruction in chronic obstructive pulmonary disease. *N. Engl. J. Med.* **2004**, *350*, 2645–2653. [CrossRef] [PubMed]
25. Gan, W.Q.; Man, S.F.; Senthilselvan, A.; Sin, D.D. Association between chronic obstructive pulmonary disease and systemic inflammation: A systematic review and a meta-analysis. *Thorax* **2004**, *59*, 574–580. [CrossRef] [PubMed]
26. Agusti, A.; Edwards, L.D.; Rennard, S.I.; MacNee, W.; Tal-Singer, R.; Miller, B.E.; Vestbo, J.; Lomas, D.A.; Calverley, P.M.; Wouters, E.; et al. Persistent systemic inflammation is associated with poor clinical outcomes in COPD: A novel phenotype. *PLoS ONE* **2012**, *7*, e37483. [CrossRef] [PubMed]
27. Garcia-Aymerich, J.; Gomez, F.P.; Benet, M.; Farrero, E.; Basagana, X.; Gayete, A.; Pare, C.; Freixa, X.; Ferrer, J.; Ferrer, A.; et al. Identification and prospective validation of clinically relevant chronic obstructive pulmonary disease (COPD) subtypes. *Thorax* **2011**, *66*, 430–437. [CrossRef] [PubMed]
28. Soriano, J.B.; Rigo, F.; Guerrero, D.; Yanez, A.; Forteza, J.F.; Frontera, G.; Togores, B.; Agusti, A. High prevalence of undiagnosed airflow limitation in patients with cardiovascular disease. *Chest* **2010**, *137*, 333–340. [CrossRef] [PubMed]
29. Behar, S.; Panosh, A.; Reicher-Reiss, H.; Zion, M.; Schlesinger, Z.; Goldbourt, U. Prevalence and prognosis of chronic obstructive pulmonary disease among 5,839 consecutive patients with acute myocardial infarction. SPRINT Study Group. *Am. J. Med.* **1992**, *93*, 637–641. [CrossRef]
30. Cazzola, M.; Calzetta, L.; Bettoncelli, G.; Cricelli, C.; Romeo, F.; Matera, M.G.; Rogliani, P. Cardiovascular disease in asthma and COPD: A population-based retrospective cross-sectional study. *Respir. Med.* **2012**, *106*, 249–256. [CrossRef] [PubMed]

31. Mota, I.L.; Sousa, A.C.S.; Almeida, M.L.D.; de Melo, E.V.; Ferreira, E.J.P.; Neto, J.B.; Matos, C.J.O.; Telino, C.; Souto, M.J.S.; Oliveira, J.L.M. Coronary lesions in patients with COPD (Global Initiative for Obstructive Lung Disease stages I-III) and suspected or confirmed coronary arterial disease. *Int. J. Chronic Obstr. Pulm. Dis.* **2018**, *13*, 1999–2006. [CrossRef] [PubMed]
32. Sin, D.D.; Man, S.F. Chronic obstructive pulmonary disease as a risk factor for cardiovascular morbidity and mortality. *Proc. Am. Thorac. Soc.* **2005**, *2*, 8–11. [CrossRef] [PubMed]
33. Anthonisen, N.R.; Connett, J.E.; Enright, P.L.; Manfreda, J.; Lung Health Study Research, G. Hospitalizations and mortality in the Lung Health Study. *Am. J. Respir. Crit. Care Med.* **2002**, *166*, 333–339. [CrossRef] [PubMed]
34. Curkendall, S.M.; DeLuise, C.; Jones, J.K.; Lanes, S.; Stang, M.R.; Goehring, E., Jr.; She, D. Cardiovascular disease in patients with chronic obstructive pulmonary disease, Saskatchewan Canada cardiovascular disease in COPD patients. *Ann. Epidemiol.* **2006**, *16*, 63–70. [CrossRef] [PubMed]
35. The Emerging Risk Factors Collaboration; Kaptoge, S.; Di Angelantonio, E.; Pennells, L.; Wood, A.M.; White, I.R.; Gao, P.; Walker, M.; Thompson, A.; Sarwar, N.; et al. C-reactive protein, fibrinogen, and cardiovascular disease prediction. *N. Engl. J. Med.* **2012**, *367*, 1310–1320. [CrossRef] [PubMed]
36. Libby, P.; Ridker, P.M.; Hansson, G.K. Progress and challenges in translating the biology of atherosclerosis. *Nature* **2011**, *473*, 317–325. [CrossRef] [PubMed]
37. The Emerging Risk Factors Collaboration; Kaptoge, S.; Di Angelantonio, E.; Lowe, G.; Pepys, M.B.; Thompson, S.G.; Collins, R.; Danesh, J. C-reactive protein concentration and risk of coronary heart disease, stroke, and mortality: An individual participant meta-analysis. *Lancet* **2010**, *375*, 132–140.
38. Kaptoge, S.; Seshasai, S.R.; Gao, P.; Freitag, D.F.; Butterworth, A.S.; Borglykke, A.; Di Angelantonio, E.; Gudnason, V.; Rumley, A.; Lowe, G.D.; et al. Inflammatory cytokines and risk of coronary heart disease: New prospective study and updated meta-analysis. *Eur. Heart J.* **2014**, *35*, 578–589. [CrossRef] [PubMed]
39. Danesh, J.; Kaptoge, S.; Mann, A.G.; Sarwar, N.; Wood, A.; Angleman, S.B.; Wensley, F.; Higgins, J.P.; Lennon, L.; Eiriksdottir, G.; et al. Long-term interleukin-6 levels and subsequent risk of coronary heart disease: Two new prospective studies and a systematic review. *PLoS Med.* **2008**, *5*, e78. [CrossRef] [PubMed]
40. Petrache, I.; Natarajan, V.; Zhen, L.; Medler, T.R.; Richter, A.T.; Cho, C.; Hubbard, W.C.; Berdyshev, E.V.; Tuder, R.M. Ceramide upregulation causes pulmonary cell apoptosis and emphysema-like disease in mice. *Nat. Med.* **2005**, *11*, 491–498. [CrossRef] [PubMed]
41. Demedts, I.K.; Demoor, T.; Bracke, K.R.; Joos, G.F.; Brusselle, G.G. Role of apoptosis in the pathogenesis of COPD and pulmonary emphysema. *Respir. Res.* **2006**, *7*, 53. [CrossRef] [PubMed]
42. Kasahara, Y.; Tuder, R.M.; Cool, C.D.; Lynch, D.A.; Flores, S.C.; Voelkel, N.F. Endothelial cell death and decreased expression of vascular endothelial growth factor and vascular endothelial growth factor receptor 2 in emphysema. *Am. J. Respir. Crit. Care Med.* **2001**, *163*, 737–744. [CrossRef] [PubMed]
43. Barr, R.G.; Mesia-Vela, S.; Austin, J.H.; Basner, R.C.; Keller, B.M.; Reeves, A.P.; Shimbo, D.; Stevenson, L. Impaired flow-mediated dilation is associated with low pulmonary function and emphysema in ex-smokers: The Emphysema and Cancer Action Project (EMCAP) Study. *Am. J. Respir. Crit. Care Med.* **2007**, *176*, 1200–1207. [CrossRef] [PubMed]
44. Barr, R.G.; Bluemke, D.A.; Ahmed, F.S.; Carr, J.J.; Enright, P.L.; Hoffman, E.A.; Jiang, R.; Kawut, S.M.; Kronmal, R.A.; Lima, J.A.; et al. Percent emphysema, airflow obstruction, and impaired left ventricular filling. *N. Engl. J. Med.* **2010**, *362*, 217–227. [CrossRef] [PubMed]
45. Barr, R.G.; Ahmed, F.S.; Carr, J.J.; Hoffman, E.A.; Jiang, R.; Kawut, S.M.; Watson, K. Subclinical atherosclerosis, airflow obstruction and emphysema: The MESA Lung Study. *Eur. Respir. J.* **2012**, *39*, 846–854. [CrossRef] [PubMed]
46. Zieman, S.J.; Melenovsky, V.; Kass, D.A. Mechanisms, pathophysiology, and therapy of arterial stiffness. *Arterioscler. Thromb. Vasc. Biol.* **2005**, *25*, 932–943. [CrossRef] [PubMed]
47. Vlachopoulos, C.; Aznaouridis, K.; Stefanadis, C. Prediction of cardiovascular events and all-cause mortality with arterial stiffness: A systematic review and meta-analysis. *J. Am. Coll. Cardiol.* **2010**, *55*, 1318–1327. [CrossRef] [PubMed]
48. Cooper, L.L.; Palmisano, J.N.; Benjamin, E.J.; Larson, M.G.; Vasan, R.S.; Mitchell, G.F.; Hamburg, N.M. Microvascular function contributes to the relation between aortic stiffness and cardiovascular events: The framingham heart study. *Circ. Cardiovasc. Imaging* **2016**, *9*. [CrossRef] [PubMed]

49. McAllister, D.A.; Maclay, J.D.; Mills, N.L.; Mair, G.; Miller, J.; Anderson, D.; Newby, D.E.; Murchison, J.T.; Macnee, W. Arterial stiffness is independently associated with emphysema severity in patients with chronic obstructive pulmonary disease. *Am. J. Respir. Crit. Care Med.* **2007**, *176*, 1208–1214. [CrossRef] [PubMed]
50. Zelt, J.T.; Jones, J.H.; Hirai, D.M.; King, T.J.; Berton, D.C.; Pyke, K.E.; O'Donnell, D.E.; Neder, J.A. Systemic vascular dysfunction is associated with emphysema burden in mild COPD. *Respir. Med.* **2018**, *136*, 29–36. [CrossRef] [PubMed]
51. Roversi, S.; Fabbri, L.M.; Sin, D.D.; Hawkins, N.M.; Agusti, A. Chronic obstructive pulmonary disease and cardiac diseases. An urgent need for integrated care. *Am. J. Respir. Crit. Care Med.* **2016**, *194*, 1319–1336. [CrossRef] [PubMed]
52. Rimm, E.B.; Appel, L.J.; Chiuve, S.E.; Djousse, L.; Engler, M.B.; Kris-Etherton, P.M.; Mozaffarian, D.; Siscovick, D.S.; Lichtenstein, A.H.; American Heart Association Nutrition Committee of the Council on Lifestyle and Cardiometabolic Health; et al. Seafood long-chain n-3 polyunsaturated fatty acids and cardiovascular disease: A science advisory from the American Heart Association. *Circulation* **2018**, *138*, e35–e47. [CrossRef] [PubMed]
53. Siscovick, D.S.; Barringer, T.A.; Fretts, A.M.; Wu, J.H.; Lichtenstein, A.H.; Costello, R.B.; Kris-Etherton, P.M.; Jacobson, T.A.; Engler, M.B.; Alger, H.M.; et al. Omega-3 polyunsaturated fatty acid (fish oil) supplementation and the prevention of clinical cardiovascular disease: A science advisory from the American Heart Association. *Circulation* **2017**, *135*, e867–e884. [CrossRef] [PubMed]
54. Abdelhamid, A.S.; Martin, N.; Bridges, C.; Brainard, J.S.; Wang, X.; Brown, T.J.; Hanson, S.; Jimoh, O.F.; Ajabnoor, S.M.; Deane, K.H.; et al. Polyunsaturated fatty acids for the primary and secondary prevention of cardiovascular disease. *Cochrane Database Syst. Rev.* **2018**, *7*, CD012345. [CrossRef] [PubMed]
55. Pizzini, A.; Lunger, L.; Demetz, E.; Hilbe, R.; Weiss, G.; Ebenbichler, C.; Tancevski, I. The role of omega-3 fatty acids in reverse cholesterol transport: A review. *Nutrients* **2017**, *9*, 1099. [CrossRef] [PubMed]
56. Back, M. Omega-3 fatty acids in atherosclerosis and coronary artery disease. *Future Sci. OA* **2017**, *3*, FSO236. [CrossRef] [PubMed]
57. Calder, P.C. n-3 polyunsaturated fatty acids, inflammation, and inflammatory diseases. *Am. J. Clin. Nutr.* **2006**, *83*, 1505S–1519S. [CrossRef] [PubMed]
58. Miles, E.A.; Calder, P.C. Influence of marine *n*-3 polyunsaturated fatty acids on immune function and a systematic review of their effects on clinical outcomes in rheumatoid arthritis. *Br. J. Nutr.* **2012**, *107*, S171–S184. [CrossRef] [PubMed]
59. Veselinovic, M.; Vasiljevic, D.; Vucic, V.; Arsic, A.; Petrovic, S.; Tomic-Lucic, A.; Savic, M.; Zivanovic, S.; Stojic, V.; Jakovljevic, V. Clinical benefits of n-3 pufa and -linolenic acid in patients with rheumatoid arthritis. *Nutrients* **2017**, *9*, 325. [CrossRef] [PubMed]
60. Stanley, J.C.; Elsom, R.L.; Calder, P.C.; Griffin, B.A.; Harris, W.S.; Jebb, S.A.; Lovegrove, J.A.; Moore, C.S.; Riemersma, R.A.; Sanders, T.A. UK Food Standards Agency Workshop Report: The effects of the dietary n-6:n-3 fatty acid ratio on cardiovascular health. *Br. J. Nutr.* **2007**, *98*, 1305–1310. [CrossRef] [PubMed]
61. Chowdhury, R.; Warnakula, S.; Kunutsor, S.; Crowe, F.; Ward, H.A.; Johnson, L.; Franco, O.H.; Butterworth, A.S.; Forouhi, N.G.; Thompson, S.G.; et al. Association of dietary, circulating, and supplement fatty acids with coronary risk: A systematic review and meta-analysis. *Ann. Int. Med.* **2014**, *160*, 398–406. [CrossRef] [PubMed]
62. Griffin, B.A. How relevant is the ratio of dietary n-6 to n-3 polyunsaturated fatty acids to cardiovascular disease risk? Evidence from the OPTILIP study. *Curr. Opin. Lipidol.* **2008**, *19*, 57–62. [CrossRef] [PubMed]
63. Sanders, T.A.; Lewis, F.; Slaughter, S.; Griffin, B.A.; Griffin, M.; Davies, I.; Millward, D.J.; Cooper, J.A.; Miller, G.J. Effect of varying the ratio of n-6 to n-3 fatty acids by increasing the dietary intake of alpha-linolenic acid, eicosapentaenoic and docosahexaenoic acid, or both on fibrinogen and clotting factors VII and XII in persons aged 45–70 y: The OPTILIP study. *Am. J. Clin. Nutr.* **2006**, *84*, 513–522. [CrossRef] [PubMed]
64. Goyens, P.L.; Spilker, M.E.; Zock, P.L.; Katan, M.B.; Mensink, R.P. Conversion of alpha-linolenic acid in humans is influenced by the absolute amounts of alpha-linolenic acid and linoleic acid in the diet and not by their ratio. *Am. J. Clin. Nutr.* **2006**, *84*, 44–53. [CrossRef] [PubMed]
65. Baker, E.J.; Yusof, M.H.; Yaqoob, P.; Miles, E.A.; Calder, P.C. Omega-3 fatty acids and leukocyte-endothelium adhesion: Novel anti-atherosclerotic actions. *Mol. Asp. Med.* **2018**, *64*, 169–181. [CrossRef] [PubMed]
66. Rosenfeld, M.E.; Palinski, W.; Yla-Herttuala, S.; Carew, T.E. Macrophages, endothelial cells, and lipoprotein oxidation in the pathogenesis of atherosclerosis. *Toxicol. Pathol.* **1990**, *18*, 560–571. [PubMed]

67. Rosenfeld, M.E.; Tsukada, T.; Chait, A.; Bierman, E.L.; Gown, A.M.; Ross, R. Fatty streak expansion and maturation in Watanabe Heritable Hyperlipemic and comparably hypercholesterolemic fat-fed rabbits. *Arteriosclerosis* **1987**, *7*, 24–34. [CrossRef] [PubMed]
68. Spite, M.; Claria, J.; Serhan, C.N. Resolvins, specialized proresolving lipid mediators, and their potential roles in metabolic diseases. *Cell Metab.* **2014**, *19*, 21–36. [CrossRef] [PubMed]
69. Norling, L.V.; Ly, L.; Dalli, J. Resolving inflammation by using nutrition therapy: Roles for specialized proresolving mediators. *Curr. Opin. Clin. Nutr. Metab. Care* **2017**, *20*, 145–152. [CrossRef] [PubMed]
70. Duvall, M.G.; Levy, B.D. DHA- and EPA-derived resolvins, protectins, and maresins in airway inflammation. *Eur. J. Pharmacol.* **2016**, *785*, 144–155. [CrossRef] [PubMed]
71. Barnig, C.; Frossard, N.; Levy, B.D. Towards targeting resolution pathways of airway inflammation in asthma. *Pharmacol. Ther.* **2018**, *186*, 98–113. [CrossRef] [PubMed]
72. Pase, M.P.; Grima, N.A.; Sarris, J. Do long-chain n-3 fatty acids reduce arterial stiffness? A meta-analysis of randomised controlled trials. *Br. J. Nutr.* **2011**, *106*, 974–980. [CrossRef] [PubMed]
73. Casanova, M.A.; Medeiros, F.; Trindade, M.; Cohen, C.; Oigman, W.; Neves, M.F. Omega-3 fatty acids supplementation improves endothelial function and arterial stiffness in hypertensive patients with hypertriglyceridemia and high cardiovascular risk. *J. Am. Soc. Hypertens.* **2017**, *11*, 10–19. [CrossRef] [PubMed]
74. Tousoulis, D.; Plastiras, A.; Siasos, G.; Oikonomou, E.; Verveniotis, A.; Kokkou, E.; Maniatis, K.; Gouliopoulos, N.; Miliou, A.; Paraskevopoulos, T.; et al. Omega-3 PUFAs improved endothelial function and arterial stiffness with a parallel antiinflammatory effect in adults with metabolic syndrome. *Atherosclerosis* **2014**, *232*, 10–16. [CrossRef] [PubMed]
75. Zhu, D.; Zhang, Y.; Li, S.; Gan, L.; Feng, H.; Nie, W. Enteral omega-3 fatty acid supplementation in adult patients with acute respiratory distress syndrome: A systematic review of randomized controlled trials with meta-analysis and trial sequential analysis. *Intensive Care Med.* **2014**, *40*, 504–512. [CrossRef] [PubMed]
76. Pontes-Arruda, A.; Demichele, S.; Seth, A.; Singer, P. The use of an inflammation-modulating diet in patients with acute lung injury or acute respiratory distress syndrome: A meta-analysis of outcome data. *J. Parenter. Enteral Nutr.* **2008**, *32*, 596–605. [CrossRef] [PubMed]
77. Sharp, D.S.; Rodriguez, B.L.; Shahar, E.; Hwang, L.J.; Burchfiel, C.M. Fish consumption may limit the damage of smoking on the lung. *Am. J. Respir. Crit. Care Med.* **1994**, *150*, 983–987. [CrossRef] [PubMed]
78. Rodriguez, B.L.; Sharp, D.S.; Abbott, R.D.; Burchfiel, C.M.; Masaki, K.; Chyou, P.H.; Huang, B.; Yano, K.; Curb, J.D. Fish intake may limit the increase in risk of coronary heart disease morbidity and mortality among heavy smokers. The Honolulu Heart Program. *Circulation* **1996**, *94*, 952–956. [CrossRef] [PubMed]
79. Shahar, E.; Folsom, A.R.; Melnick, S.L.; Tockman, M.S.; Comstock, G.W.; Gennaro, V.; Higgins, M.W.; Sorlie, P.D.; Ko, W.J.; Szklo, M. Dietary n-3 polyunsaturated fatty acids and smoking-related chronic obstructive pulmonary disease. Atherosclerosis Risk in Communities Study Investigators. *N. Engl. J. Med.* **1994**, *331*, 228–233. [CrossRef] [PubMed]
80. Shahar, E.; Folsom, A.R.; Wu, K.K.; Dennis, B.H.; Shimakawa, T.; Conlan, M.G.; Davis, C.E.; Williams, O.D. Associations of fish intake and dietary n-3 polyunsaturated fatty acids with a hypocoagulable profile. The Atherosclerosis Risk in Communities (ARIC) Study. *Arterioscler. Thromb.* **1993**, *13*, 1205–1212. [CrossRef] [PubMed]
81. Wang, L.; Folsom, A.R.; Eckfeldt, J.H. Plasma fatty acid composition and incidence of coronary heart disease in middle aged adults: The Atherosclerosis Risk in Communities (ARIC) Study. *Nutr. Metab. Cardiovasc. Dis.* **2003**, *13*, 256–266. [CrossRef]
82. Yamagishi, K.; Nettleton, J.A.; Folsom, A.R.; Investigators, A.S. Plasma fatty acid composition and incident heart failure in middle-aged adults: The Atherosclerosis Risk in Communities (ARIC) Study. *Am. Heart J.* **2008**, *156*, 965–974. [CrossRef] [PubMed]
83. Garcia-Larsen, V.; Amigo, H.; Bustos, P.; Bakolis, I.; Rona, R.J. Ventilatory function in young adults and dietary antioxidant intake. *Nutrients* **2015**, *7*, 2879–2896. [CrossRef] [PubMed]
84. Stern, D.A.; Morgan, W.J.; Wright, A.L.; Guerra, S.; Martinez, F.D. Poor airway function in early infancy and lung function by age 22 years: A non-selective longitudinal cohort study. *Lancet* **2007**, *370*, 758–764. [CrossRef]
85. Leng, S.; Picchi, M.A.; Tesfaigzi, Y.; Wu, G.; Gauderman, W.J.; Xu, F.; Gilliland, F.D.; Belinsky, S.A. Dietary nutrients associated with preservation of lung function in Hispanic and non-Hispanic white smokers from New Mexico. *Int. J. Chronic Obstr. Pulm. Dis.* **2017**, *12*, 3171–3181. [CrossRef] [PubMed]

86. Wood, L.G.; Attia, J.; McElduff, P.; McEvoy, M.; Gibson, P.G. Assessment of dietary fat intake and innate immune activation as risk factors for impaired lung function. *Eur. J. Clin. Nutr.* **2010**, *64*, 818–825. [CrossRef] [PubMed]
87. Ridker, P.M.; Rifai, N.; Stampfer, M.J.; Hennekens, C.H. Plasma concentration of interleukin-6 and the risk of future myocardial infarction among apparently healthy men. *Circulation* **2000**, *101*, 1767–1772. [CrossRef] [PubMed]
88. Scaglia, N.; Chatkin, J.; Chapman, K.R.; Ferreira, I.; Wagner, M.; Selby, P.; Allard, J.; Zamel, N. The relationship between omega-3 and smoking habit: A cross-sectional study. *Lipids Health Dis.* **2016**, *15*, 61. [CrossRef] [PubMed]
89. Matsuyama, W.; Mitsuyama, H.; Watanabe, M.; Oonakahara, K.; Higashimoto, I.; Osame, M.; Arimura, K. Effects of omega-3 polyunsaturated fatty acids on inflammatory markers in COPD. *Chest* **2005**, *128*, 3817–3827. [CrossRef] [PubMed]
90. De Batlle, J.; Sauleda, J.; Balcells, E.; Gomez, F.P.; Mendez, M.; Rodriguez, E.; Barreiro, E.; Ferrer, J.J.; Romieu, I.; Gea, J.; et al. Association between Omega3 and Omega6 fatty acid intakes and serum inflammatory markers in COPD. *J. Nutr. Biochem.* **2012**, *23*, 817–821. [CrossRef] [PubMed]
91. Broekhuizen, R.; Wouters, E.F.; Creutzberg, E.C.; Weling-Scheepers, C.A.; Schols, A.M. Polyunsaturated fatty acids improve exercise capacity in chronic obstructive pulmonary disease. *Thorax* **2005**, *60*, 376–382. [CrossRef] [PubMed]
92. Calder, P.C.; Laviano, A.; Lonnqvist, F.; Muscaritoli, M.; Ohlander, M.; Schols, A. Targeted medical nutrition for cachexia in chronic obstructive pulmonary disease: A randomized, controlled trial. *J. Cachexia Sarcopenia Muscle* **2018**, *9*, 28–40. [CrossRef] [PubMed]
93. Piepoli, M.F.; Hoes, A.W.; Agewall, S.; Albus, C.; Brotons, C.; Catapano, A.L.; Cooney, M.T.; Corra, U.; Cosyns, B.; Deaton, C.; et al. 2016 European Guidelines on cardiovascular disease prevention in clinical practice: The Sixth Joint Task Force of the European Society of Cardiology and Other Societies on Cardiovascular Disease Prevention in Clinical Practice (constituted by representatives of 10 societies and by invited experts) Developed with the special contribution of the European Association for Cardiovascular Prevention & Rehabilitation (EACPR). *Eur. Heart J.* **2016**, *37*, 2315–2381. [PubMed]
94. London, S.J.; Sacks, F.M.; Caesar, J.; Stampfer, M.J.; Siguel, E.; Willett, W.C. Fatty acid composition of subcutaneous adipose tissue and diet in postmenopausal US women. *Am. J. Clin. Nutr.* **1991**, *54*, 340–345. [CrossRef] [PubMed]
95. Silverman, D.I.; Reis, G.J.; Sacks, F.M.; Boucher, T.M.; Pasternak, R.C. Usefulness of plasma phospholipid N-3 fatty acid levels in predicting dietary fish intake in patients with coronary artery disease. *Am. J. Cardiol.* **1990**, *66*, 860–862. [CrossRef]
96. Nodari, S.; Triggiani, M.; Campia, U.; Manerba, A.; Milesi, G.; Cesana, B.M.; Gheorghiade, M.; Dei Cas, L. N-3 polyunsaturated fatty acids in the prevention of atrial fibrillation recurrences after electrical cardioversion: A prospective, randomized study. *Circulation* **2011**, *124*, 1100–1106. [CrossRef] [PubMed]
97. Rauch, B.; Schiele, R.; Schneider, S.; Diller, F.; Victor, N.; Gohlke, H.; Gottwik, M.; Steinbeck, G.; Del Castillo, U.; Sack, R.; et al. OMEGA, a randomized, placebo-controlled trial to test the effect of highly purified omega-3 fatty acids on top of modern guideline-adjusted therapy after myocardial infarction. *Circulation* **2010**, *122*, 2152–2159. [CrossRef] [PubMed]
98. Tavazzi, L.; Maggioni, A.P.; Marchioli, R.; Barlera, S.; Franzosi, M.G.; Latini, R.; Lucci, D.; Nicolosi, G.L.; Porcu, M.; Tognoni, G.; et al. Effect of n-3 polyunsaturated fatty acids in patients with chronic heart failure (the GISSI-HF trial): A randomised, double-blind, placebo-controlled trial. *Lancet* **2008**, *372*, 1223–1230. [PubMed]
99. Mozaffarian, D.; Marchioli, R.; Macchia, A.; Silletta, M.G.; Ferrazzi, P.; Gardner, T.J.; Latini, R.; Libby, P.; Lombardi, F.; O'Gara, P.T.; et al. Fish oil and postoperative atrial fibrillation: The Omega-3 Fatty Acids for Prevention of Post-operative Atrial Fibrillation (OPERA) randomized trial. *JAMA* **2012**, *308*, 2001–2011. [CrossRef] [PubMed]

5

Erucic Acid (22:1n-9) in Fish Feed, Farmed and Wild Fish and Seafood Products

Nini H. Sissener *, Robin Ørnsrud, Monica Sanden, Livar Frøyland, Sofie Remø and Anne-Katrine Lundebye

Institute of Marine Research, PO box 1870 Nordnes, N-5817 Bergen, Norway; ror@hi.no (R.Ø.); msa@hi.no (M.S.); lfr@hi.no (L.F.); sre@hi.no (S.R.); anne-katrine.lundebye@hi.no (A.-K.L.)

* Correspondence: nsi@hi.no

Abstract: The European Food Safety Authority (EFSA) published a risk assessment of erucic acid (22:1n-9) in 2016, establishing a Tolerable Daily Intake (TDI) for humans of 7 mg kg^{-1} body weight per day. This report largely excluded the contribution of erucic acid from fish and seafood, due to this fatty acid often not being reported separately in seafood. The Institute of Marine Research (IMR) in Norway analyzes erucic acid and has accumulated extensive data from analyses of fish feeds, farmed and wild fish, and seafood products. Our data show that rapeseed oil (low erucic acid varieties) and fish oil are the main sources of erucic acid in feed for farmed fish. Erucic acid content increases with total fat content, both in farmed and wild fish, and it is particularly high in fish liver, fish oil, and oily fish, such as mackerel. We show that the current TDI could be exceeded with a 200 g meal of mackerel, as at the maximum concentration analyzed, such a meal would contribute 143% to the TDI of a 60 kg person. These data cover a current knowledge gap in the scientific literature regarding the content of erucic acid in fish and seafood.

Keywords: erucic acid; fish; seafood

---

1. Introduction

The long-chain fatty acid erucic acid (22:1n-9) is a naturally occurring fatty acid, found in high concentrations in seeds of the family Brassicaceae, such as rapeseed and mustard seed. Even though natural forms of rapeseed contain high levels of erucic acid (usually more than 40% of the total fatty acids), commercially bred rapeseed cultivars today (also known as canola) typically have levels below 0.5% of total fatty acids [1]. High erucic acid cultivars are still grown for industrial, non-food purposes, while mustard oil that is sold for human consumption still may have a high content of erucic acid (up to ~50%) [2]. Low concentrations of erucic acid are naturally present in other food sources, such as fish.

The heart is the target organ for adverse effects of exposure to high concentrations of erucic acid, which may lead to lipidosis (accumulation of triacylglycerol as lipid droplets) in the heart muscle, reduced contractility, and eventually tissue damage [3]. This condition has never been documented in humans, but in both experimental and production animals, such as rats, pigs, and chicken [4]. The cause appears to be poor mitochondrial beta-oxidation of this fatty acid, especially in the heart, resulting in an accumulation of erucic acid in neutral lipid droplets. There is primarily an increase in triacylglycerol, while the levels of phospholipids and cholesterol remain relatively constant [5].

The European Food Safety Authority (EFSA) published a risk assessment of erucic acid in feed and food in 2016 [4], establishing a Tolerable Daily Intake (TDI) for humans of 7 mg/kg body weight per day based on the occurrence of cardiac lipidosis in experimental animals. The EFSA report largely excluded the contribution of erucic acid from seafood, on the following grounds: *"Besides the occurrence in oil seeds, erucic acid also occurs naturally in fish and seafood. These food groups mainly contain cetoleic acid (22:1n-11), which is usually accompanied by minor proportions of erucic acid* [6]. *It is also of importance that the database of the Max Rubner Institut provides a single value for 22:1 fatty acids, with no distinction between erucic acid (22:1n-9) and cetoleic acid (22:1n-11) or between the cis and trans isomers. Similarly, the US Department of Agriculture database does not differentiate between erucic acid and cetoleic acid, and it reports cis 22:1 as the sum of both 22:1n-9 and 22:1n-11. Therefore, information from these databases has not been included"*. Clearly, there is a knowledge gap regarding the occurrence of erucic acid in fish and seafood.

Erucic acid (22:1 n-9) and cetoleic acid (22:1 n-11) are quantified separately at the Institute of Marine Research (IMR) in Norway, with an accredited method that obtains good results in proficiency testing (ring trials). Validity tests and parameter controls are performed on a daily routine basis and our quality control systems are audited annually by Norwegian Accreditation, which is the national signatory of the European co-operation for Accreditation Multilateral Agreement (EA MLA). Through national surveillance programs of fish feed, farmed fish, wild caught fish, and commercial seafood products, our institute has extensive data on the fatty acid composition of these products, including the content of erucic acid. While some of these data are available in our seafood database [7], data on erucic acid have never been compiled for different seafood products and have not been published in a scientific journal. Furthermore, we have unpublished data on the metabolism of erucic acid in farmed fish from feeding trials with Atlantic salmon (where the main focus of previous publications has been on other fatty acids). This paper aims to fill current knowledge gaps in the scientific literature on erucic acid in seafood, by giving an overview of data on the occurrence of erucic acid in fish and seafood, and how this fatty acid is metabolized in farmed fish. The data are discussed in the context of fish and human health.

2. Materials and Methods

2.1. Feed, Fish and Seafood Samples

Data for this paper was compiled from analyses that were conducted in surveillance programs on fish feed, farmed fish, wild fish, and seafood products performed on behalf of the Norwegian Food Safety Authority. Samples of fish feed and fish feed ingredients were sampled by the Norwegian Food Safety Authority from Norwegian feed producers or at fish farms, representative of fish feed production in Norway. Before analysis, feed samples were prepared using standardized methods for the official control of feed. Samples of farmed fish were collected by official inspectors from the Norwegian Food Safety Authority from all fish-producing regions in Norway. The sampling was randomized with regard to season and geographical location. Wild fish and seafood samples were also collected through national surveillance programs in Norway.

2.2. Method of Fatty Acid Analysis

Fatty acids were analyzed by an accredited method. Briefly, lipids from the samples were extracted in chloroform/methanol (2:1, v/v), according to the method of Folch et al. [8]. The extracted lipids were filtered, saponified, and fatty acid methyl esters were prepared by boron trifluoride (12% BF_3 in methanol), as described previously [9]. Methyl esters were separated on a Thermo Finnegan Trace 2000 GC equipped with a fused silica capillary column (CP-sil 88; Chrompak Ltd., Middelburg, The Netherlands). The temperature programming was 60 °C for 1 min, 160 °C for 28 min, 190 °C for 17 min, and finally, 220 °C for 10 min, with all temperature ramps being 25 °C per min. Individual methyl esters were identified by retention time in comparison to standard mixtures of methyl esters (Nu-Chek, Elysian, Waterville, MN, USA). All of the samples were integrated using the software Chromeleon®, connected to the gas liquid chromatograph. Amount of fatty acid per gram sample was calculated using 19:0 methyl-ester as an internal standard. The separation of 22:1n-9 and 22:1n-11 is shown in Figure 1.

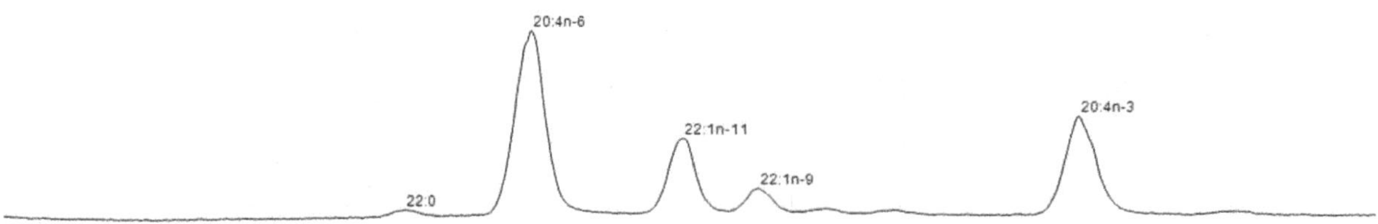

Figure 1. Chromatogram showing the separation of cetoleic acid (22:1n-11) and erucic acid (22:1n-9) in the fatty acid analysis.

2.3. Feeding Trial with Atlantic Salmon

Data are from a published feeding trial with Atlantic salmon [10], where data specifically on erucic acid were not included. Fatty acid analysis was conducted, as described above, in some cases with prior separation of the neutral and polar lipid fraction, as described by Sissener et al. [11]. Yttrium oxide for digestibility calculations was analysed in freeze dried faeces and feed samples by ICP-MS (inductively coupled plasma mass spectrometry) [12]. Digestibility was calculated as follows:

$$\text{Apparent digestibility coefficient} = 100 - (\%\ \text{yttrium in feed} \div \%\ \text{yttrium in feces}) \times (\%\ \text{nutrient in feces} \div \%\ \text{nutrient in feed}) \times 100) \quad (1)$$

Retention of erucic acid in whole fish during the experiment was calculated as follows:

$$\text{Nutrient retention} = (\text{final biomass} \times \text{final nutrient concentration} - \text{initial biomass} \times \text{initial nutrient concentration}) \times 100 \div (\text{Total feed intake} \times \text{nutrient concentration in feed}). \quad (2)$$

Linear regression analyses were conducted in GraphPad Prism 6.0 (Graphpad Software Inc., La Jolla, CA, USA).

3. Results

3.1. Content of Erucic Acid in Fish Feed Ingredients and Fish Feed

Erucic acid as a percentage of total fatty acids analyzed in fish feed ingredients in the period 2004–2008 and in fish feed from 2006, 2008, and 2012–2016 is given in Table 1. Erucic acid is present in several feed ingredients, with the highest maximum value being found in rapeseed oil (canola) at 3.2% of fatty acids, and secondly in fish oil with 2.5%. The mean values are, however, similar in fish oil, rapeseed oil, and fish silage (where the lipid fraction naturally would be similar to fish oil).

Table 1. Erucic acid (22:1n-9) as percentage of total fatty acids in fish feed and feed ingredients. The table shows the number of samples (N) for each year and matrix, the mean value of erucic acid, as well as the minimum and maximum values.

Year	Matrix	N	Mean	Min.	Max.
2004		1	1.0	1.0	1.0
2005		6	0.9	0.7	1.1
2006	Fish silage	8	1.1	1.0	1.2
2007		5	0.9	0.5	1.3
2008		2	1.0	1.0	1.0
2007		1	0.1	0.1	0.1
2008	Fish meal	4	0.6	0.1	1.3
2004		2	0.1	0.1	0.2
2005	Vegetable oil	3	0.8	0.2	1.5
2006	(uspecified)	4	0.2	0.0	0.5
2007		2	0.8	0.7	0.8
2008		1	0.7	0.7	0.7

Table 1. *Cont.*

Year	Matrix	N	Mean	Min.	Max.
2004	Rapeseed oil (canola)	3	0.6	0.2	0.8
2005		9	0.8	0.2	2.4
2006		7	1.3	0.0	3.2
2007		7	0.7	0.3	0.9
2008		7	0.7	0.2	2.7
2004	Fish oil	6	1.4	0.1	2.4
2005		10	0.6	0.1	1.8
2006		9	0.7	0.1	2.1
2007		10	0.7	0.2	1.5
2008		6	0.7	0.1	1.1
2006	Fish feed	30	0.8	0.0	1.7
2008		10	0.8	0.3	1.0
2012		13	0.6	0.2	1.1
2013		69	0.5	0.2	1.0
2014		73	0.5	0.2	0.9
2015		20	0.4	0.2	0.9
2016 [10]		20	0.3	0.2	0.5

[10], [13]. Data from the other years have not been published in reports.

Additionally, the concentration of erucic acid in mg/100 g in fish feeds from 2012–2016 is given in Table 2, while quantitative data are not available for the feed ingredients or the feed samples that were collected before 2012.

Table 2. Concentration of erucic acid (22:1n-9), given as mg fatty acid/100 g sample, in fish feed. The table shows the number of samples (N) for each year, the mean value of erucic acid, as well as the minimum and maximum values.

Year	N	Mean	Min.	Max.
Fish Feed				
2012	13	152	29	317
2013	69	138	22	250
2014	73	146	56	333
2015	20	113	53	181
2016 [5]	20	096	52	151

[5], [13].

3.2. Transfer from Feed to Fish

The digestibility of erucic acid was calculated from a previously published feeding trial with Atlantic salmon [10], with an average value of 98.1%. The digestibility was not affected by the content of erucic acid in the eight experimental feeds, which varied from 40–170 mg/100 g feed. The water temperature was 12 °C and the digestibility of erucic acid was similar to other unsaturated fatty acids of similar chain length. Fatty acid retention in salmon (the amount of a fatty acid accumulated in the fish, in percentage of the amount of the fatty acid consumed from the feed) was also calculated. The retention varied among the dietary groups, and it displayed a clear decline with increasing dietary erucic acid concentration (see Figure 2).

Values above 100% in several of the dietary groups suggest that this fatty acid, in addition to being efficiently stored in the fish, was also produced to some extent from other fatty acids, most likely from 18:1n-9, which was retained in the fish to a much lower extent. This suggests selective beta-oxidation and/or bioconversion to other fatty acids. Despite an increased storage/production of erucic acid when the dietary content was low, the absolute amount of erucic acid in the salmon fillet increased with increasing dietary content of this fatty acid (see Figure 3).

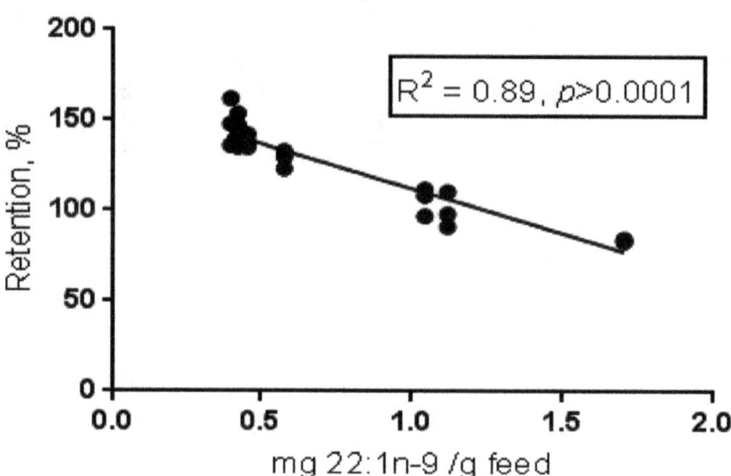

Figure 2. Retention (the amount of erucic acid accumulated in the fish during the feeding period in percentage of the amount eaten) of erucic acid in whole fish in relation to dietary content of erucic acid, in a feeding trial with Atlantic salmon [10] given eight experimental feeds ranging from 40–170 mg erucic acid/100 g feed. The adjusted *R*-value and the *p*-value for a linear regression model are given.

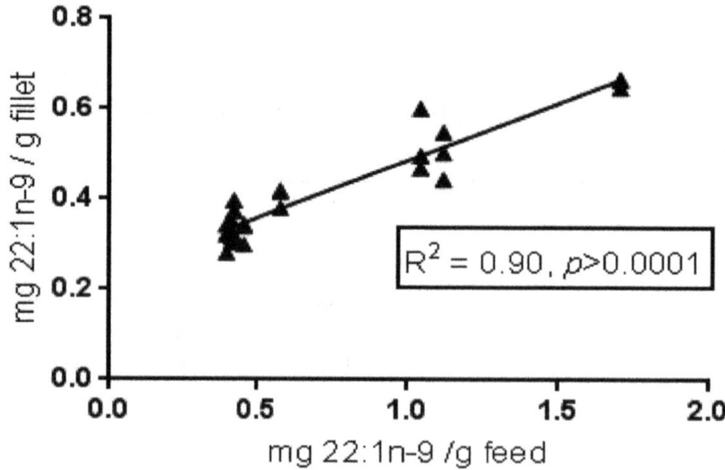

Figure 3. Content of erucic acid (22:1n-9) in salmon fillet in relation to dietary content of erucic acid, in a feeding trial with Atlantic salmon [10] given eight experimental feeds ranging from 40–170 mg erucic acid/100 g feed. The adjusted *R*-value and the *p*-value for a linear regression model are given.

In the polar lipids (cell membranes) of the heart, the content of erucic acid was mainly below the limit of detection (<0.1% of total fatty acid). This was also the case in the polar lipids of the liver. The content of erucic acid in liver neutral lipids (NL) was also low, but it increased somewhat with increasing dietary erucic acid (data not shown). Erucic acid was also low in neutral lipids in the heart, but somewhat higher than liver NL, and increased with increasing dietary erucic acid (Figure 4). There was no correlation between the total amount of neutral lipid in the heart and dietary erucic acid content ($p = 0.26$).

The feed with the highest erucic acid concentration in this trial contained 170 mg/100 g and it was a feed with a high inclusion of low erucic acid rapeseed (canola) oil (18% of the recipe/74% of added oil), while the use of other vegetable oils gave lower concentrations in the other feeds.

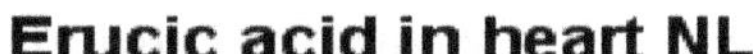

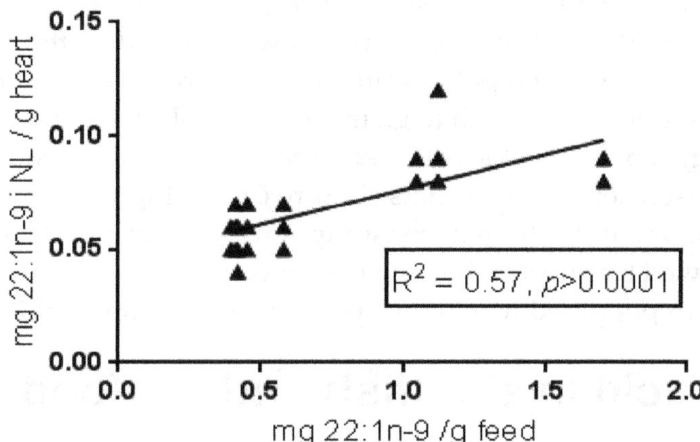

Figure 4. Content of erucic acid (22:1n-9) in neutral lipids (NL) of the heart in Atlantic salmon, in relation to the dietary content of erucic acid. The data are from a feeding trial [10] where salmon were given eight experimental feeds ranging from 40–170 mg erucic acid/100 g feed. The adjusted *R*-value and the *p*-value for a linear regression model are given.

3.3. Erucic Acid in Seafood

Concentrations of erucic acid in fish fillet, some whole fish and fish livers are given in Figure 5.

Erucic acid in fish fillet, whole fish and liver

mg eruic acid / 100 g

1000
800
600
400
200
0

Salmon, farmed
Salmon, wild
Trout
Cod
Saithe
Tusk
Ling
Blue ling
Wolf fish
Pollack
Hake
American plaice
Plaice
Halibut
Greenland halibut
Dogfish
North sea herring
NSS herring
Mackerel
Horse mackerel
Capelin, whole fish
Sprat, whole fish
Blue whiting, whole fish
Cod, liver
Saithe, liver

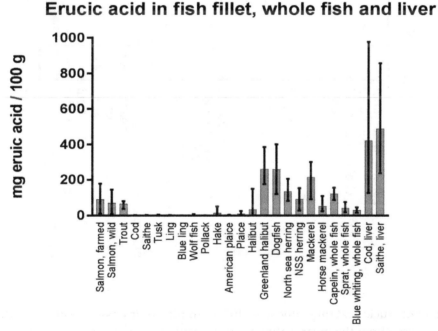

Figure 5. Content of erucic acid (22:1n-9), given as mg fatty acid/100 g sample in fish (in fillets if not otherwise specified, as well as some data for whole fish and fish livers towards the right of the figure). The bars show the mean values of erucic acid, as well as the minimum and maximum values. The number of samples analyzed for each category (N) are as follows; salmon, farmed n = 590, salmon, wild n = 99, trout n = 16, cod n = 60, saithe n = 40, tusk n = 63, ling n = 70, blue ling n = 10, wold fish n = 3, pollack n = 50, hake n = 46, American plaice n = 5, plaice n = 20, halibut n = 68, Greenland halibut n = 18, dogfish n = 15, North sea herring n = 19, NSS herring n = 30, mackerel n = 20, horse mackerel n = 21, capelin (whole fish) n = 10, sprat (whole fish) n = 8, blue whiting (whole fish) n = 10, cod liver n = 51, saithe liver n = 30. Many of the values were below the level of quantification (LOQ) for the analytical method, which is 1mg/100g. When some values were below the LOQ, 0 was used in calculation of the mean (lowerbound LOQ). Source of data: from the Institute of Marine Research' seafood database [7].

The content of erucic acid was highly variable, among both species and individual samples within the same species. In farmed salmon, the mean concentration of erucic acid was 89.4 mg/100 g, with a range from 11.5 to 179.0 mg/100 g. Low levels were found in the fillets of lean fish species (e.g., cod, saithe, tusk, ling, wolf fish, and pollock, mean values from <LOQ–3.7 mg/100 g), as compared to the much higher levels in fillets of oily fish (e.g., mackerel, halibut, herring, and salmon, mean values from 33.8–260.4 mg/100 g). The highest levels were detected in liver of cod and saithe (mean values >400 mg/100 g). In processed seafood products (Figure 6), the highest concentrations of erucic acid were found in fish oil supplements for human consumption (mean value 371.3 mg/100 g and maximum value 678 mg/100 g), followed by mustard herring (mean value 334.4 mg/100 g) and different mackerel products (~250 mg/100 g in peppered mackerel, spiced mackerel, and cold- smoked mackerel).

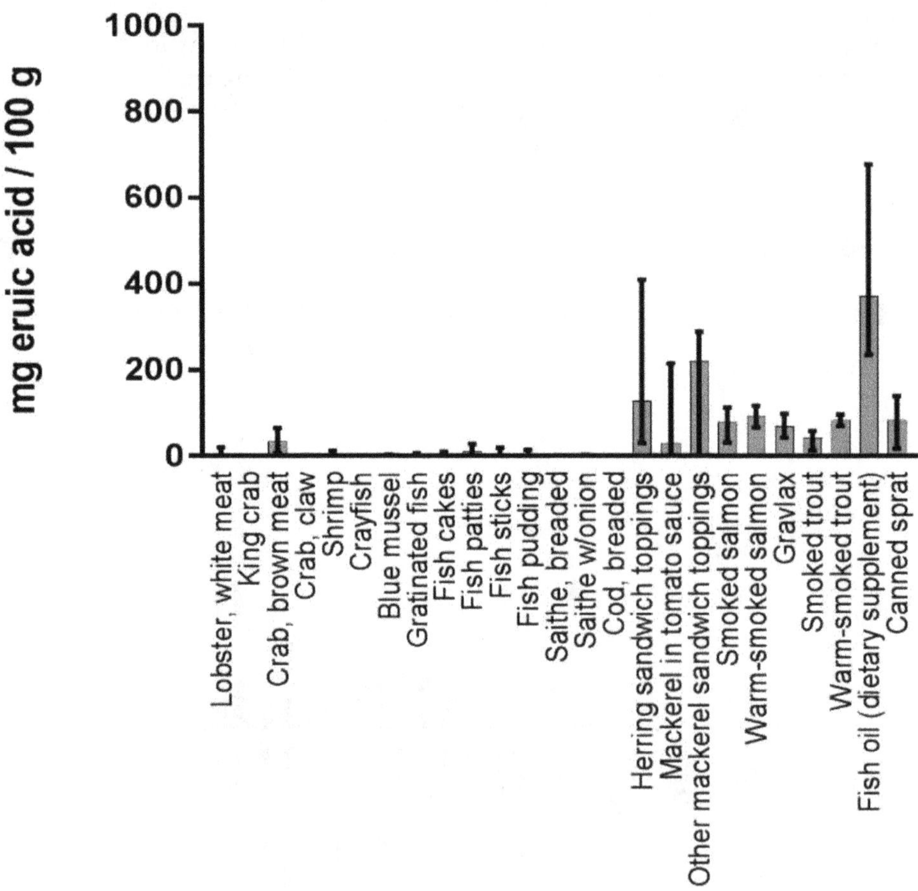

Figure 6. Content of erucic acid (mg fatty acid/100 g sample) in processed seafood products sampled in Norway. The bars show the mean value of erucic acid, as well as the minimum and maximum values. The number of samples for each category were as follows; lobster, white meat $n = 15$, king crab $n = 151$, crab, brown meat $n = 10$, crab, claw $n = 10$, shrimp $n = 11$, crayfish $n = 52$, blue mussel $n = 12$, gratinated fish $n = 5$, fish cakes $n = 5$, fish patties $n = 5$, fish sticks $n = 5$, fish pudding $n = 5$, breaded saithe $n = 2$, saithe w/onion $n = 5$, breaded cod $n = 3$, herring sandwich toppings $n = 44$, mackerel in tomato sauce $n = 11$, other mackerel sandwich toppings $n = 13$, smoked salmon $n = 18$, warm-smoked salmon $n = 3$, gravlax $n = 6$, smoked trout $n = 4$, fish oil (dietary supplement) $n = 17$, canned sprat $n = 8$.

Many of the values were below the level of quantification (LOQ) for the analytical method, which is 1 mg/100 g. When some values were below the LOQ, 0 was used in calculation of the mean (lowerbound LOQ). Source of the data: the Institute of Marine Research' seafood database [7].

3.4. Human Consumption

The human intake of erucic acid from seafood depends on the amount of seafood consumed and the concentration of erucic acid in that seafood. Table 3 gives examples of erucic acid intake associated with consumption of a 200 g portion of different fish and the contribution to the TDI for a person with a body weight of 60 kg. A 200 g portion of farmed salmon with the mean analyzed concentration of erucic acid would contribute with 43% of the TDI in a 60 kg person, while 200 g of mackerel would cover the entire TDI (102%). However, at the maximum analyzed concentrations in these species, a 200 g portion of farmed salmon or mackerel would contribute 85% and 143% of the TDI, respectively.

Table 3. Intake of erucic acid (22:1n-9) when consuming 200 g fish and the proportion of the Tolerable Daily Intake (TDI) of 7 mg per kg bodyweight per day, for a 60 kg person, using the mean and the maximum value for the respective fish species.

Species	Mean Value mg Erucic Acid	% TDI	Max Value mg Erucic Acid	% TDI
Farmed salmon	179	43	358	85
Wild salmon	141	34	290	69
North sea herring	271	65	411	98
Mackerel	429	102	601	143

4. Discussion

The ubiquitous presence of erucic acid in the lipids of fish and shellfish indicates that this fatty acid is naturally present in the marine food chain. Our data clearly show a relationship between the lipid content and the erucic acid content in various fish species, with a higher content in fish fillets with a high lipid level. These data support the limited data set on seafood from the EFSA report, showing the highest seafood levels of erucic acid in the oily fish species halibut, salmon, herring, sprat, and mackerel, with maximum values between 220–430 mg/100 g [4]. Average levels of erucic acid reported by the EFSA for salmon and trout' samples (~100 mg/kg), were also comparable to those that were found in the present study. Higher concentration of erucic acid in farmed as compared to wild salmon probably reflect the higher lipid content in farmed salmon, which was reported to be almost twice as high in the farmed salmon [14]. Our data show that both fish oil and rapeseed oil are sources of erucic acid in commercial feeds for farmed salmon, contributing similar amounts. For fish oils, the geographical origin of the oil might affect erucic acid content, since long chain monounsaturated fatty acids are particularly high in oily fish species from the Northern hemisphere, such as capelin. However, the origin of the fish oils was not specified for the oils in the current dataset. In a previous salmon feeding trial that used capelin oil as the lipid source, the experimental feed contained 440 mg erucic acid/100 g feed [15], exceeding the levels of erucic acid in all of the commercial feeds that were analysed in the surveillance programme. This was gradually reduced to 120 mg/100 g with increasing replacement of the capelin oil by low erucic acid rapeseed oil (25–100% replacement). This shows that certain fish oils can be a greater source of erucic acid in fish feeds than rapeseed oil. However, high inclusion of fish oil is not a common feeding strategy used in commercial salmon feeds. Currently, commercial salmon feeds in Norway contain on average about two-thirds rapeseed oil (low erucic acid varieties) and one-third fish oil [16].

The main adverse effect of erucic acid found in various animal species is accumulation of lipid droplets (neutral lipids) in myocardial cells. This is a reversible effect, but high doses of erucic acid may cause degenerative lesions in the muscle fibers, followed by necrosis of the myocardial tissue [3]. A feeding study with high erucic acid rapeseed oil (HEAR) was conducted in Atlantic salmon [17], where both HEAR, low erucic acid rapeseed oil (LEAR), and soybean oil were used to replace capelin oil, resulting in dietary erucic acid concentrations varying from 0.3 to 28.1% of total fatty acids. There was no effect on weight gain, unlike observations in warm-blooded animals, possibly indicating a higher tolerance for this fatty acids in fish [17]. The lack of significant differences in heart lipid content after two and four weeks of feeding was probably due to low n and high variation (as there were large numerical differences), while heart lesions were not investigated. Heart lesions have been reported in Atlantic salmon fed sunflower oil [18], compared to few such lesions in fish fed a fish oil diet. While dietary erucic acid level was not reported in that paper, it is likely to have been higher in the fish oil diet. Consequently, the dietary content of erucic acid was not a likely cause of these lesions. The presence of lesions in the coronary artery have been investigated in both a short term study in salmon fed with diets containing fish oil, rapeseed oil, or 50:50 fish oil and rapeseed oil [19], and in a long-term study where fish oil was compared with a blend of vegetable oils [20]. There were no apparent effects on lesions in the coronary artery of fish oil versus vegetable oil fed fish in either study. In the feeding trial described in the current paper, there was no correlation between the total amount of neutral lipid in the heart and dietary erucic acid content, and hence no indication that erucic acid causes an accumulation of neutral lipids in the heart at these low dietary levels. In another study, increased level of TAG was found in the heart of salmon fed vegetable oil when compared to salmon fed fish oil, while the content of erucic acid in both heart tissue and muscle tissue was the same in both dietary groups (erucic acid levels were not reported for the diets) [21]. To sum up, there is limited information on how erucic acid might affect lipid accumulation in the heart, development of lesions or other health parameters in farmed fish, but the available information does not indicate such effects at the concentrations of erucic acid present in commercial salmon feeds.

Salmon and other fish are capable of both chain elongation and beta-oxidation of fatty acids, and are hence able to produce erucic acid from shorter chain fatty acids, such as oleic acid (18:1n-9) and gondoic acid (20:1n-9), as well as from longer chain fatty acids, such as nevronic acid (24:1n-9). Fish are also able to desaturate fatty acids, including the insertion of double bonds in the n-9 position of the carbon chain, and are thus theoretically able to produce erucic acid from saturated fatty acids. Although the retention of erucic acid (possibly including some in vivo production) appeared to increase with decreasing dietary levels in the present feeding trial, total erucic acid levels in the fish decreased with decreasing dietary levels. The retention of this fatty acid is also likely to be dependent on feed concentrations, as most other fatty acids are retained in salmon to a high extent when low levels are provided in the feed (like for erucic acid in the present trial), while the retention is much lower when feed concentrations are high [22]. In support of this, fish that were fed a HEAR diet (with erucic acid constituting 28.1% of dietary fatty acids) for 18 weeks, had only 6.5% erucic acid of the total fatty acids in heart triacylglycerols and 11.5% in muscle triacylglycerols [17]. If one would want to reduce the amount of erucic acid in farmed fish as compared to current levels, this could easily be achieved by utilizing other lipid sources than fish oils and rapeseed oil, for instance, other vegetable oils.

Our data indicate that seafood consumption might contribute considerably to the TDI, especially for population groups with a high intake of oily fish. One may even exceed the TDI by eating a single 200 g portion of mackerel. Based on the maximum erucic acid concentration found in cod liver, a 50 g serving would exceed the TDI for a 60 kg person. However, it must be taken into account that the TDI is a chronic health-based guidance value and includes an uncertainty factor of 100. It is more correct to compare the TDI with chronic exposure rather than intake from a single meal. In the EFSA report, the contribution of "fish meat" to total erucic acid exposure was important in some adult populations in different dietary surveys, with contributions up to 41% of the total exposure [4]. Higher contributions than this could be expected in certain population groups in Norway (and high consumption population groups in other European countries), due to the consumption of oily fish, fish liver, and the intake of fish oil supplements, such as cod liver oil. In Norway, the mean consumption of fish in two-year old's is 16 g/day, and the 95th percentile consumption is 36 g/day; for adults, the mean consumption of fish is 52 g/day and the 95th percentile consumption is 201 g fish /day [23]. Mean consumption of fish oils and cod liver oil in two-year-old's was 2 g/day, while the 95th percentile was 6 g/day; in adults, the mean consumption of fish oils and cod liver oil was 3 g/day and the 95th percentile was 10 g/day [23]. However, these data are not detailed enough to regarding distribution of fish species etc to assess erucic acid exposure, which should be included in future risk-benefit assessments of seafood.

Despite the potentially high contribution of oily fish to erucic acid intake, there are few indications that seafood intake, and, in particular, oily fish, has a negative impact on cardio-vascular health in humans. On the contrary, the risk of cardiovascular disease was reported to be reduced by the intake of oily fish, see, e.g. [24]. The Norwegian Scientific Committee for Food Safety (VKM) has conducted risk-benefit evaluations of fish consumption in the Norwegian diet and recommends that most people should increase their consumption due to the health benefits [23]. However, erucic acid exposure has not been specifically addressed in these risk-benefit evaluations. Increased levels of 22:1 fatty acids in plasma phospholipids have been associated with a higher incidence of congestive heart failure in two independent cohorts [25]. However, fish consumption seemed to lower the risk of congestive heart failure in both of these cohorts [26,27]. In another cohort, higher levels of erucic acid in erythrocytes was associated with lower incidence of coronary heart disease, leading the authors to conclude on a cardioprotective effect [28]. Another study on patients with coronary artery disease found no association between erucic acid in erythrocytes and all-cause mortality or CVD-mortality [29]. Indian studies have shown positive effects of mustard seed oil, which is high in erucic acid, on ischemic heart disease, and myocardial infarction [30,31]. These positive effects are more likely to be associated with the high content of α-linolenic acid (18:3n-3) in mustard seed oil in a population with a generally low seafood intake, but at least they occurred despite the high content of erucic acid.

There are currently a number of knowledge gaps regarding erucic acid, and especially erucic acid from seafood. Data on health effects of erucic acid in humans is scarce, and the TDI set by EFSA is based on effects that were observed in animal studies [4]. Exposure should be assessed in population groups with a high consumption of oily fish and/or fish oil, and erucic acid should be specifically included in future risk-benefit assessments regarding seafood intake.

5. Conclusions

The concentrations of erucic acid in fish and other seafood varies considerably among species and individual samples, with the highest concentrations being found in fish liver, fish oil, and in the fillet of oily fish. Consumption of a 200 g portion of oily fish contributes significantly to the TDI set by EFSA in 2016, and may even exceed it.

There are currently many knowledge gaps regarding erucic acid, and further studies regarding its metabolism and its health effects in fish and humans are warranted. This paper contributes with new knowledge on the presence of erucic acid fish feeds, fish, and seafood products.

Author Contributions: Conceptualization, R.Ø., L.F. and A.-K.L.; Data curation, N.H.S., M.S. and A.-K.L.; Formal analysis, N.H.S. and M.S.; Project administration, R.Ø. and A.-K.L.; Writing—original draft, N.H.S.; Writing—review & editing, R.Ø., M.S., L.F., S.R. and A.-K.L.

References

1. Friedt, W.; Snowdon, R. Oilseed Rape. In *Oil Crops*; Vollmann, J., Rajcan, I., Eds.; Springer New York: New York, NY, USA, 2010; pp. 91–126.
2. Wendlinger, C.; Hammann, S.; Vetter, W. Various concentrations of erucic acid in mustard oil and mustard. *Food Chem.* **2014**, *153*, 393–397. [CrossRef] [PubMed]
3. Bremer, J.; Norum, K.R. Metabolism of very long-chain monounsaturated fatty acids (22:1) and the adaptation to their presence in the diet. *J. Lipid Res.* **1982**, *23*, 243–256. [PubMed]
4. EFSA. Scientific opinion on erucic acid in feed and food. *EFSA J.* **2016**, *14*, 1–173.
5. Houtsmuller, U.M.T.; Struijk, C.B.; Van der Beek, A. Decrease in rate of ATP synthesis of Isolated rat heart mitochondria induced by dietary erucic acid. *Biochim. Biophys. Acta. Lipids Lipid Metab.* **1970**, *218*, 564–566. [CrossRef]

6. Ackman, R.G. Fatty Acids in Fish and Shellfish. In *Fatty Acids in Foods and Their Health Implications*; Chow, C.K., Ed.; CRC Press, Tylor & Francis Group: London, UK, 2008.
7. Sjømatdata. Available online: https://sjomatdata.hi.no/#search/ (accessed on 30 September 2018).
8. Folch, J.; Lees, M.; Sloane-Stanley, G.H. A simple method for the isolation and purification of total lipids from animal tissues. *J. Biol Chem*, **1957**, *226*, 497–509.
9. Lie, Ø.; Lambertsen, G. Fatty-acid composition of glycerophospholipids in 7 tissues of cod (*Gadus morhua*), determined by combined high-performance liquid-chromotography and gas-chromotography. *J. Chromatogr Biomed. Appl.* **1991**, *565*, 119–129. [CrossRef]
10. Sissener, N.H.; Sanden, M.; Torstensen, B.E.; Waagbø, R.; Stubhaug, I.; Rosenlund, G. High dietary 18:2n-6 does not inhibit elongation and desaturation of 18:3n-3 to EPA and DHA in Atlantic salmon. *Aquac. Nutr.* **2017**, *23*, 899–909. [CrossRef]
11. Sissener, N.H.; Torstensen, B.E.; Stubhaug, I.; Rosenlund, G. Long-term feeding of Atlantic salmon in seawater with low dietary long-chain n-3 fatty acids affects tissue status of brain, retina and red blood cells. *Br. J. Nutr.* **2016**, *115*, 1919–1929. [CrossRef] [PubMed]
12. Julshamn, K.; Brenna, J.; Holland, R.; Tanner, S. Plasma source mass spectrometry—New developments and applications. *R Soc. Chem.* **1999**, *241*, 167–172.
13. Sanden, M.; Hemre, G.; Måge, A.; Lunestad, B.; Espe, M.; Lundebye, A.; Amlund, H.; Ørnsrud, R. Program for overvåking av fiskefôr. *Årsrapport Prøver Innsamlet 2016* **2017**, 1–51. Available online: https://www.researchgate.net/profile/Monica_Sanden/publication/322597959_Overvaking_av_fiskefor_Arsrapport_for_prover_innsamlet_i_2016/links/5a61e3d6aca272a1581770f6/Overvaking-av-fiskefor-Arsrapport-for-prover-innsamlet-i-2016.pdf (accessed on 30 September 2018).
14. Lundebye, A.-K.; Lock, E.-J.; Rasinger, J.D.; Nøstbakken, O.J.; Hannisdal, R.; Karlsbakk, E.; Wennevik, V.; Madhun, A.S.; Madsen, L.; Graff, I.E.; et al. Lower levels of Persistent Organic Pollutants, metals and the marine omega 3-fatty acid DHA in farmed compared to wild Atlantic salmon (*Salmo salar*). *Environ. Res.* **2017**, *155*, 49–59. [CrossRef] [PubMed]
15. Torstensen, B.E.; Frøyland, L.; Ørnsrud, R.; Lie, Ø. Tailoring of a cardioprotective muscle fatty acid composition of Atlantic salmon (*Salmo salar*) fed vegetable oils. *Food Chem.* **2004**, *87*, 567–580. [CrossRef]
16. Ytrestøyl, T.; Aas, T.S.; Åsgård, T. Utilisation of feed resources in production of Atlantic salmon (*Salmo salar*) in Norway. *Aquaculture* **2015**, *448*, 365–374. [CrossRef]
17. Thomassen, M.S.; Røsjø, C. Different fats in feed for salmon: Influence on sensory parameters, growth rate and fatty acids in muscle and heart. *Aquaculture* **1989**, *79*, 129–135. [CrossRef]
18. Bell, J.; McVicar, A.; Park, M.; Sargent, J.R. High dietary linoleic-acid affects the fatty-acid compositions of individual phospholipids from tissues of Atlantic salmon (Salmo salar)—Association with stress susceptibility and cardiac lesion. *J. Nutr.* **1991**, *121*, 1163–1172. [CrossRef] [PubMed]
19. Seierstad, S.L.; Seljeflot, I.; Johansen, O.; Hansen, R.; Haugen, M.; Rosenlund, G.; Frøyland, L.; Arnesen, H. Dietary intake of differently fed salmon; the influence on markers of human atherosclerosis. *Eur. J. Clin. Invest.* **2005**, *35*, 52–59. [CrossRef] [PubMed]
20. Seierstad, S.L.; Svindland, A.; Larsen, S.; Rosenlund, G.; Torstensen, B.E.; Evensen, Ø. Development of intimal thickening of coronary arteries over the lifetime of Atlantic salmon, *Salmo salar* L., fed different lipid sources. *J. Fish. Dis.* **2008**, *31*, 401–413.
21. Remø, S.C.; Hevrøy, E.M.; Olsvik, P.A.; Fontanillas, R.; Breck, O.; Waagbø, R. Dietary histidine requirement to reduce the risk and severity of cataracts is higher than the requirement for growth in Atlantic salmon smolts, independently of the dietary lipid source. *Br. J. Nutr.* **2014**, *111*, 1759–1772. [CrossRef] [PubMed]
22. Sissener, N.H. Are we what we eat? Changes to the feed fatty acid composition of farmed salmon and its effects through the food chain. *J. Exp. Biol.* **2018**, *221*, jeb161521. [PubMed]
23. Skåre, J.U.; Brantsæter, A.L.; Frøyland, L.; Hemre, G.I.; Knutsen, H.K.; Lillegaard, I.T.L.; Torstensen, B. Benefit-risk assessment of fish and fish products in the Norwegian diet—An update. Opinion of the Scientific Steering Committee of the Norwegian Scientific Committee for Food Safety. *VKM Report.* **2014**, *4*, 1–293.
24. EFSA. Scientific opinion on dietary reference values for fats, including saturated fatty acids, polyunsaturated fatty acids, monounsaturated fatty acids, trans fatty acids, and cholesterol. *EFSA J.* **2010**, *8*, 197.
25. Imamura, F.; Lemaitre, R.; King, I.; Song, X.; Steffen, L.; Folsom, A.; Siscovick, D.; Mozaffarian, D. Long-chain monounsaturated fatty acids and incidence of congestive heart failure in 2 prospective cohorts. *Circulation* **2013**, *127*, 1512–1521. [CrossRef] [PubMed]

26. Nettleton, J.; Steffen, L.; Loehr, L.; Rosamond, W.; Folsom, A. Incident heart failure is associated with lower whole-grain intake and greater high-fat dairy and egg intake in theatherosclerosis risk in communities (aric) study. *J. Am. Diet. Assoc.* **2008**, *108*, 1881–1887. [CrossRef]
27. Mozaffarian, D.; Bryson, C.; Lemaitre, R.; Burke, G.; Siscovick, D. Fish intake and risk of incident heart failure. *J. Am. Coll. Cardiol.* **2005**, *45*, 2015–2021. [CrossRef] [PubMed]
28. Matsumoto, C.; Matthan, N.R.; Lichtenstein, A.H.; Gaziano, J.M.; Djoussé, L. Red blood cell MUFAs and risk of coronary artery disease in the Physicians' Health Study. *Am. J. Clin. Nutr.* **2013**, *98*, 749–754. [CrossRef] [PubMed]
29. Li, Z.; Zhang, Y.; Su, D.; Lv, X.; Wang, M.; Ding, D.; Ma, J.; Xia, M.; Wang, D.; Yang, Y.; et al. The opposite associations of long-chain versus very long-chain monounsaturated fatty acids with mortality among patients with coronary artery disease. *Heart* **2014**, *100*, 1597–1605. [CrossRef] [PubMed]
30. Singh, R.B.; Niaz, M.A.; Sharma, J.P.; Kumar, R.; Rastogi, V.; Moshiri, M. Randomized, double-blind, placebo-controlled trial of fish oil and mustard oil in patients with suspected acute myocardial infarction: The Indian experiment of infarct survival. *Cardiovasc. Drugs Ther.* **1997**, *11*, 485–491. [CrossRef] [PubMed]
31. Rastogi, T.; Reddy, K.S.; Vaz, M.; Spiegelman, D.; Prabhakaran, D.; Willett, W.C.; Stampfer, M.J.; Ascherio, A. Diet and risk of ischemic heart disease in India. *Am. J. Clin. Nutr.* **2004**, *79*, 582–592. [CrossRef] [PubMed]

6

Genes and Dietary Fatty Acids in Regulation of Fatty Acid Composition of Plasma and Erythrocyte Membranes

Maria Lankinen [1,*], Matti Uusitupa [1] and Ursula Schwab [1,2]

1 Institute of Public Health and Clinical Nutrition, University of Eastern Finland, 70211 Kuopio, Finland; matti.uusitupa@uef.fi (M.U.); ursula.schwab@uef.fi (U.S.)

2 Department of Medicine, Endocrinology and Clinical Nutrition, Kuopio University Hospital, 70210 Kuopio, Finland

* Correspondence: maria.lankinen@uef.fi

Abstract: The fatty acid compositions of plasma lipids and cell membranes of certain tissues are modified by dietary fatty acid composition. Furthermore, many other factors (age, sex, ethnicity, health status, genes, and gene × diet interactions) affect the fatty acid composition of cell membranes or plasma lipid compartments. Therefore, it is of great importance to understand the complexity of mechanisms that may modify fatty acid compositions of plasma or tissues. We carried out an extensive literature survey of gene × diet interaction in the regulation of fatty acid compositions. Most of the related studies have been observational studies, but there are also a few intervention trials that tend to confirm that true interactions exist. Most of the studies deal with the desaturase enzyme cluster (*FADS1, FADS2*) in chromosome 11 and elongase enzymes. We expect that new genetic variants are being found that are linked with the genetic regulation of plasma or tissue fatty acid composition. This information is of great help to understanding the contribution of dietary fatty acids and their endogenic metabolism to the development of some chronic diseases.

Keywords: fatty acid; diet; genotype; human; *FADS*

---

1. Introduction

Traditionally, the fatty acid compositions of plasma and its components (triglycerides (TG), phospholipids (PL), cholesteryl esters (CE)) have been used as biomarkers of dietary intake of certain fatty acids. Furthermore, the fatty acid compositions of adipose tissue and erythrocyte and platelet membranes reflect the dietary intakes of different fatty acids [1–4]. In particular, proportions of omega-3 long-chain unsaturated fatty acids in CE and in erythrocyte and platelet membranes reflect quite well the intakes of these fatty acids, e.g., from fatty fish. On the contrary, the major dietary saturated fatty acid, palmitic acid, is more problematic as a biomarker of saturated fatty acid intake due to its rapid desaturation and elongation to longer-chain fatty acids in the body and due to its endogenous de novo lipogenesis [5]. Still, based on long-term trial evidence, the palmitic acid content of CE also reflects dietary intake [4]. Odd-chain fatty acids (15:0 and 17:0) have been used as biomarkers for dairy fat intake, but they are also produced from gut-derived propionate [6] and exist in fish [7–9]. Moreover, the measured contents of given fatty acids in different biomarkers indicate only relative patterns of the fatty acids in the diet, and, e.g., incorporation of omega-3 polyunsaturated fatty acids (PUFAs) into various biomarkers may vary considerably [10,11]. Various fatty acid biomarkers reflect dietary intakes from a few days even to years, as does adipose tissue fatty acid composition [11]. Furthermore, well-known competition occurs between *n*-6 and *n*-3 PUFA; the higher the intakes and proportions of eicosapentaenoic acid (EPA) and docosahexaenoic acid (DHA) are, the lower the relative linoleic acid content of biomarkers [12,13]. Endogenous fatty acid metabolism is also quite complex, and some studies suggest, e.g., retroconversion of DHA to EPA and that DHA also interferes with linoleic acid metabolism [10]. Another example is that trans-fatty acid 18:1t incorporates markedly higher into TG and PL than CE and may result in a decreased conversion of linoleic acid to its more unsaturated metabolites [14]. Oleic acid (18:1*n*-9) is the dominant fatty acid in TGs, whereas linoleic acid (18:2*n*-6) is very abundant in CE fraction [15].

Postprandial fatty acid metabolism and fatty acid composition of biomarkers may be modified by other dietary components and factors related to glucose and insulin metabolism and cardio-metabolic health in general [16,17]. Finally, the fatty acid composition of various biomarkers is under genetic regulation [18,19]. Figure 1 summarizes the major factors affecting the fatty acid composition of serum lipids and cell membranes.

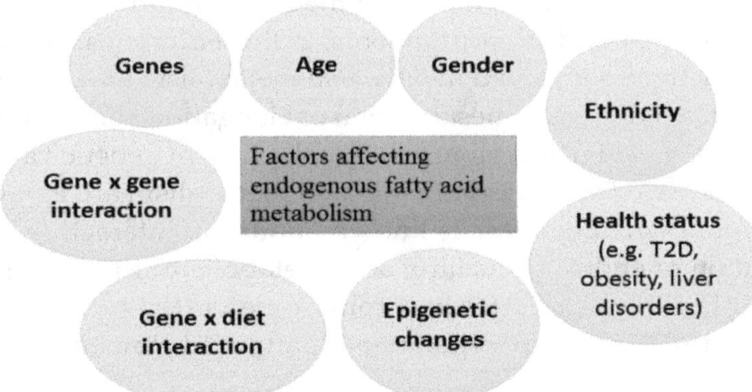

Figure 1. Factors affecting endogenous fatty acid metabolism. T2D, type 2 diabetes.

We became interested in the genetic regulation of fatty acid metabolism over 20 years ago when we examined whether polymorphism of the fatty acid binding protein 2 gene (*FABP2*) that is expressed in intestinal enterocytes modified postprandial lipemic response in humans [20]. In our oral fat-loading test, we examined postprandial triglyceride, chylomicron, and very-low-density lipoprotein TG in individuals homozygous for the Ala encoding allele (wild type) and individuals homozygous for the Thr54 allele variant. The Thr54 genetic variant was suggested to result in an increased absorption and processing of fatty acids in the intestine and showed an association with higher lipid oxidation and insulin resistance in Pima Indians [21] and with insulin resistance and increased intra-abdominal fat mass in Japanese men [22]. We found a markedly higher postprandial lipemic response in Finnish individuals homozygous for the Thr54 allele. Consequently, we also found an increased postprandial response of C14–C18 fatty acids in chylomicron and very-low-density lipoprotein (VLDL) TG in study persons homozygous for Thr54 variant [20]. However, we did not find any relative differences in the amounts of individual fatty acids introduced to these lipid fractions between these two genotype groups [23]. This particular genetic variant may also affect the postprandial TG content of high-density lipoprotein (HDL) in visceral obese individuals heterozygous for the Thr54 allele [24], and, interestingly, it may associate with reduced delta-6 desaturase (D6D) activity and lowered arachidonic acid (AA, 18:2*n*-6) content in obese children homozygous for Thr54 allele D [25]. In a clinical trial in patients with type 2 diabetes (T2D), individuals homozygous for the Thr54 allele showed an increased postprandial response of mono- and polyunsaturated fatty acids as an indication of increased fatty acid absorption [26]. In some other studies, postprandial lipemic response has not been related to this genetic polymorphism [16]. Nevertheless, these results on *FABP2* genetic variation, along with rapidly increasing knowledge about genes involved in fatty acid desaturation and elongation, indicate that fatty acid absorption and metabolism are under tight genetic regulation, and there may occur gene–diet interaction in fatty acid metabolism [19].

2. Methods

We carried out a literature survey of genes and diet in the context of the regulation of fatty acid compositions in PubMed. We used the following search term: (genotype OR gene OR fads OR elovl) AND fatty acid AND (diet OR dietary intake OR nutrition) AND (plasma OR erythrocyte membrane) AND human NOT animal. The search was performed on 3 July 2018 and it gave 553 hits altogether. Relevant articles were selected based on their abstracts (n = 32).

3. Genetic Variants of Fatty Acid Metabolism and Disease Risk

Figure 2 illustrates how a given genetic variant of fatty acid metabolism could modify endogenous fatty acid metabolism, their downstream metabolites, and, finally, risk of diseases. Principally, genetic variation may increase or decrease the activity of certain steps in endogenous fatty acid metabolism, affecting either desaturation or elongation processes. This effect is also modified by other factors, as shown in Figure 1. Altogether, modified fatty acid metabolism can be demonstrated by examining the fatty acid content of plasma and its components, cell membranes, or adipose tissue. In most studies [15,27,28], enzyme activities involved in fatty acid metabolism have been estimated by different ratios of certain fatty acids reflecting either desaturation or elongation of fatty acids to their longer chain metabolites (Figure 3 and Table 1). Furthermore, most of the known genetic variants (single-nucleotide polymorphisms, SNPs) associated with altered fatty acid metabolism are in fact genetic markers and their exact function is unknown. Even less is known about the interaction of genes and diet with regard to genetic regulation of endogenous fatty acid metabolism. In particular, genetic variants of the fatty acid desaturase (*FADS*) gene cluster in chromosome 11 (*FADS1*, *FADS2*) and elongases (e.g., *ELOVL2* and *ELOVL5*) are involved in the regulation of fatty acid metabolism.

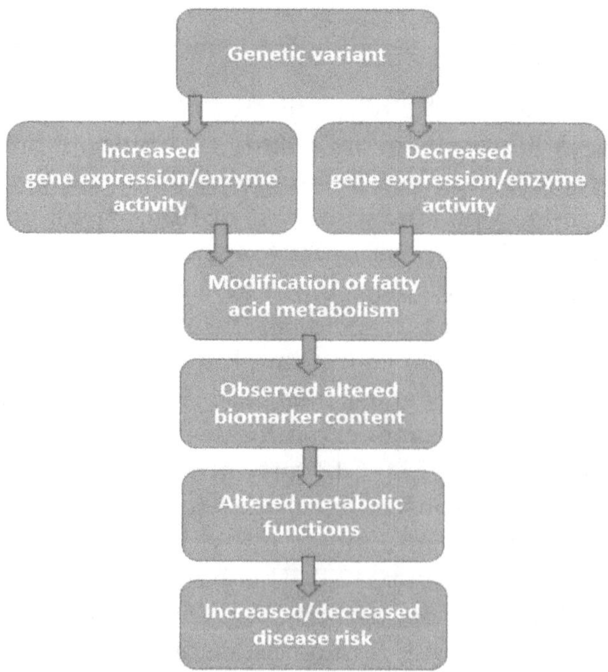

Figure 2. Impacts of genetic variants regulating fatty acid metabolism in the body.

Table 1. Fatty acid ratios used for the estimation of desaturase and elongase activities.

Estimated Desaturase/Elongase	Fatty Acid Ratio
Stearoyl-CoA desaturase 1 (SCD1)	16:1n-7/16:0
Delta-6-delta (D6D)	18:3n-6/18:2n-6
Delta-5-delta (D5D)	20:4n-6/20:3n-6
Elongase	18:1n-7/16:1n-7

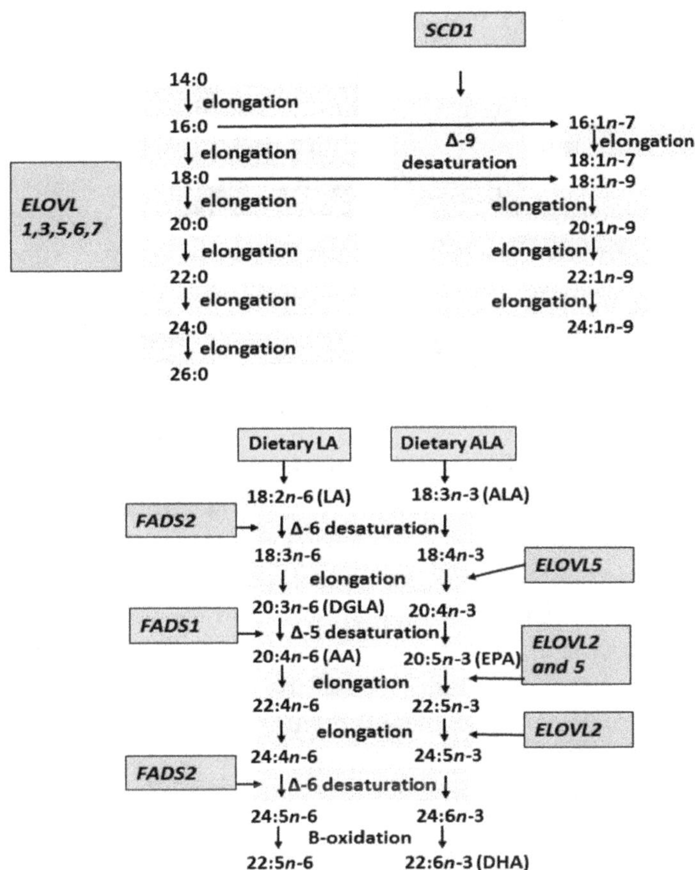

Figure 3. Simplified figure of the synthesis of fatty acids in the human body including key enzymes regulating fatty acid metabolism and genes coding them. AA, arachidonic acid; ALA, alpha-linolenic acid; DGLA, Di-homo-gamma linolenic acid; DHA docosahexaenoic acid; ELOVL, fatty acid elongase; EPA, eicosapentaenoic acid; FADS, fatty acid desaturase; LA, linoleic acid; SCD, stearoyl-CoA desaturase 1.

Many studies suggest that delta-5-desaturase (D5D) activity (*FADS1*) is associated with a lower risk of T2D [29], while stearoyl-CoA desaturase 1 (SCD1) [27] and delta-6-desaturase (D6D, FADS2) variants are linked with insulin resistance and worsening of glucose tolerance or an increased risk of T2D [15,29–32]. In the longitudinal Finnish Diabetes Prevention Study, we confirmed the preventive effect of D5D activity on future T2D risk, and we showed that a higher insulin sensitivity may explain this finding [33]. Furthermore, based on the Metabolic Syndrome in Men (METSIM) study population where erythrocyte membrane fatty acids were analyzed, high estimated elongase activity was associated with a beneficial effect on glucose tolerance [30]. In another study carried out with the METSIM study population where the fatty acid compositions of serum lipids from TG, CE, and PL were analyzed, D6D activity predicted a worsening of glycemia, whereas elongase activity had an opposite effect on glycemia [15]. Furthermore, it is not surprising that genetic markers of the *FADS* cluster are also associated with lipid metabolism, in particular with HDL and triglyceride metabolism [34], but the data on cardiovascular disease (CVD) risk are lacking. In a meta-analysis studying associations between omega-3 fatty acid biomarkers and coronary heart disease (CHD), there was no significant interaction identified by *FADS* variant for incident CHD events [35]. Interestingly, in a genome-wide association study (GWAS) of Greenland Inuits, *ELOVL2* showed an association with sleep duration, age, and DNA methylation, and *ELOVL5* coding mutations may lead to spinocerebellar ataxia; as an example of epigenetic effect, epigenetic markers were associated with depression and suicide risk [19]. Disease per se may also modify enzyme activities involved in endogenous fatty acid metabolism. For instance, non-alcoholic steatohepatitis was found to affect desaturase enzyme activities in the liver in a cross-sectional study [36].

4. Genetic Regulation of Endogenous Fatty Acid Metabolism

Figure 3 summarizes the key enzymes regulating fatty acid metabolism in the body. Recently, many new genetic variants have been identified that may modify endogenous fatty acid metabolism and, consequently, the profile of fatty acid composition in different plasma components or tissues. In particular, the knowledge of genes participating in elongation processes has increased rapidly. We expect that new genetic variants linked with biomarkers reflecting the fatty acid composition of plasma components or cell membranes will be identified in the future. Some of these novel genetic variants are listed and briefly discussed in Table 2A–C and the next chapter.

There has been huge progress in research into fatty acid metabolism over the last 20 years. Both single-nucleotide polymorphism studies and GWAS have focused on enzymes regulating endogenous fatty acid metabolism (Figure 3). Specifically, these enzymes regulate both desaturation and elongation processes in fatty acid metabolism. Their genetic variations are associated with altered accumulation of long-chain PUFAs in the cell membranes of tissues and plasma lipid components [19]. Epigenetic variation of these genes may also play a role in this context [37,38]. In the present review based on a literature survey and our own studies, we focus on studies investigating the genetic regulation of plasma and membrane fatty acids in relation to the putative interaction between dietary fat and fatty acid incorporation into different biomarkers used to evaluate the quality of dietary fat in observational and intervention studies.

Table 2 summarizes the current knowledge about the genetic variants that have been associated with endogenous fatty acid metabolism. Most of the studies deal with individual SNPs of the *FADS* cluster (Table 2B) or elongases, and only some of them are based on GWAS (Table 2A). Among them, only a couple studies are true intervention trials (Table 2C), most without a specific hypothesis, and others are observational trials.

A GWAS based on the Invecchiare in Chianti (InCHIANTI) study population and Genetics of Lipid Lowering Drugs and Diet Network (GOLDN) study population used for replication observed that the *FADS* genetic cluster located in chromosome 11 was associated with AA, eisosadienoic acid (EDA), and EPA, and the *EVOLV2* genetic variant in chromosome 6 with EPA concentrations, but in the replication study, the association with EPA was not confirmed [18] (Table 2A). A few years earlier, two cross-sectional studies from Germany reported that haplotypes of the *FADS1* and *FADS2* region was associated with AA and many other longer-chain fatty acids of both the *n*-6 and *n*-3 series [39] (Table 2B); specifically, minor alleles of *FADS1/FADS2* showed mostly an association with decreased levels of plasma phospholipids. In a later study [40], associations between *FADS1/FADS2* haplotypes and fatty acids in phospholipids were replicated, and this study also showed similar associations with phospholipids of erythrocyte membranes, but only regarding omega-6 PUFAs (Table 2B). In 2011, Lemaitre and co-authors [41] published an important GWAS from five cohorts comprising altogether 8866 individuals of European ancestry, and smaller African, Chinese, and Hispanic populations were also examined. In line with previous studies, minor alleles of *FADS1* and *FADS2* were associated with higher ALA but lower EPA and docosapentaenoic acid (DPA), while minor alleles of *ELOVL2* were associated with higher EPA and DPA but lower DHA content. The results on *FADS1* were replicated in other ancestries examined. Furthermore, this study reported a novel association of DPA with several SNPs in *GCKR*.

With regard to interaction, ethnicity may also have an impact on gene–diet interactions. In a study on Inuits applying GWAS, several SNPs were examined in relation to erythrocyte membrane fatty acids [42]. Novel genes and polymorphisms that modified fatty acid composition were identified (Table 2A). This study also suggests that genetic and physiological adaptation to the intake of a diet rich in omega-3 PUFAs could happen with time.

5. Interaction between Genes and Dietary Fatty Acids

Most of the studies on interactions between genes and dietary fat in terms of the regulation of fatty acid composition of plasma or erythrocyte membranes are based on observational studies in various study populations. These studies have limitations relating to the accuracy of dietary data collection and possible weaknesses associated with controlling confounding factors (e.g., age, sex, ethnicity, lifestyle factors, liver status, and cardiometabolic health). Furthermore, genetic effect on fatty acid composition may vary depending on the fatty acid biomarker used. Therefore, intervention studies may give more comprehensive data on the variation of biomarker fatty acid composition according to the genetic background. Intervention studies also have limitations. They are laborious to carry out and without a pre-genotyped study population, the screening, especially regarding rare gene variants, is demanding. In our studies, we have been able to invite participants from the large METSIM cohort with wide genotype and phenotype data [43]. A big limitation related to experimental studies with a prior hypothesis is that in intervention studies, only one preselected genetic marker can be examined at a time. Furthermore, a highly experimental diet may not reflect the effects achieved with habitual diet, and adherence to an experimental diet may remain insufficient in free-living conditions in longer-term interventions. In large-scale observational studies, a multitude of genetic variations can be examined at the same time, and it is possible to combine the data collected from different study populations or the results may be confirmed in other study populations.

Zietemann and co-authors examined the fatty acid composition of erythrocyte membranes and estimated desaturase activities in relation to the rs174546 *FADS* genotype variant in their cross-sectional study [44] (Table 2B). The estimated activities of *FADS1* and *FADS2* were strongly decreased in individuals with the minor allele, and in principle, fatty acid compositions reported were in line with earlier observations. Furthermore, this study described an interaction with diet, i.e., the dietary fatty acid *n*-6 to *n*-3 ratio was suggested to modify the association between the *FADS1* and *FADS2* genotype and estimated D5D activity calculated from measured fatty acids (see Table 1). In one study [45] (Table 2B), 309 pregnant women in the Netherlands were examined at the 36th gestational week and then one month postpartum. Both plasma phospholipids and milk fat composition postpartum were examined in relation to high fish or fish oil intakes. The results were divergent in phospholipids and milk: a higher omega-3 PUFA intake from fish or fish oil compensated for the lower DHA in plasma phospholipids irrespective of genotype, but the proportion of DHA in excreted milk remained unchanged in women who were homozygous for minor alleles of *FADS1*/*FADS2*. This study suggests that there may even be tissue-specific interactions regarding genes regulating fatty acid metabolism. Porenta and co-authors [46] (Table 2C) randomized 108 individuals with increased risk for colon cancer into the Mediterranean type diet or the Healthy Eating diet for 6 months. Serum and colonic mucosa fatty acid compositions were examined in relation to selected *FADS1*/*FADS2* alleles. In individuals with major alleles of the *FADS* cluster, interaction was suggested between the diets and colonic AA content that remained unchanged after the Mediterranean diet. In a small intervention study on putative interaction between fish oil supplementation and the *FADS* cluster, no significant interaction was found, but fish oil supplementation resulted in greater increases in erythrocyte EPA levels in minor allele carriers of *FADS1*/*FADS2* variants [47] (Table 2C).

In a large updated meta-analysis of the Cohorts for Heart and Aging Research in Genomic Epidemiology (CHARGE) consortium [48] (Table 2B), interaction between dietary PUFAs and 5 different genes affecting fatty acid composition was examined. However, no significant interactions were found after corrections. Interestingly, the results varied according to the compartments used. Specifically, regarding the *FADS1* interaction term for ALA, even opposite effects were found in proportions of fatty acids between plasma and erythrocyte membranes.

In a small randomized cross-over trial [49], individuals homozygous for the minor allele of *FADS1*/*FADS2* had a lower plasma AA and AA/LA ratio when compared with the major allele carriers after each diet, while *ELOVL2* had no effect on PUFAs. Furthermore, flaxseed oil, which is rich in ALA, resulted in increased plasma composition of EPA beyond that of major allele homozygotes consuming a typical "western" diet (Table 2C). While very sophisticated methodologies were applied, the study design was quite complicated in this particular study.

Table 2. Studies on the relation between genetic polymorphism and biomarkers of dietary fatty acids and reported interaction between diets and genetic variants regulating fatty acid metabolism. Part A includes genome-wide association studies (GWAS), Part B includes a priori selected genes, and Part C includes intervention studies.

Study	Study Population and Design	Fatty Acid Biomarkers Examined	Main Findings	Comment
A) GWAS Studies				
Tanaka T et al. PLoS Genet 2009. [18]	InCHIANTI Study (Chianti region of Tuscana, Italy, n = 1075) and GOLDN (predominantly Caucasian, n = 1076) replication study	PUFAs in plasma in CHIANTI study and in erythrocytes in GOLDN study	*FADS* genetic cluster marker (*FADS1, FADS2, FADS3*) in chromosome 11 associated with AA, EDA, and EPA, and *EVOLV2* genetic marker in chromosome 6 with EPA.	First GWAS with replication data. The *ELOVL2* SNP was associated with DPA and DHA but not with EPA in GOLDN replication study.
Lemaitre RN et al. PLoS Genet 2011. [41]	Five cohorts (n = 8866) of European ancestry (CHARGE consortium). In addition, African (n = 2547), Chinese (n = 633), and Hispanic ancestry (n = 661) study populations were examined.	Four major n-3 PUFAs (ALA, EPA, DPA, DHA) in plasma PL	Minor alleles of *FADS1* and *FADS2* associated with higher ALA, but lower EPA and DPA. Minor alleles of SNPs in *ELOVL2* were associated with higher EPA and DPA and lower DHA content.	A novel association of DPA with several SNPs in *GCKR* (glucokinase regulator) was reported. Results on *FADS1* were similar regardless of ancestry studied.
Wu et al. Circ Cardiovasc Genet 2013. CHARGE consortium [50]	European Ancestry (n = 8961)	Plasma levels of 16:0, 18:0, 16:1n-7, 18:1n-9	*ALG14* polymorphisms were associated with higher 16:0 and lower 18:0. *FADS1* and *FADS2* polymorphisms were associated with higher 16:1n-7 and 18:1n-9 and lower 18:0. *LPGAT1* polymorphisms were associated with lower 18:0. *GCKR* and *HIF1AN* polymorphisms were associated with higher 16:1n-7, whereas *PKD2L1* and a locus on chromosome 2 (not near known genes) were associated with lower 16:1n-7.	Polymorphisms in 7 novel loci were associated with circulating levels of $\geq$1 of 16:0, 18:0, 16:1n-7, 18:1n-9.
Guan et al. Circ Cardiovasc Genet 2014. [51]	White adults (n = 8631)	Total plasma or plasma PL n-6 PUFAs	Novel regions were identified on chromosome 10 associated with LA (rs10740118; near *NRBF2*); on chromosome 16 with LA, GLA, dihomo-GLA, and AA (rs16966952; *NTAN1*); and on chromosome 6 with adrenic acid after adjustment for AA (rs3134950; *AGPAT1*). Previous findings of the *FADS* cluster on chromosome 11 with LA and AA were confirmed.	
Dorajoo R et al. Genes Nutr. 2015. [52]	Singaporean Chinese population (n = 1361)	Plasma PUFAs	Genome-wide associations with ALA, all four n-6 PUFAs, and delta-6 desaturase activity at the *FADS1/FADS2* locus. These associations were independent of dietary intake of PUFAs.	Genetic loci that influence plasma concentrations of n-3 and n-6 PUFAs are shared across different ethnic groups.

Table 2. *Cont.*

Study	Study Population and Design	Fatty Acid Biomarkers Examined	Genes Examined	Main Findings	Comment
Fumagalli M et al. Science 2015. [42]	Inuits (n = 191), European (n = 60), and Han Chinese (n = 44) individuals	Erythrocyte membrane fatty acids		*FADS1*, *FADS2*, *FADS3*, and SNPs 7115739, rs174570 (among others) had positive association with ETA, but negative associations with EPA and DPA; no effect on DHA content.	Novel genes and polymorphisms were identified in Inuits that may suggest genetic and physiological adaptation to a high-omega-3-PUFA diet; associations with height and weight were also found.
Lemaitre et al. J Lipid Res 2015. [53]	European ancestry (n = 10,129)	Plasma PL and Erythrocyte levels of VLSFA (20:0, 22:0, 24:0)		The *SPTLC3* (serine palmitoyl-transferase long-chain base subunit 3) variant at rs680379 was associated with higher 20:0. The *CERS4* (ceramide synthase 4) variant at rs2100944 was associated with higher levels of 20:0 and in analyses that adjusted for 20:0, with lower levels of 22:0 and 24:0.	*SPTLC3* is a gene involved in the rate-limiting step of de novo sphingolipid synthesis.
Mozaffarian et al. Am J Clin Nutr 2015. CHARGE consortium [54]	Meta-analysis of GWA studies (n = 8013)	Erythrocyte of PL trans fatty acids and 31 SNPs in or near the *FADS1* and *FADS2* cluster		Genetic regulation of cis/trans-18:2 by the *FADS1/2* cluster.	Trans fatty acids.
Tintle NL et al. Prostaglandins Leukot Essent Fatty Acids 2015. [55]	Framingham Offspring Study (n = 2633)	14 red blood cell fatty acids		Novel associations between (1) AA and *PCOLCE2* (regulates apoA-I maturation and modulates apoA-I levels), and (2) oleic and linoleic acid and *LPCAT3* (mediates the transfer of fatty acids between glycerolipids). Also, previously identified strong associations between SNPs in the *FADS* and *ELOVL* regions were replicated.	Multiple SNPs explained 8–14% of the variation in 3 high-abundance (>11%) fatty acids, but only 1–3% in 4 low-abundance (<3%) fatty acids, with the notable exception of DGLA acid with 53% of variance explained by SNPs.
de Oliveira Otto MC et al. CHARGE consortium. PLoS One 2018. [56]	Meta-analysis of GWA studies (n = 11,494); individuals of European descent	15:0, 17:0, 19:0, and 23:0 (OCSFA) in plasma PL and erythrocytes		SNP *MYO10* rs 13361131 associated with 17:0 level, *DLEU1* rs12874278 and rs 17363566 associated with 19:0 level. Using candidate gene approach, a few other SNPs also associated with 17:0 and 23:0 levels.	Circulating levels of OCSFA are predominantly influenced by nongenetic factors.
B) Candidate Gene Studies					
Study	**Study Population and Design**	**Fatty Acid Biomarkers Examined**	**Genes Examined**	**Main Findings**	**Comment**
Schaeffer L et al. Hum Mol Genet 2006. [39]	N = 727 from Erfurt, Germany, from The European Community Respiratory Health Survey I (ECRHS I), cross-sectional	PUFAs in plasma PL	Haplotypes of FADS1 and *FADS2* region	Haplotypes of *FADS1* and *FADS2* region associated with AA and many other long-chain n-6 and n-3 fatty acids (e.g., LA, GLA, and EPA and DPA.	Mostly decreased levels of PUFAs associated with minor alleles of *FADS1* and *FADS2*.

Table 2. *Cont.*

Xie L and Innis SM. J Nutr 2008. [57]	69 pregnant women in Canada and breast milk for a subset of 54 women exclusively breast-feeding at 1 month postpartum, cross-sectional	Plasma phospholipid and erythrocyte ethanolamine phosphoglyceride (EPG) (n-6) and (n-3) fatty acids	*FADS1/FADS2* rs174553, rs99780, rs174575, and rs174583	Minor allele homozygotes of rs174553 (GG), rs99780 (TT), and rs174583 (TT) had lower AA but higher LA in plasma phospholipids and erythrocyte EPG and decreased (n-6) and (n-3) fatty acid product/precursor ratios at 16 and 36 weeks of gestation.	Breast milk fatty acids were influenced by genotype, with significantly lower 14:0, AA, and EPA but higher 20:2(n-6) in the minor allele homozygotes of rs174553, rs99780, and rs174583 and lower AA, EPA, DPA, and DHA in the minor allele homozygotes of rs174575.
Rzehak P et al. Br J Nutr 2009. [40]	Bavarian Nutrition survey II, Germany, cross-sectional, (n = 163 and n = 535)	Phospholipid PUFA in plasma (n = 163), erythrocyte membranes (n = 535)	*FADS1* and *FADS2* haplotypes	Replication of *FADS1* and *FADS2* haplotypes associations in phospholipids (Schaeffer et al. 2006) and associations with PUFA in membranes.	Association with cell membranes was a novel finding. No associations with omega-3 PUFA.
Molto-Puigmarti C et al. Am J Clin Nutr 2010. [45]	KOALA Birth Cohort Study in the Netherlands. Plasma samples were collected at 36th gestational week in pregnant women (N = 309) and milk samples at 1 month postpartum.	Plasma phospholipids and milk DHA proportion	*FADS1* rs174561, *FADS2* rs174575, and intergenic rs3834458	A higher fish (or fish oil) intake compensated for the lower DHA proportions in plasma phospholipids irrespective of genotype but not in the milk from women with minor allele carriers of selected gene variants.	The study confirms earlier studies with regard to PUFA associations with minor allele carriers. Novelty of this study was gene–diet interaction regarding milk fat; DHA content remained unchanged with increasing fish/fish oil intake in women homozygous for minor allele.
Zietemann V et al. Br J Nutr 2010. [44]	A random sample of 2066 participants from the European Prospective Investigation into Cancer and Nutrition-Potsdam study, cross-sectional	Erythrocyte membrane fatty acids and estimated desaturase activity	rs174546 genetic variation (reflecting genetic variation in the *FADS1/FADS2* gene cluster)	Higher proportions of LA, EDA, and DGLA and lower proportions of GLA, AA, and DTA for the minor allele carriers. The estimated activities of *FADS1* and *FADS2* strongly decreased with minor T-allele.	Interaction with diet; dietary n-6/n-3 ratio was suggested to modify the association between the *FADS1*/ *FADS2* genotype and the estimated D5D activity.
Dumont J et al. J Nutr 2011. [58]	European adolescents, HELENA study (n = 573), cross-sectional	Dietary intake of LA and ALA ALA, PUFA levels in serum PL Serum concentrations of TG, cholesterol, and lipoproteins	FADS1 rs174546	The associations between *FADS1* rs174546 and concentrations of PUFA, TG, cholesterol, and lipoproteins were not affected by dietary LA intake. Similarly, the association between the *FADS1* rs174546 polymorphism and serum phospholipid concentrations of ALA or EPA was not modified by dietary ALA intake. In contrast, the rs174546 minor allele was associated with lower total cholesterol concentrations and non-HDL cholesterol concentrations in the high-ALA-intake group but not in the low-ALA-intake group.	These results suggest that dietary ALA intake modulates the association between *FADS1* rs174546 and serum total and non-HDL cholesterol concentrations at a young age.

Table 2. *Cont.*

Merino et al. Mol Genet Metab. 2011. [59]	Toronto Nutrigenomics and Health study, (Caucasians $n = 78$, Asian, $n = 69$), cross-sectional	Plasma fatty acids	*FADS1* and *FADS2* genotypes (19 SNPs)	The most significant association was between the *FADS1* rs174547 and AA/LA in both Caucasians and Asians. Although the minor allele for this SNP differed between Caucasians (T) and Asians (C), carriers of the C allele had a lower desaturase activity than carriers of the T allele in both groups.	
Hong et al. Clin Interv Aging 2013. [60]	3 years follow-up study, nonobese men in South Korea ($n = 122$)	Serum PL PUFAs	near *FADS1* rs174537; *FEN1* rs174537G; *FADS2* rs174575 and rs2727270; *FADS3* rs1000778	The minor variants of rs174537 and rs2727270 were significantly associated with lower concentrations of long-chain PUFAs.	*FADS* polymorphisms can affect age-associated changes in serum phospholipid long-chain PUFAs, Δ5-desaturase activity, and oxidative stress.
Roke K et al. Prostaglandins Leukot Essent Fatty Acids 2013. [61]	Cross-sectional study, healthy young adults in Canada ($n = 878$)	Plasma levels of LA, GLA, DGLA, and AA	*FADS1/2* rs174579, rs174593, rs174626, rs526126, rs968567 and rs17831757	Several SNPs were associated with circulating levels of individual FAs and desaturase indices, with minor allele carriers having lower AA levels and reduced desaturase indices.	A single SNP in *FADS2* (rs526126) was weakly associated with hsCRP.
Huang et al. Nutrition 2014. [62]	T2DM patients ($n = 758$) and healthy individuals ($n = 400$) in Han Chinese, cross-sectional	Erythrocyte PL Fatty acids	Genetic variants in the *FADS* gene cluster	Minor allele homozygotes and heterozygotes of rs174575 and rs174537 had lower AA levels in healthy individuals. Minor allele homozygotes and heterozygotes of rs174455 in *FADS3* gene had lower levels of DPA, AA, and Δ5desaturase activity in patients with T2DM.	
Smith CE et al. Mol Nutr Food Res 2015. [48]	Updated meta-analysis of CHARGE consortium ($n = 11{,}668$) evaluating interactions between dietary PUFAs and selected genetic variants of 5 genes	Total plasma, phospholipids or erythrocyte membranes ALA, EPA, DHA, and DPA Dietary PUFA	*FADS1* rs174538 and rs174548; *AGPAT3* rs7435; *PDXDC1* rs4985167; *GCKR* rs780094; *ELOVL2* rs3734398	Primary aim was to examine gene–diet interactions regarding PUFAs. No significant interactions were found after corrections.	Fatty acid compartments affected the results, and, e.g., *FADS1* interaction terms for dietary ALA vs plasma phospholipids (negative) and erythrocytes (positive) were opposite.
Andersen et al. PLoS Genet 2016. [63]	Cross-sectional, Greenlanders ($n = 2626$)	22 FAs in the PL fraction in erythrocytemembranes	*ACSL6* rs76430747; *DTD1* rs6035106; *CPT1A* rs80356779; *FADS2* rs174570; *LPCAT3* rs2110073; *CERS4* rs11881630	Novel loci were identified on chromosomes 5 and 11, showing strongest association with oleic acid (*ACSL6*) and DHA (*DTD1*), respectively. For a missense variant (in *CPT1A*), a number of novel FA associations were identified; the strongest with 11-eicosenoic acid.	Novel loci associating with FAs in the PL fraction of erythrocytemembranes were identified in Greenlanders. For variants in *FADS2*, *LPCAT3*, and *CERS4*, known FA associations were replicated.

Table 2. *Cont.*

Takkunen M et al. Mol Nutr Food Res 2016. [64]	962 men from the METSIM study and Kuopio Obesity Surgery Study participants (n = 240) in Finland, cross-sectional	Fatty acid composition in erythrocyte and plasma PL, CE, and TG	Hepatic expression of *FADS1* (rs174547/rs174550)	A common *FADS1* variant (rs 174550) showed nominally significant gene–diet interactions between EPA in erythrocytes, and plasma CE and TG and dietary intakes.	Minor allele (C) of *FADS1* (rs174547) was strongly associated with reduced hepatic mRNA expression. High intake of EPA and DHA may reduce D5D activity in the liver.
de la Garza Puentes A et al. PLoS ONE 2017. [65]	PREOBE cohort in Spain (n = 180), 24 weeks of gestation, cross-sectional	Plasma PL FAs	7 SNPs in *FADS1*, 5 in *FADS2*, 3 in *ELOVL2* and 2 in *ELOVL5*	Normal-weight women who were minor allele carriers of *FADS* SNPs had lower levels of AA, lower AA/DGLA and AA/LA indices, and higher levels of DGLA compared to major homozygotes. Among minor allele carriers of *FADS2* and *ELOVL2* SNPs, overweight/obese women showed a higher DHA/EPA index than the normal-weight group.	Maternal weight modifies the effect of genotype on FA levels.
Guo H et al. Lipids Health Dis 2017. [66]	951 Chinese adults, cross-sectional	Plasma PL FAs *FADS1* rs174547	*FADS1* rs174547	The rs174547 C minor allele was associated with a higher proportion of LA, lower AA and DHA, as well as lower delta-6-desaturase and delta-5-desaturase activities.	Confirms earlier finding in Chinese population.
Kim et al. Prostaglandins Leukot Essent Fatty Acids 2018. [67]	Three-year prospective cohort study in Korea, 287 healthy subjects	Plasma PUFA levels	*FADS1* rs174547	The minor allele of the *FADS1* rs174547 associated with age-related decrease in the EPA/AA ratio among overweight subjects.	The minor allele of the *FADS* 1 rs174547 associated with increase in arterial stiffness among overweight subjects.
Li et al. Am J Clin Nutr 2018. [68]	1504 healthy Chinese adults, cross-sectional	Plasma PUFA concentration	FADS2 rs66698963	The rs66698963 genotype is associated with AA concentration and AA to EPA+DHA ratio.	Genotype also affected triglyceride and HDL cholesterol concentrations.
C) Intervention Studies					
Study	**Study Population and Design**	**Fatty Acid Biomarkers Examined**	**Genes Examined**	**Main Findings**	**COMMENT**
Al-Hilal M et al. J Lipid Res 2013. [69]	RCT in United Kingdom (n = 310) Supplementation of EPA + DHA 1) 0.45 g/day 2) 0.9 g/day 3) 1.8 g/day 4) placebo for 6 months	Plasma and erythrocyte PUFAs	*FADS1/FADS2* rs174537, rs174561, and rs3834458	s174537, rs174561, and rs3834458 in the *FADS1–FADS2* gene cluster were strongly associated with proportions of LC-PUFAs and desaturase activities estimated in plasma and Ery. In a randomized controlled dietary intervention, increasing EPA and docosahexaenoic acid DHA intake significantly increased D5D and decreased D6D activity after doses of 0.45, 0.9, and 1.8 g/day for six months. Interaction of rs174537 genotype with treatment was a determinant of D5D activity estimated in plasma.	Different sites at the *FADS1–FADS2* locus appear to influence D5D and D6D activity, and rs174537 genotype interacts with dietary EPA+DHA to modulate D5D.

Table 2. *Cont.*

Gillingham LG et al. Am J Clin Nutr 2013. [49]	36 hyperlipidemic individuals in Canada, randomized cross-over design with 3 experimental diets for 4 weeks 1) Flax seed oil 2) High canola oil 3) Western diet Only a few persons with minor allele of a given gene	Plasma FAs and (U-^{13}C) ALA metabolism	SNPs for *FADS1*, *FADS2* and *ELOVL2*	Subjects homozygous for the minor allele of *FADS1*/*FADS2* had lower plasma composition of AA and AA/LA ratio in comparison with the major allele carriers after consumption of each experimental diet. *ELOVL2* had no effect on PUFAs.	Increasing ALA intake with a diet enriched in flaxseed oil in minor allele homozygotes resulted in an increased plasma composition of EPA beyond that of major allele homozygotes consuming a typical western diet.
Porenta SR et al. Cancer Prev Res (Phila) 2013. [46]	108 individuals with increased risk of colon cancer in USA, RCT for 6 months with two intervention diets: 1) Mediterranean type (MedD) 2) Heathy Eating Diet	Serum and colonic mucosa fatty acids	*FADS1*/ *FADS2* minor allele SNPs (rs174556, rs174561, rs174537, rs3834458)	At 6 months, an increase in colonic AA in the Healthy Eating diet arm was found, while colon AA concentrations remained fairly constant in the MedD group in persons with major alleles in the *FADS1*/*2* gene cluster.	These results suggest gene–diet interaction in fatty acid metabolism related to different response to diets, but in individuals with major alleles of the *FADS* cluster.
Roke K and Mutch DM. Nutrients 2014. [47]	12 young men in Canada, 12 week intervention with fish oil capsules with 8 week wash-out; no control group	Fatty acid analysis from serum and erythrocytes	*FADS1*/*FADS2* (rs174537, rs174576)	Marked increase in serum and erythrocyte EPA and DHA. Elevation in RBC was sustained for 8 weeks during wash-out.	No significant gene × fish oil interaction, but % change in minor allele carriers of *FADS1*/*FADS2* had a greater increase in RBC EPA levels.
Scholtz SA et al. Prostaglandins Leukot Essent Fatty Acids 2015. [70]	Intervention, pregnant women (n = 205) in USA 1) Supplementation with 600 mg per day of DHA 2) Placebo for the last two trimesters of pregnancy	Plasma and RBC PL AA and DHA	*FADS1* rs174533 and *FADS2* rs174575	DHA but not the placebo decreased the AA status of minor allele homozygotes of both *FADS* SNPs but not major allele homozygotes at delivery.	
Lankinen et al. Am J Clin Nutr 2018. (in press)	Intervention, men with *FADS1* rs174550 TT or CC genotype (n = 59) in Finland High-LA diet for 4 weeks	Plasma PL and CE fatty acids	*FADS1* rs174550	There was a significant increase in the LA proportion in PL and CE in both genotype groups. A significant interaction between intervention and genotype was observed in AA, (decreased in CC genotype, but remained unchanged (in PL) or decreased only slightly (in CE) in TT genotype).	The response to higher LA intake in hsCRP was different between the genotypes. Individuals with the rs174550-TT genotype had a trend towards decreased hsCRP, while individuals with the rs174550-CC genotype had a trend towards increased hsCRP (significant diet × genotype interaction).

Abbreviations: AA, arachidonic acid (20:4*n*-6); ALA, alpha-linolenic acid (18:3*n*-3); DGLA; Di-homo-gamma linolenic acid (20:3*n*-6); DPA, docosapentaenoic acid (22:5*n*-3); EDA, eicosadienoic acid (20:2*n*-6); EPA, eicosapentaenoic acid (20:5*n*-3); Ery, erythrocyte membranes; ETA, eicosatetraenoic acid (20:4*n*-3); hsCRP; high-sensitivity C-reactive protein; GLA, gamma-linolenic acid (18:3*n*-6); LA, linoleic acid (18:2*n*-6), OCSFA; odd-chain saturated fatty acids; PL, phospholipid; PUFA, polyunsaturated fatty acid; RBC, red blood cell; RCT, randomized controlled trial; SNP, single-nucleotide polymorphism; T2D, type 2 diabetes; VLSFA, very-long-chain saturated fatty acids.

In one of our own cross-sectional studies [64], we reported a nominally significant gene–diet interaction between EPA in erythrocytes, CE and TG, and dietary intake of EPA in 962 men who were participating in the METSIM study (Table 2B). Interestingly, exclusion of fish oil supplement users strengthened the observed interaction with diet. We also confirmed that the minor allele of rs174550 of *FADS1* (C allele) was strongly associated with a lower hepatic mRNA expression, as observed recently by Wang et al. in their cross-sectional study [71]. Thus, we concluded that the observed interaction could be explained by divergent activity of the liver D5D enzyme in the genetic variants of *FADS* examined in our study.

Ideally, gene–diet interaction would be studied using an intervention design with participants with pre-selected genotypes. In our recent trial (Lankinen et al., Am J Clin Nutr 2018, in press), our aim was to test the hypothesis that the *FADS1* rs174550 genotype modifies the effect of dietary LA intake on the fatty acid composition of plasma lipids. Altogether, 59 men who were homozygotes for *FADS1* rs174550 SNP (TT or CC) completed the 4-week dietary intervention with a diet enriched in LA. During the 4-week intervention period, participants consumed their habitual diet with a supplement of 30 mL, 40 mL, or 50 mL (27–45 g) sunflower oil daily depending on their BMI. The doses of sunflower oil provided 17–28 g (6 E%) LA daily on top of the average intake of approximately 10–12 g (4.5 E%). The response in the proportion of AA in plasma phospholipids and cholesteryl esters differed between the genotype groups (Table 2C). The proportion of AA decreased in participants with the CC genotype, but remained unchanged (in PL) or decreased only slightly (in CE) in participants with the TT genotype. We also found that the *FADS1* genotype modified the lipid mediator profile (including eicosanoids and oxylipins) and inflammatory response, measured as serum high-sensitivity C-reactive protein, to an LA-rich diet.

6. Concluding Remarks

In this review, we aimed to summarize the current evidence regarding genes and dietary fatty acids in the regulation of the fatty acid composition of plasma lipids and erythrocyte membranes. The knowledge related to this topic has increased markedly during recent years, but there is no earlier review article compiling it together. The fatty acid composition of blood lipids and tissues is modified by dietary intake, but endogenous metabolism of fatty acids, which is strongly genetically regulated, also has an important role. In particular, genetic variants of the *FADS* gene cluster in chromosome 11 and elongases (*ELOVLs*) are involved in the regulation of fatty acid metabolism. In recent years, some new genetic variants have been shown to be associated with the fatty acid composition of plasma lipids or erythrocytes, and we expect that new variants will be identified in the near future. Many of the known genetic variants are quite common. Therefore, it is important to understand better how the enzymes regulating fatty acid metabolism, and the genes coding them, modify the effect of dietary intake of fatty acids on metabolism, low-grade inflammation, and metabolic diseases such as T2D. This understanding may help us to move towards personalized nutrition. It is also noteworthy that ethnicity may have an impact on gene–diet interactions. Most of the studies on interactions between genes and dietary fat in the regulation of fatty acid composition of plasma lipids are observational. Study designs and data collection should be carefully considered in the interpretation of the results. There are only a few intervention trials regarding this topic, and most of them were performed without pre-selected genotypes. Definite answers regarding true gene × diet interactions may need well-planned intervention studies with specific hypotheses and pre-selected genotypes.

Author Contributions: All authors were involved in the literature research, writing, reviewing, and editing of the manuscript.

References

1. Farquhar, J.W.; Ahrens, E.H., Jr. Effects of dietary fats on human erythrocyte fatty acid patterns. *J. Clin. Investig.* **1963**, *42*, 675–685. [CrossRef] [PubMed]
2. Hunter, D. Biochemical indicators of dietary fat. In *Nutritional Epidemiology*; Willett, W., Ed.; Oxford University Press: Oxford, UK, 1990.
3. Vessby, B.; Lithell, H.; Gustafsson, I.B.; Boberg, J. Changes in the fatty acid composition of the plasma lipid esters during lipid-lowering treatment with diet, clofibrate and niceritrol. reduction of the proportion of linoleate by clofibrate but not by niceritrol. *Atherosclerosis* **1980**, *35*, 51–65. [CrossRef]
4. Sarkkinen, E.S.; Agren, J.J.; Ahola, I.; Ovaskainen, M.L.; Uusitupa, M.I. Fatty acid composition of serum cholesterol esters, and erythrocyte and platelet membranes as indicators of long-term adherence to fat-modified diets. *Am. J. Clin. Nutr.* **1994**, *59*, 364–370. [CrossRef] [PubMed]
5. Carta, G.; Murru, E.; Banni, S.; Manca, C. Palmitic acid: Physiological role, metabolism and nutritional implications. *Front. Physiol.* **2017**, *8*, 902. [CrossRef] [PubMed]
6. Weitkunat, K.; Schumann, S.; Nickel, D.; Hornemann, S.; Petzke, K.J.; Schulze, M.B.; Pfeiffer, A.F.; Klaus, S. Odd-Chain Fatty acids as a biomarker for dietary fiber intake: A novel pathway for endogenous production from propionate. *Am. J. Clin. Nutr.* **2017**, *105*, 1544–1551. [CrossRef] [PubMed]
7. Saadatian-Elahi, M.; Slimani, N.; Chajes, V.; Jenab, M.; Goudable, J.; Biessy, C.; Ferrari, P.; Byrnes, G.; Autier, P.; Peeters, P.H.; et al. Plasma phospholipid fatty acid profiles and their association with food intakes: Results from a cross-sectional study within the european prospective investigation into cancer and nutrition. *Am. J. Clin. Nutr.* **2009**, *89*, 331–346. [CrossRef] [PubMed]
8. Ozogul, Y.; Ozogul, F.; Cicek, E.; Polat, A.; Kuley, E. Fat content and fatty acid compositions of 34 marine water fish species from the mediterranean sea. *Int. J. Food Sci. Nutr.* **2008**, *60*, 464–475. [CrossRef] [PubMed]
9. Aggelousis, G.; Lazos, E.S. Fatty acid composition of the lipids from eight freshwater fish species from greece. *J. Food Compos. Anal.* **1991**, *4*, 68–76. [CrossRef]
10. Vidgren, H.M.; Agren, J.J.; Schwab, U.; Rissanen, T.; Hanninen, O.; Uusitupa, M.I. Incorporation of n-3 fatty acids into plasma lipid fractions, and erythrocyte membranes and platelets during dietary supplementation with fish, fish oil, and docosahexaenoic acid-rich oil among healthy young men. *Lipids* **1997**, *32*, 697–705. [CrossRef] [PubMed]
11. Katan, M.B.; Deslypere, J.P.; van Birgelen, A.P.; Penders, M.; Zegwaard, M. Kinetics of the incorporation of dietary fatty acids into serum cholesteryl esters, erythrocyte membranes, and adipose tissue: An 18-month controlled study. *J. Lipid Res.* **1997**, *38*, 2012–2022. [PubMed]
12. Rodriguez, A.; Sarda, P.; Nessmann, C.; Boulot, P.; Leger, C.L.; Descomps, B. Delta6- and delta5-desaturase activities in the human fetal liver: Kinetic aspects. *J. Lipid Res.* **1998**, *39*, 1825–1832. [PubMed]
13. Takkunen, M.; Agren, J.; Kuusisto, J.; Laakso, M.; Uusitupa, M.; Schwab, U. Dietary fat in relation to erythrocyte fatty acid composition in men. *Lipids* **2013**, *48*, 1093–1102. [CrossRef] [PubMed]
14. Vidgren, H.M.; Louheranta, A.M.; Agren, J.J.; Schwab, U.S.; Uusitupa, M.I. Divergent incorporation of dietary trans fatty acids in different serum lipid fractions. *Lipids* **1998**, *33*, 955–962. [CrossRef] [PubMed]
15. Lankinen, M.A.; Stancakova, A.; Uusitupa, M.; Agren, J.; Pihlajamaki, J.; Kuusisto, J.; Schwab, U.; Laakso, M. Plasma fatty acids as predictors of glycaemia and type 2 diabetes. *Diabetologia* **2015**, *58*, 2533–2544. [CrossRef] [PubMed]
16. Lopez-Miranda, J.; Williams, C.; Lairon, D. Dietary, physiological, genetic and pathological influences on postprandial lipid metabolism. *Br. J. Nutr.* **2007**, *98*, 458–473. [CrossRef] [PubMed]
17. Smith, C.E.; Ordovas, J.M. Fatty acid interactions with genetic polymorphisms for cardiovascular disease. *Curr. Opin. Clin. Nutr. Metab. Care* **2010**, *13*, 139–144. [CrossRef] [PubMed]
18. Tanaka, T.; Shen, J.; Abecasis, G.R.; Kisialiou, A.; Ordovas, J.M.; Guralnik, J.M.; Singleton, A.; Bandinelli, S.; Cherubini, A.; Arnett, D.; et al. Genome-wide association study of plasma polyunsaturated fatty acids in the inchianti study. *PLoS Genet.* **2009**, *5*, e1000338. [CrossRef] [PubMed]
19. Zhang, J.Y.; Kothapalli, K.S.; Brenna, J.T. Desaturase and elongase-limiting endogenous long-chain polyunsaturated fatty acid biosynthesis. *Curr. Opin. Clin. Nutr. Metab. Care* **2016**, *19*, 103–110. [CrossRef] [PubMed]

20. Agren, J.J.; Valve, R.; Vidgren, H.; Laakso, M.; Uusitupa, M. Postprandial lipemic response is modified by the polymorphism at codon 54 of the fatty acid-binding protein 2 gene. *Arterioscler. Thromb. Vasc. Biol.* **1998**, *18*, 1606–1610. [CrossRef] [PubMed]
21. Baier, L.J.; Sacchettini, J.C.; Knowler, W.C.; Eads, J.; Paolisso, G.; Tataranni, P.A.; Mochizuki, H.; Bennett, P.H.; Bogardus, C.; Prochazka, M. An amino acid substitution in the human intestinal fatty acid binding protein is associated with increased fatty acid binding, increased fat oxidation, and insulin resistance. *J. Clin. Investig.* **1995**, *95*, 1281–1287. [CrossRef] [PubMed]
22. Yamada, K.; Yuan, X.; Ishiyama, S.; Koyama, K.; Ichikawa, F.; Koyanagi, A.; Koyama, W.; Nonaka, K. Association between Ala54Thr substitution of the fatty acid-binding protein 2 gene with insulin resistance and intra-abdominal fat thickness in japanese men. *Diabetologia* **1997**, *40*, 706–710. [CrossRef] [PubMed]
23. Agren, J.J.; Vidgren, H.M.; Valve, R.S.; Laakso, M.; Uusitupa, M.I. Postprandial responses of individual fatty acids in subjects homozygous for the threonine- or alanine-encoding allele in codon 54 of the intestinal fatty acid binding protein 2 gene. *Am. J. Clin. Nutr.* **2001**, *73*, 31–35. [CrossRef] [PubMed]
24. Berthier, M.T.; Couillard, C.; Prud'homme, D.; Nadeau, A.; Bergeron, J.; Tremblay, A.; Despres, J.P.; Vohl, M.C. Effects of the FABP2 A54T mutation on triglyceride metabolism of viscerally obese men. *Obes. Res.* **2001**, *9*, 668–675. [CrossRef] [PubMed]
25. Okada, T.; Sato, N.F.; Kuromori, Y.; Miyashita, M.; Iwata, F.; Hara, M.; Harada, K.; Hattori, H. Thr-Encoding allele homozygosity at codon 54 of fabp 2 gene may be associated with impaired delta 6 desatruase activity and reduced plasma arachidonic acid in obese children. *J. Atheroscler. Thromb.* **2006**, *13*, 192–196. [CrossRef] [PubMed]
26. Almeida, J.C.; Gross, J.L.; Canani, L.H.; Zelmanovitz, T.; Perassolo, M.S.; Azevedo, M.J. The Ala54Thr polymorphism of the fabp2 gene influences the postprandial fatty acids in patients with type 2 diabetes. *J. Clin. Endocrinol. Metab.* **2010**, *95*, 3909–3917. [CrossRef] [PubMed]
27. Sjogren, P.; Sierra-Johnson, J.; Gertow, K.; Rosell, M.; Vessby, B.; de Faire, U.; Hamsten, A.; Hellenius, M.L.; Fisher, R.M. Fatty acid desaturases in human adipose tissue: Relationships between gene expression, desaturation indexes and insulin resistance. *Diabetologia* **2008**, *51*, 328–335. [CrossRef] [PubMed]
28. Warensjo, E.; Rosell, M.; Hellenius, M.L.; Vessby, B.; De Faire, U.; Riserus, U. Associations between estimated fatty acid desaturase activities in serum lipids and adipose tissue in humans: Links to obesity and insulin resistance. *Lipids Health. Dis.* **2009**, *8*, 37. [CrossRef] [PubMed]
29. Kroger, J.; Schulze, M.B. Recent insights into the relation of delta5 desaturase and delta6 desaturase activity to the development of type 2 diabetes. *Curr. Opin. Lipidol.* **2012**, *23*, 4–10. [CrossRef] [PubMed]
30. Mahendran, Y.; Agren, J.; Uusitupa, M.; Cederberg, H.; Vangipurapu, J.; Stancakova, A.; Schwab, U.; Kuusisto, J.; Laakso, M. Association of erythrocyte membrane fatty acids with changes in glycemia and risk of type 2 diabetes. *Am. J. Clin. Nutr.* **2014**, *99*, 79–85. [CrossRef] [PubMed]
31. Jacobs, S.; Schiller, K.; Jansen, E.H.; Boeing, H.; Schulze, M.B.; Kroger, J. Evaluation of various biomarkers as potential mediators of the association between delta5 desaturase, delta6 desaturase, and stearoyl-coa desaturase activity and incident type 2 diabetes in the european prospective investigation into cancer and nutrition-potsdam study. *Am. J. Clin. Nutr.* **2015**, *102*, 155–164. [PubMed]
32. Yary, T.; Voutilainen, S.; Tuomainen, T.P.; Ruusunen, A.; Nurmi, T.; Virtanen, J.K. Serum N-6 polyunsaturated fatty acids, delta5- and delta6-desaturase activities, and risk of incident type 2 diabetes in men: The kuopio ischaemic heart disease risk factor study. *Am. J. Clin. Nutr.* **2016**, *103*, 1337–1343. [CrossRef] [PubMed]
33. Takkunen, M.J.; Schwab, U.S.; de Mello, V.D.; Eriksson, J.G.; Lindstrom, J.; Tuomilehto, J.; Uusitupa, M.I.; DPS Study Group. Longitudinal associations of serum fatty acid composition with type 2 diabetes risk and markers of insulin secretion and sensitivity in the finnish diabetes prevention study. *Eur. J. Nutr.* **2016**, *55*, 967–979. [CrossRef] [PubMed]
34. Willer, C.J.; Schmidt, E.M.; Sengupta, S.; Peloso, G.M.; Gustafsson, S.; Kanoni, S.; Ganna, A.; Chen, J.; Buchkovich, M.L.; Mora, S.; et al. Discovery and refinement of loci associated with lipid levels. *Nat. Genet.* **2013**, *45*, 1274–1283. [CrossRef] [PubMed]
35. Del Gobbo, L.C.; Imamura, F.; Aslibekyan, S.; Marklund, M.; Virtanen, J.K.; Wennberg, M.; Yakoob, M.Y.; Chiuve, S.E.; Dela Cruz, L.; Frazier-Wood, A.C.; et al. Omega-3 polyunsaturated fatty acid biomarkers and coronary heart disease: Pooling project of 19 cohort studies. *JAMA Intern. Med.* **2016**, *176*, 1155–1166. [CrossRef] [PubMed]

36. Vaittinen, M.; Mannisto, V.; Kakela, P.; Agren, J.; Tiainen, M.; Schwab, U.; Pihlajamaki, J. Interorgan cross talk between fatty acid metabolism, tissue inflammation, and fads2 genotype in humans with obesity. *Obesity (Silver Spring)* **2017**, *25*, 545–552. [CrossRef] [PubMed]
37. Howard, T.D.; Mathias, R.A.; Seeds, M.C.; Herrington, D.M.; Hixson, J.E.; Shimmin, L.C.; Hawkins, G.A.; Sellers, M.; Ainsworth, H.C.; Sergeant, S.; et al. DNA methylation in an enhancer region of the fads cluster is associated with fads activity in human liver. *PLoS ONE* **2014**, *9*, e97510. [CrossRef] [PubMed]
38. Reynolds, L.M.; Howard, T.D.; Ruczinski, I.; Kanchan, K.; Seeds, M.C.; Mathias, R.A.; Chilton, F.H. Tissue-specific impact of fads cluster variants on fads1 and fads2 gene expression. *PLoS ONE* **2018**, *13*, e0194610. [CrossRef] [PubMed]
39. Schaeffer, L.; Gohlke, H.; Muller, M.; Heid, I.M.; Palmer, L.J.; Kompauer, I.; Demmelmair, H.; Illig, T.; Koletzko, B.; Heinrich, J. Common genetic variants of the fads1 fads2 gene cluster and their reconstructed haplotypes are associated with the fatty acid composition in phospholipids. *Hum. Mol. Genet.* **2006**, *15*, 1745–1756. [CrossRef] [PubMed]
40. Rzehak, P.; Heinrich, J.; Klopp, N.; Schaeffer, L.; Hoff, S.; Wolfram, G.; Illig, T.; Linseisen, J. Evidence for an association between genetic variants of the fatty acid desaturase 1 fatty acid desaturase 2 (FADS1 FADS2) gene cluster and the fatty acid composition of erythrocyte membranes. *Br. J. Nutr.* **2009**, *101*, 20–26. [CrossRef] [PubMed]
41. Lemaitre, R.N.; Tanaka, T.; Tang, W.; Manichaikul, A.; Foy, M.; Kabagambe, E.K.; Nettleton, J.A.; King, I.B.; Weng, L.C.; Bhattacharya, S.; et al. Genetic loci associated with plasma phospholipid n-3 fatty acids: A meta-analysis of genome-wide association studies from the CHARGE consortium. *PLoS Genet.* **2011**, *7*, e1002193. [CrossRef] [PubMed]
42. Fumagalli, M.; Moltke, I.; Grarup, N.; Racimo, F.; Bjerregaard, P.; Jorgensen, M.E.; Korneliussen, T.S.; Gerbault, P.; Skotte, L.; Linneberg, A.; et al. Greenlandic inuit show genetic signatures of diet and climate adaptation. *Science* **2015**, *349*, 1343–1347. [CrossRef] [PubMed]
43. Pihlajamaki, J.; Schwab, U.; Kaminska, D.; Agren, J.; Kuusisto, J.; Kolehmainen, M.; Paananen, J.; Laakso, M.; Uusitupa, M. Dietary polyunsaturated fatty acids and the pro12ala polymorphisms of pparg regulate serum lipids through divergent pathways: A randomized crossover clinical trial. *Genes Nutr.* **2015**, *10*. [CrossRef] [PubMed]
44. Zietemann, V.; Kroger, J.; Enzenbach, C.; Jansen, E.; Fritsche, A.; Weikert, C.; Boeing, H.; Schulze, M.B. Genetic variation of the FADS1 FADS2 gene cluster and N-6 PUFA composition in erythrocyte membranes in the european prospective investigation into cancer and nutrition-potsdam study. *Br. J. Nutr.* **2010**, *104*, 1748–1759. [CrossRef] [PubMed]
45. Molto-Puigmarti, C.; Plat, J.; Mensink, R.P.; Muller, A.; Jansen, E.; Zeegers, M.P.; Thijs, C. FADS1 FADS2 gene variants modify the association between fish intake and the docosahexaenoic acid proportions in human milk. *Am. J. Clin. Nutr.* **2010**, *91*, 1368–1376. [CrossRef] [PubMed]
46. Porenta, S.R.; Ko, Y.A.; Gruber, S.B.; Mukherjee, B.; Baylin, A.; Ren, J.; Djuric, Z. Interaction of fatty acid genotype and diet on changes in colonic fatty acids in a mediterranean diet intervention study. *Cancer Prev. Res. (Phila)* **2013**, *6*, 1212–1221. [CrossRef] [PubMed]
47. Roke, K.; Mutch, D.M. The role of FADS1/2 polymorphisms on cardiometabolic markers and fatty acid profiles in young adults consuming fish oil supplements. *Nutrients* **2014**, *6*, 2290–2304. [CrossRef] [PubMed]
48. Smith, C.E.; Follis, J.L.; Nettleton, J.A.; Foy, M.; Wu, J.H.; Ma, Y.; Tanaka, T.; Manichakul, A.W.; Wu, H.; Chu, A.Y.; et al. Dietary fatty acids modulate associations between genetic variants and circulating fatty acids in plasma and erythrocyte membranes: Meta-analysis of nine studies in the charge consortium. *Mol. Nutr. Food Res.* **2015**, *59*, 1373–1383. [CrossRef] [PubMed]
49. Gillingham, L.G.; Harding, S.V.; Rideout, T.C.; Yurkova, N.; Cunnane, S.C.; Eck, P.K.; Jones, P.J. Dietary oils and FADS1-FADS2 genetic variants modulate [13C] alpha-linolenic acid metabolism and plasma fatty acid composition. *Am. J. Clin. Nutr.* **2013**, *97*, 195–207. [CrossRef] [PubMed]
50. Wu, J.H.; Lemaitre, R.N.; Manichaikul, A.; Guan, W.; Tanaka, T.; Foy, M.; Kabagambe, E.K.; Djousse, L.; Siscovick, D.; Fretts, A.M.; et al. Genome-wide association study identifies novel loci associated with concentrations of four plasma phospholipid fatty acids in the de novo lipogenesis pathway: Results from the cohorts for heart and aging research in genomic epidemiology (CHARGE) consortium. *Circ. Cardiovasc. Genet.* **2013**, *6*, 171–183. [CrossRef] [PubMed]

51. Guan, W.; Steffen, B.T.; Lemaitre, R.N.; Wu, J.H.; Tanaka, T.; Manichaikul, A.; Foy, M.; Rich, S.S.; Wang, L.; Nettleton, J.A.; et al. Genome-wide association study of plasma n6 polyunsaturated fatty acids within the cohorts for heart and aging research in genomic epidemiology consortium. *Circ. Cardiovasc. Genet.* **2014**, *7*, 321–331. [CrossRef] [PubMed]
52. Dorajoo, R.; Sun, Y.; Han, Y.; Ke, T.; Burger, A.; Chang, X.; Low, H.Q.; Guan, W.; Lemaitre, R.N.; Khor, C.C.; et al. A genome-wide association study of n-3 and n-6 plasma fatty acids in a singaporean chinese population. *Genes Nutr.* **2015**, *10*. [CrossRef] [PubMed]
53. Lemaitre, R.N.; King, I.B.; Kabagambe, E.K.; Wu, J.H.; McKnight, B.; Manichaikul, A.; Guan, W.; Sun, Q.; Chasman, D.I.; Foy, M.; et al. Genetic loci associated with circulating levels of very long-chain saturated fatty acids. *J. Lipid Res.* **2015**, *56*, 176–184. [CrossRef] [PubMed]
54. Mozaffarian, D.; Kabagambe, E.K.; Johnson, C.O.; Lemaitre, R.N.; Manichaikul, A.; Sun, Q.; Foy, M.; Wang, L.; Wiener, H.; Irvin, M.R.; et al. Genetic loci associated with circulating phospholipid trans fatty acids: A meta-analysis of genome-wide association studies from the CHARGE consortium. *Am. J. Clin. Nutr.* **2015**, *101*, 398–406. [CrossRef] [PubMed]
55. Tintle, N.L.; Pottala, J.V.; Lacey, S.; Ramachandran, V.; Westra, J.; Rogers, A.; Clark, J.; Olthoff, B.; Larson, M.; Harris, W.; et al. A genome-wide association study of saturated, mono- and polyunsaturated red blood cell fatty acids in the framingham heart offspring study. prostaglandins leukot. essent. *Fatty Acids* **2015**, *94*, 65–72. [CrossRef] [PubMed]
56. de Oliveira Otto, M.C.; Lemaitre, R.N.; Sun, Q.; King, I.B.; Wu, J.H.Y.; Manichaikul, A.; Rich, S.S.; Tsai, M.Y.; Chen, Y.D.; Fornage, M.; et al. Genome-wide association meta-analysis of circulating odd-numbered chain saturated fatty acids: Results from the CHARGE consortium. *PLoS ONE* **2018**, *13*, e0196951. [CrossRef] [PubMed]
57. Xie, L.; Innis, S.M. Genetic variants of the FADS1 FADS2 gene cluster are ASSOCIATED with altered (N-6) and (N-3) essential fatty acids in plasma and erythrocyte phospholipids in women during pregnancy and in breast milk during lactation. *J. Nutr.* **2008**, *138*, 2222–2228. [CrossRef] [PubMed]
58. Dumont, J.; Huybrechts, I.; Spinneker, A.; Gottrand, F.; Grammatikaki, E.; Bevilacqua, N.; Vyncke, K.; Widhalm, K.; Kafatos, A.; Molnar, D.; et al. FADS1 genetic variability interacts with dietary alpha-linolenic acid intake to affect serum Non-HDL-Cholesterol concentrations in european adolescents. *J. Nutr.* **2011**, *141*, 1247–1253. [CrossRef] [PubMed]
59. Merino, D.M.; Johnston, H.; Clarke, S.; Roke, K.; Nielsen, D.; Badawi, A.; El-Sohemy, A.; Ma, D.W.; Mutch, D.M. Polymorphisms in FADS1 and FADS2 alter desaturase activity in young caucasian and asian adults. *Mol. Genet. Metab.* **2011**, *103*, 171–178. [CrossRef] [PubMed]
60. Hong, S.H.; Kwak, J.H.; Paik, J.K.; Chae, J.S.; Lee, J.H. Association of polymorphisms in FADS gene with age-related changes in serum phospholipid polyunsaturated fatty acids and oxidative stress markers in middle-aged nonobese men. *Clin. Interv. Aging* **2013**, *8*, 585–596. [PubMed]
61. Roke, K.; Ralston, J.C.; Abdelmagid, S.; Nielsen, D.E.; Badawi, A.; El-Sohemy, A.; Ma, D.W.; Mutch, D.M. Variation in the FADS1/2 gene cluster alters plasma n-6 PUFA and is weakly associated with hsCRP levels in healthy young adults. *Prostaglandins Leukot. Essent. Fatty Acids* **2013**, *89*, 257–263. [CrossRef] [PubMed]
62. Huang, T.; Sun, J.; Chen, Y.; Xie, H.; Xu, D.; Huang, J.; Li, D. Genetic variants in desaturase gene, erythrocyte fatty acids, and risk for type 2 diabetes in chinese hans. *Nutrition* **2014**, *30*, 897–902. [CrossRef] [PubMed]
63. Andersen, M.K.; Jorsboe, E.; Sandholt, C.H.; Grarup, N.; Jorgensen, M.E.; Faergeman, N.J.; Bjerregaard, P.; Pedersen, O.; Moltke, I.; Hansen, T.; et al. Identification of novel genetic determinants of erythrocyte membrane fatty acid composition among greenlanders. *PLoS Genet.* **2016**, *12*, e1006119. [CrossRef] [PubMed]
64. Takkunen, M.J.; de Mello, V.D.; Schwab, U.S.; Kuusisto, J.; Vaittinen, M.; Agren, J.J.; Laakso, M.; Pihlajamaki, J.; Uusitupa, M.I. Gene-diet interaction of a common fads1 variant with marine polyunsaturated fatty acids for fatty acid composition in plasma and erythrocytes among men. *Mol. Nutr. Food Res.* **2016**, *60*, 381–389. [CrossRef] [PubMed]
65. de la Garza Puentes, A.; Montes Goyanes, R.; Chisaguano Tonato, A.M.; Torres-Espinola, F.J.; Arias Garcia, M.; de Almeida, L.; Bonilla Aguirre, M.; Guerendiain, M.; Castellote Bargallo, A.I.; Segura Moreno, M.; et al. Association of maternal weight with fads and elovl genetic variants and fatty acid levels- the PREOBE follow-up. *PLoS ONE* **2017**, *12*, e0179135. [CrossRef] [PubMed]

66. Guo, H.; Zhang, L.; Zhu, C.; Yang, F.; Wang, S.; Zhu, S.; Ma, X. A single nucleotide polymorphism in the FADS1 gene is associated with plasma fatty acid and lipid profiles and might explain gender difference in body fat distribution. *Lipids Health. Dis.* **2017**, *16*. [CrossRef]
67. Kim, M.; Kim, M.; Yoo, H.J.; Lee, A.; Jeong, S.; Lee, J.H. Associations among FADS1 rs174547, eicosapentaenoic acid/arachidonic acid ratio, and arterial stiffness in overweight subjects. *Prostaglandins Leukot. Essent. Fatty Acids* **2018**, *130*, 11–18. [CrossRef] [PubMed]
68. Li, P.; Zhao, J.; Kothapalli, K.S.D.; Li, X.; Li, H.; Han, Y.; Mi, S.; Zhao, W.; Li, Q.; Zhang, H.; et al. A regulatory insertion-deletion polymorphism in the fads gene cluster influences PUFA and lipid profiles among chinese adults: A population-based study. *Am. J. Clin. Nutr.* **2018**, *107*, 867–875. [CrossRef] [PubMed]
69. Al-Hilal, M.; Alsaleh, A.; Maniou, Z.; Lewis, F.J.; Hall, W.L.; Sanders, T.A.; O'Dell, S.D.; MARINA study team. Genetic variation at the FADS1-FADS2 gene locus influences delta-5 desaturase activity and LC-PUFA proportions after fish oil supplement. *J. Lipid Res.* **2013**, *54*, 542–551. [CrossRef] [PubMed]
70. Scholtz, S.A.; Kerling, E.H.; Shaddy, D.J.; Li, S.; Thodosoff, J.M.; Colombo, J.; Carlson, S.E. Docosahexaenoic acid (DHA) supplementation in pregnancy differentially modulates arachidonic acid and DHA status across FADS genotypes in pregnancy. *Prostaglandins Leukot. Essent. Fatty Acids* **2015**, *94*, 29–33. [CrossRef] [PubMed]
71. Wang, L.; Athinarayanan, S.; Jiang, G.; Chalasani, N.; Zhang, M.; Liu, W. Fatty acid desaturase 1 gene polymorphisms control human hepatic lipid composition. *Hepatology* **2015**, *61*, 119–128. [CrossRef] [PubMed]

7

Fish Oil Supplementation Reduces Inflammation but does not Restore Renal Function and Klotho Expression in an Adenine-Induced CKD Model

Juan S. Henao Agudelo [1], Leandro C. Baia [1,2], Milene S. Ormanji [1], Amandda R. P. Santos [1], Juliana R. Machado [3], Niels O. Saraiva Câmara [1,4], Gerjan J. Navis [2], Martin H. de Borst [2] and Ita P. Heilberg [1,*]

1 Division of Nephrology, Federal University of São Paulo (UNIFESP), Rua Botucatu 740, 04023-900 São Paulo, Brazil; juanelmono17@hotmail.com (J.S.H.A.); leandronut@yahoo.com.br (L.C.B.); milene.ormanji@gmail.com (M.S.O.); amandda.rpds@gmail.com (A.R.P.S.); niels@icb.usp.br (N.O.S.C.)
2 Division of Nephrology, University of Groningen, University Medical Centre Groningen (UMCG), P.O. Box 30.001, 9700 RB Groningen, The Netherlands; g.j.navis@umcg.nl (G.J.N.); m.h.de.borst@umcg.nl (M.H.d.B.)
3 Tropical Medicine & Public Health, Federal University of Goiás (UFG), Rua 235 s/n-University Sector, 74605-050 Goiânia, Brazil; juliana.patologiageral@gmail.com
4 Department of Immunology, Institute of Biomedical Sciences, University of São Paulo (USP), Av. Prof. Lineu Prestes 1730, ICB IV, Sala 238, 05508-000 São Paulo, Brazil
* Correspondence: ita.heilberg@gmail.com

Abstract: Background: Chronic kidney disease and inflammation promote loss of Klotho expression. Given the well-established anti-inflammatory effects of omega-3 fatty acids, we aimed to investigate the effect of fish oil supplementation in a model of CKD. Methods: Male C57BL/6 mice received supplementation with an adenine-enriched diet (AD, $n = 5$) or standard diet (CTL, $n = 5$) for 10 days. Two other experimental groups were kept under the adenine diet for 10 days. Following adenine withdrawal on the 11th day, the animals returned to a standard diet supplemented with fish oil (Post AD-Fish oil, $n = 9$) or not (Post AD-CTL, $n = 9$) for an additional period of 7 days. Results: Adenine mice exhibited significantly higher mean serum urea, creatinine, and renal expression of the pro-inflammatory markers Interleukin-6 (IL-6), C-X-C motif chemokine 10 (CXCL10), and Interleukin-1β (IL-1β), in addition to prominent renal fibrosis and reduced renal Klotho gene expression compared to the control. Post AD-Fish oil animals demonstrated a significant reduction of IL-6, C-X-C motif chemokine 9 (CXCL9), and IL-1β compared to Post AD-CTL animals. However, serum creatinine, renal fibrosis, and Klotho were not significantly different in the fish oil-treated group. Furthermore, renal histomorphological changes such as tubular dilatation and interstitial infiltration persisted despite treatment. Conclusions: Fish oil supplementation reduced renal pro-inflammatory markers but was not able to restore renal function nor Klotho expression in an adenine-induced CKD model.

Keywords: klotho; CKD; fish oil; fibrosis; inflammation

---

1. Introduction

Inflammation plays a central role in the pathogenesis and progression of chronic kidney disease (CKD). The activation of innate and adaptive arms of immune response leads to cell infiltration (mainly macrophages) and the production of proinflammatory molecules that ultimately lead to collagen deposition and loss of renal function [1].

The α-Klotho protein was originally identified as an anti-aging gene in 1997 and was later recognized as a transmembrane co-receptor of fibroblast growth factor (FGF23) [2]. Under healthy conditions, Klotho is a protein highly expressed in the renal distal convolute tubule [3], which under homeostatic conditions may also be present in soluble form in the blood, urine and cerebrospinal fluid. Soluble Klotho has several endocrine functions like anti-senescence, anti-oxidative, anti-renal angiotensin–aldosterone system (RAAS), and anti-inflammatory modulation [4]. Klotho deficiency is associated with reduced renal function, hyperphosphatemia, increased FGF23 levels, RAAS activation, and chronic complications such as ectopic calcification, cardiac hypertrophy, secondary hyperparathyroidism, and progression of CKD [4,5]. Klotho-deficient rodents exhibit manifestations of CKD and conversely, rodent CKD models show markedly reduced *Klotho* mRNA expression [4].The reasons why Klotho is reduced in patients with CKD are not completely understood, but it seems that inflammation could be one of the underlying mechanisms. The exogenous administration of TWEAK (Tumor Necrosis Factor-like weak inducer of apoptosis) decreased renal expression of Klotho and the blockade of TWEAK by neutralizing antibodies restored renal expression of Klotho [6]. These data suggest the existence of a bidirectional relationship between Klotho and inflammation. Therefore, treatment strategies targeting renal inflammation could potentially restore Klotho expression, reducing renal damage and preventing the associated comorbidities.

Omega-3 fatty acids such as docosahexaenoic (DHA) and eicosapentaenoic (EPA) exert anti-inflammatory effects and may have reno-protective properties in kidney diseases [7,8]. Experimental data showed reduced tubulointerstitial cell infiltration, pro-inflammatory mediators such as Cyclooxygenase-2 (COX-2) and Monocyte chemoattractant protein-1 (MCP-1), and attenuation of fibrosis [9]. In addition, we previously observed that higher intake of EPA–DHA was independently associated with lower levels of FGF23 in renal transplant recipients [10], suggesting that omega-3 fatty acids could favorably affect the FGF23–Klotho axis. In the present study, we investigated whether fish oil, rich in omega-3 fatty acids, increases renal Klotho expression and reduces renal inflammation and fibrosis in a mouse model of inflammatory CKD.

2. Materials and Methods

2.1. Animal Model

C57BL/6 wild-type mice, aged 8 to 12 weeks, were obtained from a local facility. All the procedures were developed according to international guidelines for care of laboratory animals and approved by the Animal Ethics Committee of the Federal University of São Paulo (CEUA, 1558280214). In order to ensure that renal inflammation and fibrosis were induced in this adenine CKD model, initial experiments were conducted over 10 days in two groups, which received either a standard diet (7.0% soy oil, CTL group, n = 5), or the same diet enriched with 0.25% adenine (AD group, n = 5). Once the renal inflammation and fibrosis were confirmed in the model, two additional experimental groups were initiated to evaluate the effects of fish oil supplementation. Both groups received adenine supplementation to the standard diet for 10 days. From the 11th day on, adenine administration was discontinued and the animals were either switched back to their standard diet (7.0% soy oil, Post AD-CTL group, n = 9), or started supplementation with fish oil (6.3%, Post AD-Fish oil group, n = 9), for 7 additional days (see experimental design in Figure 1a). The diets were purchased from Rhoster, Araçoiaba da Serra, Brazil and were in accordance with the American Institute of Nutrition recommendations (AIN 93G). At the end of the study, the animals were anesthetized with xylazine (10 mg/kg) and ketamine (50 mg/kg) by intra-peritoneal injection for blood sample collection by cardiac puncture and euthanized thereafter. The kidneys were harvested and immediately dissected, washed with saline, embedded in paraffin, sectioned longitudinally, and processed routinely for histologic examination. The remaining part was snap frozen in liquid nitrogen and stored at −80 °C. Serum creatinine was measured by the Jaffe modified method, and serum urea was measured using a Labtest Kit (Minas Gerais, Brazil) according to the manufacturer's instructions.

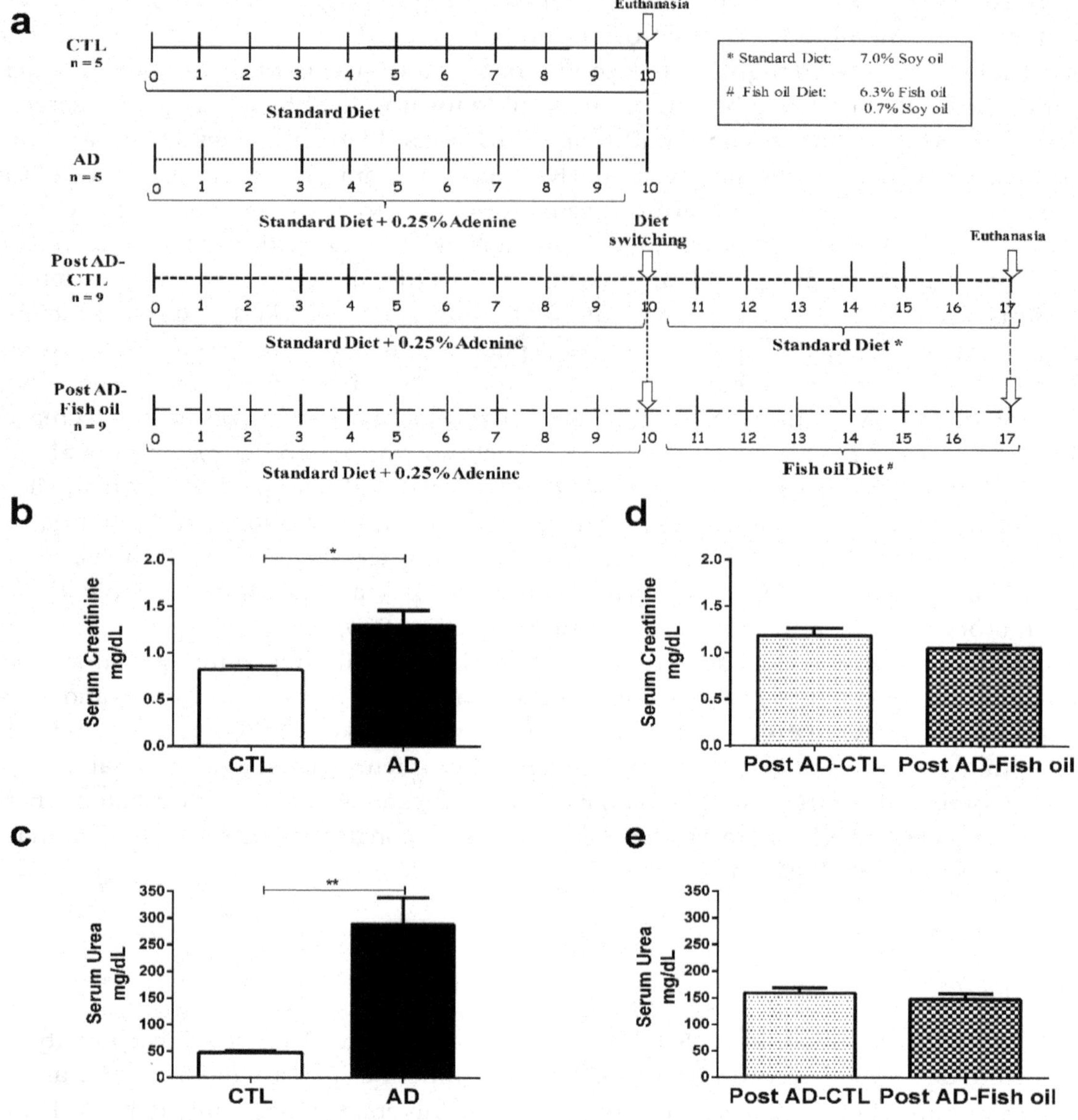

Figure 1. Experimental design and assessment of renal function: (**a**) experimental design, (**b**) serum creatinine, and (**c**) urea from the standard diet (CTL) and adenine (AD) mice. (**d**,**e**) Serum creatinine urea of Post AD-CTL and Post AD-Fish oil animals. (* $p < 0.05$, ** $p < 0.01$).

2.2. Real-Time PCR

IL-6 (Mm00446190_m1), IL-1β (Mm00434228_m1), TGF-β (Mm01178820_m1), HPRT (Mm00446968_m1), CXCL10, CXCL9, and *Klotho* gene expressions were assessed by real-time RT-Polymerase Chain Reaction (PCR). Renal tissues were crushed and homogenized, and the RNeasy Mini Purification Kit (Qiagen, Valencia, CA, USA) was used to extract RNA from all samples. RNA quantification was carried out using a NanoDrop Spectrophotometer (NanoDrop ND-1000 Spectrophotometer; Thermo Scientific, Wilmington, DE, USA). Nucleic acid concentration was determined using ultraviolet spectrophotometry at 260 nm and purity was determined using the absorbance ratios of 260/280 and 260/230. RNA was reverse transcribed using the QuantiTec SYBR Green Kit (Qiagen) and the manufacturer's instructions were followed. Reverse transcription and Real-Time PCR were performed using commercially available reagents and a 7500 Fast Real-Time Thermocycler (Applied Biosystems, Carlsbad, CA, USA). For relative quantification of message expression (ΔCT Method), target gene expression was normalized to Hypoxanthine Phosphoribosyltransferase (*HPRT*) gene expression.

The following primers were assessed for quantitative Syber Green RT-PCR:

KLOTHO fw: GGTGTCCATTGCCCTAAGCTC; KLOTHO rev: TCGGTCATTCTTCGAGGATTGA. CXCL9 fw: 5-TGCACGATGCTCCTGCA-3; CXCL9 rev:5-AGGTCTTTGAGGGATTTGTAGTGG-3. CXCL10 fw:5-GACGGTCCGCTGCAACTG-3; CXCL10 rev: 5-GCTTCCCTATGGCCCTCATT-3.

2.3. Histological Evaluation

Formaldehyde-fixed paraffin kidney sections (3 m) were dewaxed and stained with Picrosirius solution. Sections were immersed in saturated picric acid solution for 15 min and then in Picrosirius for 20 more minutes. Counter-staining was carried out with Harris hematoxylin. Picrosirius-stained sections were analyzed by an Olympus BX50 microscope (Olympus, Feasterville, PA, USA) with an Olympus camera attached. Manual shots were taken of the cortex, magnified 40X, and observed under polarized light. Photos of at least five different fields in each slide were taken, and structures such as the glomeruli, subcapsular cortex, large vessels, and medulla were excluded. The pictures were digitalized in a HP Scanjet 2400 (Hewllet Packard, Barueri, São Paulo, Brazil) and then the interstitial volume of collagen in the cortex compared to the overall cortex area was quantified by morphometry. For the morphometric analysis, the Image Processing and Analysis in Java (Image J—image processing program, National Institutes of Health, Maryland, MD, USA) was used. The result of the analysis is represented as a percentage of cortical interstitial collagen volume relative to the total cortical interstitial volume. Subsequently, the arithmetic mean of the analyzed fields was calculated for each slide. Collagen type I was associated with yellow/red birefringence and type III with green color, according to the description of Montes GS and Junqueira LC [11]. The assessment of the interstitial fibrosis volume obtained by morphometric analysis of the digital image stained with picrosirius was based on previous studies [12].

2.4. Western Blotting

Here, 50 ug of total protein was obtained from kidney lysate of CTL, AD, Post AD-CTL, and Post AD-Fish oil mice. The protein extract was denatured by heating at 5 min at 95 °C and separated by 10% polyacrylamide gel electrophoresis (SDS-PAGE). Subsequently, protein extract was transferred into nitrocellulose membrane and next, the immunostaining was performed with the following primary antibodies: E-cadherin (Dako: M3612, Santa Clara, CA, USA), alpha smooth muscle actin (α-SMA, DAKO: M0851, Santa Clara, CA, USA), Klotho: (CosmoBIO: K0603, Carlsbad, CA, USA), and α-tubulin (InVitrogen: 32-2500, Sunnyvale, CA, USA). Then, nitrocellulose membrane was incubated with conjugated secondary antibodies (anti-rabbit or anti-mouse peroxidase/1: 125.0000, Sigma-Aldrich, St. Louis, MO, USA) and revealed by chemiluminescence methods using an ECL kit (Millipore, Burlington, MA, USA). Finally, the image was acquired on Amersham Imager 600 (GE Healthcare, Marlborough, MA, USA) and analyzed with Image J.

2.5. Statistical Analyses

Differences between AD versus CTL and Post AD-CTL versus Post AD-Fish oil groups were assessed using Student's t-test. All statistical analyses were performed using GraphPad Prism version 5.0 (GraphPad Software, La Jolla, CA, USA). The results are presented as mean and SD for parametric variables. Differences were considered significant if $p < 0.05$.

3. Results

3.1. Adenine Supplementation Induces Inflammation, Loss of Renal Function, and Klotho Reduction

Animals fed with adenine for 10 days exhibited higher mean levels of serum creatinine and urea when compared with the control group (Figure 1b,c). AD mice exhibited significantly higher renal expression of IL-6, IL-1β, and CXCL10 versus CTL (Figure 2a,b,d). Finally, we noted that *Klotho* mRNA expression was at least six-fold lower in the renal tissues of AD mice when compared with CTL

(Figure 3a) (0.163 ± 0.01 vs. 1.001 ± 0.02), which was also confirmed by Western blot (Figure 4a,d). In summary, these data indicate that experimental adenine-induced CKD was associated with impaired renal function, increased pro-inflammatory mediators, and decreased *Klotho* expression.

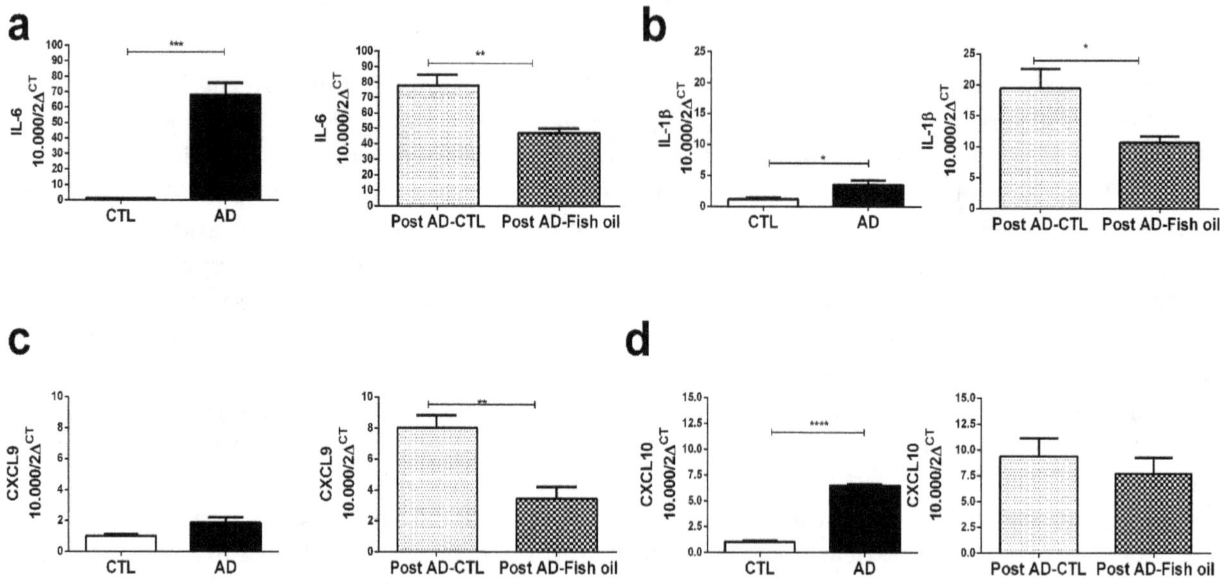

Figure 2. Pro-inflammatory markers: (**a**) IL-6, (**b**) IL-1b, (**c**) CXCL9 and (**d**) CXCL10 in the CTL/AD and Post AD-CTL and Post AD-Fish oil groups (* $p < 0.05$, ** $p < 0.01$, *** $p < 0.001$, **** $p < 0.0001$).

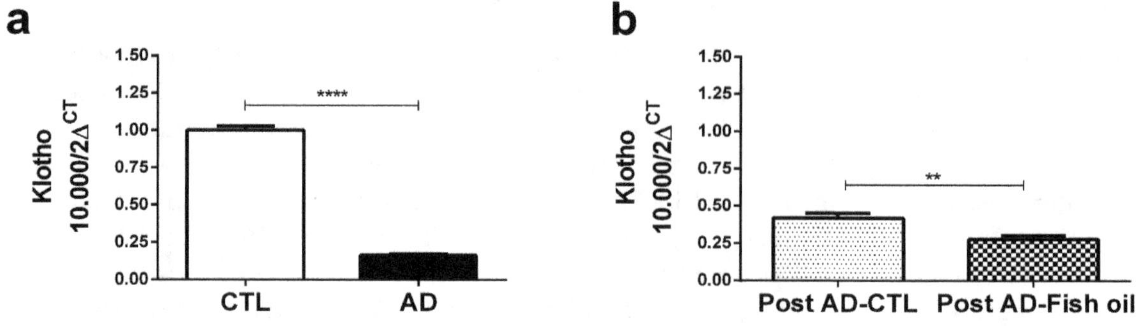

Figure 3. mRNA *Klotho* by PCR: (**a**) CTL/AD and (**b**) Post AD-CTL and Post AD-Fish oil mice (** $p < 0.01$, **** $p < 0.0001$).

3.2. Fish Oil Supplementation Reduces Pro-Inflammatory Markers but Does Not Improve Renal Function

Fish oil treatment promoted reduction of renal IL-6, IL-1β, and CXCL9 expression (Figure 2a–c). The reduction of CXCL10 by fish oil did not reach statistical significance (Figure 2d). Interestingly, the expression of IL-1β and CXCL9 was even higher in the Post AD-CTL group when compared descriptively with group AD (Figure 2b,c). Such an increase of inflammatory mediators in Post AD-CTL indicated that following the withdrawal of adenine on the 10th day, the process of inflammation continued to be active for the next 7 days during which the animals returned to the standard diet. Present findings suggested that treatment with fish oil exerted some renal anti-inflammatory effects on CKD animals subjected to adenine supplementation. However, the Post AD-Fish oil and Post AD-CTL animals did not differ statistically with respect to renal function (Figure 1d,e).

3.3. Fish Oil Supplementation Does Not Revert Progressive Renal Fibrosis

The deposition of crystals in tubular lumens from the kidneys of AD mice, coupled with tubular dilatation, interstitial infiltrate and hyaline cylindersresulting in tubular damage was confirmed by histomorphological analysis (Figure 5a). Furthermore, renal deposition of types I and III collagens, revealed by Picrosirius staining, were evidenced in AD mice (Figure 5b). In addition, other pro-fibrotic markers such as transforming growth factor beta (TGFβ) expression (Figure 5d) and alpha smooth muscle actin (α-SMA) evaluated by Western blot, were significantly higher in AD mice compared with CTL (Figure 4a,b). These data confirm that mice fed with adenine for 10 days had tubulointerstitial inflammation with progressive fibrosis.

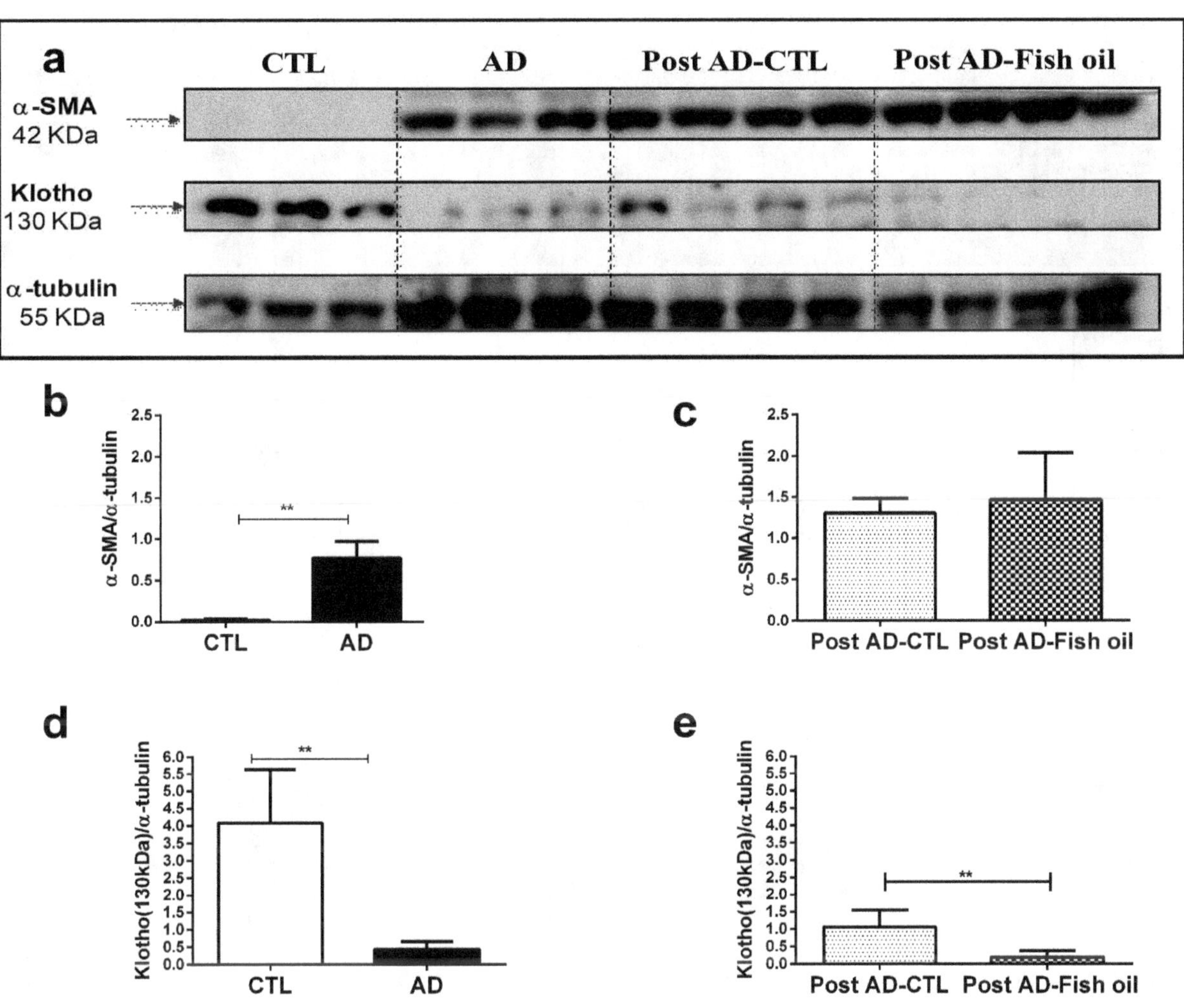

Figure 4. Klotho and alpha smooth muscle actin (α-SMA) expression by Western blot: (**a**) α-SMA and Klotho expression in renal tissue, normalized by α-tubulin in the CTL, AD, Post AD-CTL, and Post AD-Fish oil groups. Relative quantification of α-SMA (**b**,**c**) and Klotho (**d**,**e**) in the CTL, AD, Post AD-CTL and Post AD-Fish oil groups (** $p < 0.01$).

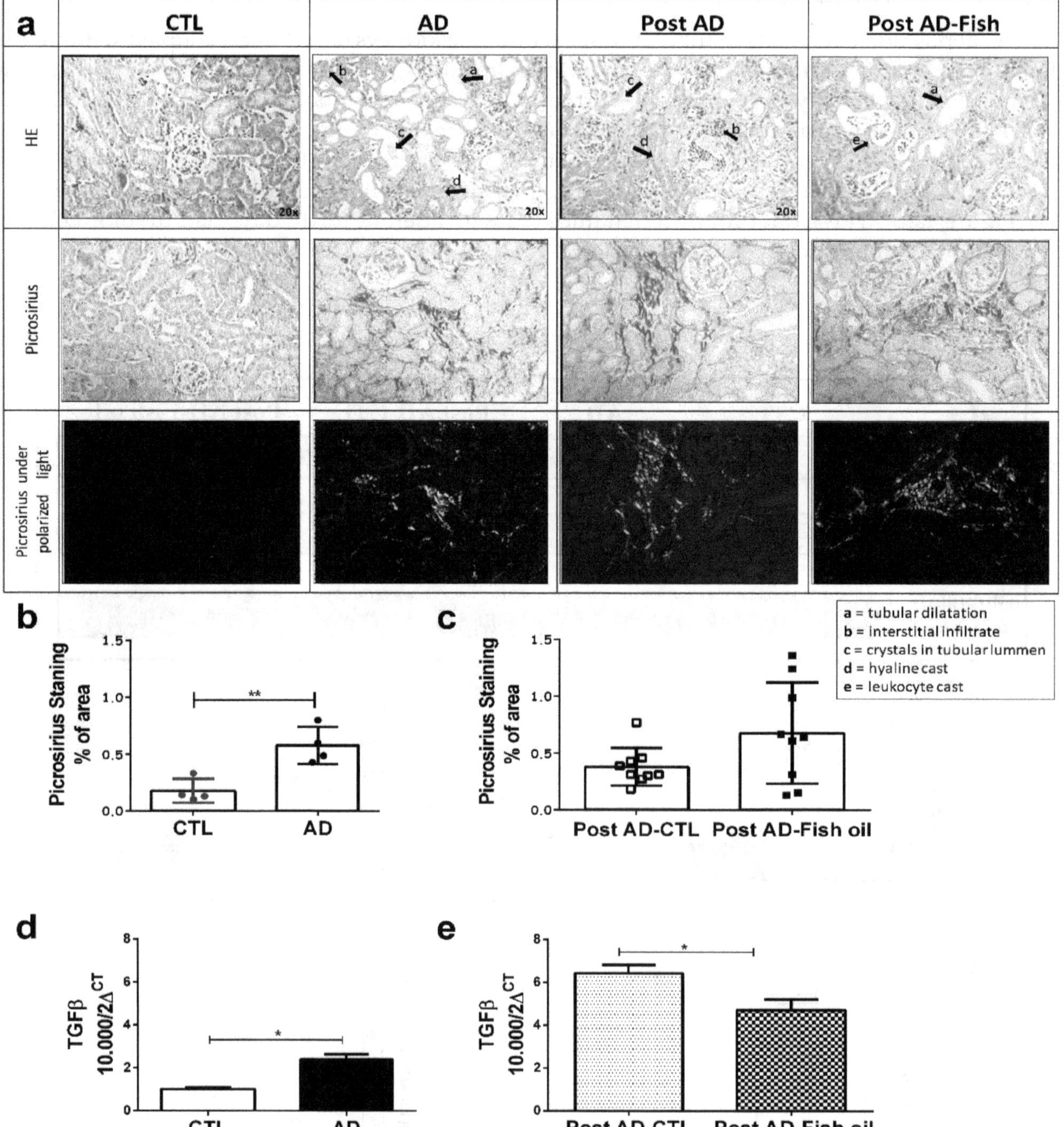

Figure 5. Fibrosis evaluation through picrosirius and transforming growth factor beta (TGFβ): (**a**) Images from Hematoxylin and eosin (HE) stain and picrosirius the kidney samples of CTL/AD and Post AD-CTL and Post AD-Fish oil groups. Graphical quantification of fibrosis observed by picrosirius in (**b**) CTL/AD and (**c**) Post AD-CTL and Post AD-Fish oil groups. TGF-β expression in (**d**) CTL/AD and (**e**) Post AD-CTL and Post AD-Fish oil groups (* $p < 0.05$, ** $p < 0.01$).

Both Post AD-CTL and Post AD-Fish oil mice showed the same degree of renal tissue injury as observed in AD mice. (Figure 5a). Similarly, interstitial deposition of types I and III collagen was not statistically different between Post AD-Fish oil and Post AD-CTL mice (Figure 5c). Although TGFβ expression was reduced in Post AD-Fish oil versus Post AD-CTL mice (Figure 5e), we showed that protein expression of α-SMA was not different between both groups (Figure 4a,c). Taken together, these results suggest that fibrosis was not ameliorated by fish oil in this CKD model.

3.4. Fish Oil Does Not Restore Renal Klotho

The expression of *Klotho* mRNA (Figure 3b) and transmembrane Klotho expression, shown by Western blot (Figure 4a,e) could not be restored by fish oil treatment; Klotho expression in Post AD-Fish oil was even slightly lower than in Post AD-CTL mice. Nevertheless, this difference did not seem to yield an important biological effect, given that some consequences such as impact on renal function and magnitude of fibrosis observed in both groups were quite similar.

4. Discussion

Several factors contribute to downregulate Klotho expression in CKD, including uremic toxins, vitamin D deficiency, phosphate overload, activation of RAAS, oxidative stress, and inflammation [4,5]. In the same way, experimental studies have shown that exogenous Klotho supplementation or its transgenic overexpression attenuates renal injury [4,13]. In various mice models of inflammatory disease, renal Klotho expression is suppressed [6,14–16] and Klotho possesses anti-inflammatory properties as well [17,18]. Given the potential anti-inflammatory effects of omega-3 fatty acids, largely shown in vitro and in vivo [19,20], we hypothesized that fish oil could restore the downregulation of Klotho in an adenine-induced CKD mice model. We found that fish oil supplementation reduced intra-renal inflammation but was not enough to ameliorate renal function and interstitial fibrosis nor retrieved kidney Klotho expression. The rationale for choosing the experimental model of adenine-induced tubulointerstitial nephritis [21] relied on the characteristic features of progressive renal dysfunction and interstitial fibrosis of this model [22] coupled with an intense local tissue inflammation with high expression of pro-inflammatory cytokines [12] which ultimately leads to progression of the disease. The model resembles the adenine phosphoribosyl transferase (APRT) deficiency, a rare human monogenic disease in which adenine cannot be salvaged to adenosine monophosphate, but is catabolized instead to 2,8-DHA in which crystals deposition leads to irreversible renal failure [23,24]. In the present study, aiming to determine the therapeutic rather than the preventive effects of fish oil on the amelioration of the renal inflammatory damage, adenine feeding was withdrawn at the 10th day, when according to our experimental design, the animals were either returned to a standard diet or switched to the fish oil-supplemented one. In the first set of experiments, we found that compared to controls, adenine-fed animals exhibited significantly higher renal expressions of inflammatory markers such as IL-6 and IL-1β, and of CXCL10 (a chemokine responsible for leucocyte recruitment), as well as increased renal tissue expressions of α-SMA (indicating myofibroblast deposition), and of TGF-β (a surrogate marker of fibrosis). Histomorphological analyses confirmed the presence of crystals in tubular lumen, tubular dilatation, interstitial infiltration, and leukocyte casts. Fibrosis was clearly evident by picrosirius staining as well. All these findings agreed well with other studies employing the adenine TIN mouse model [12,22,25]. As might be expected, renal function was also reduced in adenine-fed mice groups, as evidenced by the rises in serum urea and creatinine, in agreement with previous reports [12,21,22,25]. Although the elevation of serum creatinine level in this model has been described in a time-dependent manner, this parameter is already significantly higher after 7 days following the initiation of adenine feeding [22]. Moreover, previous data from our group have shown that the inflammatory process and enhanced cellular infiltration accompanied by collagen deposition leading to a progressive renal dysfunction is readily installed at 10 days after adenine supplementation [12]. In view of the presence of CKD [4,26,27], inflammation [15,16], or both, current experiments disclosed a marked reduction in renal Klotho expression in these adenine-fed animals, corroborating previously published data who showed extremely low levels of serum and renal Klotho after 4 and 6 weeks of adenine feeding [25,28]. Of note, our findings revealed an even earlier Klotho loss, at 10 days. A precocious Klotho deficiency has been described at the earliest stage of CKD (stage 1) when Glomerular Filtration Rate (GFR) is still normal [29]. Animal experiments have demonstrated that EPA and DHA provide benefits in a range of models of inflammatory conditions [30]. Nevertheless, the results of human clinical trials on prevention of inflammation-driven diseases using fish oil have been heterogeneous, with no overall clear evidence of efficacy [31]. With respect to kidney function, a small beneficial effect of an additional amount of 400 mg EPA–DHA per day on kidney function in patients with a history of myocardial infarction and a low habitual EPA–DHA intake has been observed [8]. However, no beneficial effect on inflammation markers such as high-sensitivity C-reactive protein (hsCRP) was further obtained [32]. Dose-dependent actions of marine omega−3 Polyunsaturated Fatty Acids (PUFAs) on inflammatory responses have not been well described, but it appears that a dose of at least 2 g per day is necessary to achieve an anti-inflammatory effect, an unlikely quantity to obtain from the diet [31]. Although other randomized controlled trials employing higher doses of omega-3 fatty acids also did not show a significant effect on circulating parameters of inflammation [33,34], an effect on intra-renal inflammation could not be ruled out by clinical studies.

In the present study, fish oil promoted a reduction in renal expression of IL-6, IL-1β, and CXCL9, reflecting, at least in part, diminished intra-renal inflammation. This is in accordance with experimental data in rodents dealing with other types of renal injuries such as tacrolimus-induced nephrotoxicity and polycystic kidney disease [35,36]. Despite of the decreased inflammation markers, we observed no restoration of renal expression of Klotho in the fish oil group. As reduced Klotho expression level in the kidney may sensitize the kidneys to injury and aggravation of renal interstitial fibrosis [37,38], hence accelerating renal disease progression, a vicious cycle may ensue.

Several other reasons might also explain why renal Klotho expression could not be restored. Given the persistence of loss of renal function in our model, irrespective of the fish oil administration, Klotho deficiency is expected, since the kidneys produce/release α-Klotho into the circulation and help clearing it [27]. Moreover, in the CKD setting, over production of reactive oxygen species [39], elevation of uremic toxins [40], high serum phosphate/excess FGF23 [41], and low serum 1,25-dihydroxy vitamin D3 (1,25 Vit D3) are expected to further suppress Klotho production [37,42,43]. Unfortunately, parameters of mineral metabolism such as phosphate, FGF23, and 1,25 Vit D3 have not been measured in the present study.

Other factors which could account for by renal Klotho deficiency in some circumstances depend on its epigenetic modulation. Methylation of the *Klotho* gene promoter, which has been shown to reduce its activity up to 40%, may inhibit Klotho gene expression in CKD [39,44,45] and TGF-β is known to induce global changes in DNA methylation [46]. Accordingly, demethylation of *Klotho* gene promoter remarkably reversed renal Klotho deficiency and reduced renal fibrosis [25]. The hyperacetylation of histone in the *Klotho* promoter also may contribute to Klotho underexpression [6]. In summary, decreased Klotho expression may result from an epigenetic response to inflammation inside or outside the kidney [47]. The possibility of a time delay in the response to local inflammation in our model cannot be ruled out. One could argue that a persistent uremic environment has not been fully accomplished in 10 days, but an irreversible renal failure after 2 weeks has been achieved in rats [48]. Given that the progression of renal failure is faster in mice, and that the current histomorphometric results obtained 7 days after the withdrawal of adenine feeding (17th day from baseline) showed a still important interstitial fibrosis, indeed suggest that the latter might have been responsible for the lack of Klotho restoration.

The present study had several limitations as well as strengths. The first concerns with the length of adenine administration/fish oil treatment and the eventual concomitancy of both supplementations. Had fish oil treatment been simultaneously administered with the adenine-supplemented diet, no inflammation or a shorter period of inflammation could have occurred, hence preventing the progression of fibrosis and loss of renal function. In this scenario, Klotho reduction could have even been averted. However, as discussed above, we aimed to determine the therapeutic rather than the preventive effects of fish oil on inflammation, given that in the clinical practice, the exact moment of initiation of a renal insult cannot be predicted. Second, higher doses of fish oil to achieve a more potent anti-inflammatory effect could have been employed. Nevertheless, few dose finding experimental and clinical studies have been performed to help determine optimal dose-response effects. A third limitation of the present study was that adhesion molecule expression and leucocyte chemotaxis

(CXCL8 and MCP1) have not been currently determined in our model to more properly assess both the magnitude and recovery of inflammation. The lack of measurement of parameters of mineral metabolism such as phosphate, FGF23, and 1,25 Vit D3, which are involved in Klotho regulation, compromised a further discussion of the absence of Klotho recovery. Finally, we are aware that the current model represents a specific tubulointerstitial insult with no glomerular injury, thus not reflecting all types of CKD.More studies employing different timing and dose of fish oil treatment in this and other models of CKD are still warranted in order to better understand the link between Klotho reduction and inflammation, fibrosis, and renal dysfunction.

5. Conclusions

The present study suggested that fish oil supplementation reduces renal expression of pro-inflammatory markers, but was not able to restore renal function or Klotho expression in an inflammatory model of CKD.

Author Contributions: Conceptualization, J.S.H.A., L.C.B., N.O.S.C., M.H.B., and I.P.H.; Methodology, J.S.H.A., L.C.B., A.R.P.S., N.O.S.C., and I.P.H.; Validation, J.S.H.A., M.S.O., N.O.S.C., and I.P.H.; Formal Analysis, J.S.H.A., A.R.P.S., N.O.S.C., and I.P.H.; Investigation, J.S.H.A., L.C.B., M.S.O., A.R.P.S., J.R.M., N.O.S.C., and I.P.H.; Writing—Original Draft Preparation, J.S.H.A., N.O.S.C., M.H.B., and I.P.H.; Writing—Review and Editing, N.O.S.C., G.J.N., M.H.B., and I.P.H.; Supervision, N.O.S.C., G.J.N., M.H.B., and I.P.H.; Funding Acquisition, N.O.S.C., M.H.B., and I.P.H.

References

1. Braga, T.T.; Agudelo, J.S.; Camara, N.O. Macrophages during the fibrotic process: M2 as friend and foe. *Front. Immunol.* **2015**, *6*, 602. [CrossRef] [PubMed]
2. Kuro-o, M.; Matsumura, Y.; Aizawa, H.; Kawaguchi, H.; Suga, T.; Utsugi, T.; Ohyama, Y.; Kurabayashi, M.; Kaname, T.; Kume, E.; et al. Mutation of the mouse klotho gene leads to a syndrome resembling ageing. *Nature* **1997**, *390*, 45–51. [CrossRef] [PubMed]
3. Hu, M.C.; Shi, M.; Zhang, J.; Pastor, J.; Nakatani, T.; Lanske, B.; Razzaque, M.S.; Rosenblatt, K.P.; Baum, M.G.; Kuro-o, M.; et al. Klotho: A novel phosphaturic substance acting as an autocrine enzyme in the renal proximal tubule. *FASEB J.* **2010**, *24*, 3438–3450. [CrossRef] [PubMed]
4. Hu, M.C.; Kuro-o, M.; Moe, O.W. Klotho and chronic kidney disease. *Contrib. Nephrol.* **2013**, *180*, 47–63. [PubMed]
5. De Borst, M.H.; Vervloet, M.G.; ter Wee, P.M.; Navis, G. Cross talk between the renin-angiotensin-aldosterone system and vitamin D-FGF23-klotho in chronic kidney disease. *J. Am. Soc. Nephrol.* **2011**, *22*, 1603–1609. [CrossRef] [PubMed]
6. Moreno, J.A.; Izquierdo, M.C.; Sanchez-Nino, M.D.; Suarez-Alvarez, B.; Lopez-Larrea, C.; Jakubowski, A.; Blanco, J.; Ramirez, R.; Selgas, R.; Ruiz-Ortega, M.; et al. The inflammatory cytokines TWEAK and TNFα reduce renal klotho expression through NFkB. *J. Am. Soc. Nephrol.* **2011**, *22*, 1315–1325. [CrossRef] [PubMed]
7. Fassett, R.G.; Gobe, G.C.; Peake, J.M.; Coombes, J.S. Omega-3 polyunsaturated fatty acids in the treatment of kidney disease. *Am. J. Kidney Dis.* **2010**, *56*, 728–742. [CrossRef] [PubMed]
8. Hoogeveen, E.K.; Geleijnse, J.M.; Kromhout, D.; Stijnen, T.; Gemen, E.F.; Kusters, R.; Giltay, E.J. Effect of omega-3 fatty acids on kidney function after myocardial infarction: The alpha omega trial. *Clin. J. Am. Soc. Nephrol.* **2014**, *9*, 1676–1683. [CrossRef] [PubMed]
9. An, W.S.; Kim, H.J.; Cho, K.H.; Vaziri, N.D. Omega-3 fatty acid supplementation attenuates oxidative stress, inflammation, and tubulointerstitial fibrosis in the remnant kidney. *Am. J. Physiol. Ren. Physiol.* **2009**, *297*, F895–F903. [CrossRef] [PubMed]

10. Baia, L.C.; Van den Berg, E.; Vervloet, M.G.; Heilberg, I.P.; Navis, G.; Bakker, S.J.; Geleijnse, J.M.; Kromhout, D.; Soedamah-Muthu, S.S.; De Borst, M.H.; et al. Fish and omega-3 fatty acid intake in relation to circulating fibroblast growth factor 23 levels in renal transplant recipients. *Nutr. Metab. Cardiovasc. Dis.* **2014**, *24*, 1310–1316. [CrossRef] [PubMed]
11. Montes, G.S.; Junqueira, L.C. The use of the picrosirius-polarization method for the study of the biopathology of collagen. *Memórias do Instituto Oswaldo Cruz* **1991**, *86* (Suppl. 3), 1–11. [CrossRef] [PubMed]
12. Correa-Costa, M.; Braga, T.T.; Semedo, P.; Hayashida, C.Y.; Bechara, L.R.; Elias, R.M.; Barreto, C.R.; Silva-Cunha, C.; Hyane, M.I.; Goncalves, G.M.; et al. Pivotal role of toll-like receptors 2 and 4, its adaptor molecule Myd88, and inflammasome complex in experimental tubule-interstitial nephritis. *PLoS ONE* **2011**, *6*, e29004. [CrossRef] [PubMed]
13. Mitani, H.; Ishizaka, N.; Aizawa, T.; Ohno, M.; Usui, S.; Suzuki, T.; Amaki, T.; Mori, I.; Nakamura, Y.; Sato, M.; et al. In vivo klotho gene transfer ameliorates angiotensin II-induced renal damage. *Hypertension* **2002**, *39*, 838–843. [CrossRef] [PubMed]
14. Sanz, A.B.; Izquierdo, M.C.; Sanchez-Nino, M.D.; Ucero, A.C.; Egido, J.; Ruiz-Ortega, M.; Ramos, A.M.; Putterman, C.; Ortiz, A. TWEAK and the progression of renal disease: Clinical translation. *Nephrol. Dial Transplant.* **2014**, *29* (Suppl. 1), i54–i62. [CrossRef]
15. Ohyama, Y.; Kurabayashi, M.; Masuda, H.; Nakamura, T.; Aihara, Y.; Kaname, T.; Suga, T.; Arai, M.; Aizawa, H.; Matsumura, Y.; et al. Molecular cloning of rat klotho cdna: Markedly decreased expression of klotho by acute inflammatory stress. *Biochem. Biophys. Res. Commun.* **1998**, *251*, 920–925. [CrossRef] [PubMed]
16. Feger, M.; Mia, S.; Pakladok, T.; Nicolay, J.P.; Alesutan, I.; Schneider, S.W.; Voelkl, J.; Lang, F. Down-regulation of renal klotho expression by shiga toxin 2. *Kidney Blood Press. Res.* **2014**, *39*, 441–449. [CrossRef] [PubMed]
17. Zhao, Y.; Banerjee, S.; Dey, N.; LeJeune, W.S.; Sarkar, P.S.; Brobey, R.; Rosenblatt, K.P.; Tilton, R.G.; Choudhary, S. Klotho depletion contributes to increased inflammation in kidney of the db/db mouse model of diabetes via rela (serine)536 phosphorylation. *Diabetes* **2011**, *60*, 1907–1916. [CrossRef] [PubMed]
18. Maekawa, Y.; Ishikawa, K.; Yasuda, O.; Oguro, R.; Hanasaki, H.; Kida, I.; Takemura, Y.; Ohishi, M.; Katsuya, T.; Rakugi, H. Klotho suppresses TNF-alpha-induced expression of adhesion molecules in the endothelium and attenuates nf-kappab activation. *Endocrine* **2009**, *35*, 341–346. [CrossRef] [PubMed]
19. Li, H.; Ruan, X.Z.; Powis, S.H.; Fernando, R.; Mon, W.Y.; Wheeler, D.C.; Moorhead, J.F.; Varghese, Z. Epa and dha reduce LPS-induced inflammation responses in hk-2 cells: Evidence for a ppar-gamma-dependent mechanism. *Kidney Int.* **2005**, *67*, 867–874. [CrossRef] [PubMed]
20. Li, C.C.; Yang, H.T.; Hou, Y.C.; Chiu, Y.S.; Chiu, W.C. Dietary fish oil reduces systemic inflammation and ameliorates sepsis-induced liver injury by up-regulating the peroxisome proliferator-activated receptor gamma-mediated pathway in septic mice. *J. Nutr. Biochem.* **2014**, *25*, 19–25. [CrossRef] [PubMed]
21. Jia, T.; Olauson, H.; Lindberg, K.; Amin, R.; Edvardsson, K.; Lindholm, B.; Andersson, G.; Wernerson, A.; Sabbagh, Y.; Schiavi, S.; et al. A novel model of adenine-induced tubulointerstitial nephropathy in mice. *BMC Nephrol.* **2013**, *14*, 116. [CrossRef] [PubMed]
22. Tamura, M.; Aizawa, R.; Hori, M.; Ozaki, H. Progressive renal dysfunction and macrophage infiltration in interstitial fibrosis in an adenine-induced tubulointerstitial nephritis mouse model. *Histochem. Cell Biol.* **2009**, *131*, 483–490. [CrossRef] [PubMed]
23. Edvardsson, V.; Palsson, R.; Olafsson, I.; Hjaltadottir, G.; Laxdal, T. Clinical features and genotype of adenine phosphoribosyltransferase deficiency in iceland. *Am. J. Kidney Dis.* **2001**, *38*, 473–480. [CrossRef] [PubMed]
24. Engle, S.J.; Stockelman, M.G.; Chen, J.; Boivin, G.; Yum, M.N.; Davies, P.M.; Ying, M.Y.; Sahota, A.; Simmonds, H.A.; Stambrook, P.J.; et al. Adenine phosphoribosyltransferase-deficient mice develop 2,8-dihydroxyadenine nephrolithiasis. *Proc. Natl. Acad. Sci. USA* **1996**, *93*, 5307–5312. [CrossRef] [PubMed]
25. Zhang, Q.; Liu, L.; Lin, W.; Yin, S.; Duan, A.; Liu, Z.; Cao, W. Rhein reverses klotho repression via promoter demethylation and protects against kidney and bone injuries in mice with chronic kidney disease. *Kidney Int.* **2017**, *91*, 144–156. [CrossRef] [PubMed]
26. Koh, N.; Fujimori, T.; Nishiguchi, S.; Tamori, A.; Shiomi, S.; Nakatani, T.; Sugimura, K.; Kishimoto, T.; Kinoshita, S.; Kuroki, T.; et al. Severely reduced production of klotho in human chronic renal failure kidney. *Biochem. Biophys. Res. Commun.* **2001**, *280*, 1015–1020. [CrossRef] [PubMed]

27. Hu, M.C.; Shi, M.; Zhang, J.; Addo, T.; Cho, H.J.; Barker, S.L.; Ravikumar, P.; Gillings, N.; Bian, A.; Sidhu, S.S.; et al. Renal production, uptake, and handling of circulating αklotho. *J. Am. Soc. Nephrol.* **2016**, *27*, 79–90. [CrossRef] [PubMed]
28. Lin, W.; Li, Y.; Chen, F.; Yin, S.; Liu, Z.; Cao, W. Klotho preservation via histone deacetylase inhibition attenuates chronic kidney disease-associated bone injury in mice. *Sci. Rep.* **2017**, *7*, 46195. [CrossRef] [PubMed]
29. Hu, M.C.; Shi, M.; Zhang, J.; Quinones, H.; Griffith, C.; Kuro-o, M.; Moe, O.W. Klotho deficiency causes vascular calcification in chronic kidney disease. *J. Am. Soc. Nephrol.* **2011**, *22*, 124–136. [CrossRef] [PubMed]
30. Calder, P.C. Omega-3 fatty acids and inflammatory processes: From molecules to man. *Biochem. Soc. Trans.* **2017**, *45*, 1105–1115. [CrossRef] [PubMed]
31. Calder, P.C. Omega-3 polyunsaturated fatty acids and inflammatory processes: Nutrition or pharmacology? *Br. J. Clin. Pharmacol.* **2013**, *75*, 645–662. [CrossRef] [PubMed]
32. Hoogeveen, E.K.; Geleijnse, J.M.; Kromhout, D.; Giltay, E.J. No effect of n-3 fatty acids on high-sensitivity c-reactive protein after myocardial infarction: The alpha omega trial. *Eur. J. Prev. Cardiol.* **2014**, *21*, 1429–1436. [CrossRef] [PubMed]
33. Geelen, A.; Brouwer, I.A.; Schouten, E.G.; Kluft, C.; Katan, M.B.; Zock, P.L. Intake of n-3 fatty acids from fish does not lower serum concentrations of c-reactive protein in healthy subjects. *Eur. J. Clin. Nutr.* **2004**, *58*, 1440–1442. [CrossRef] [PubMed]
34. Madsen, T.; Schmidt, E.B.; Christensen, J.H. The effect of n-3 fatty acids on c-reactive protein levels in patients with chronic renal failure. *J. Ren. Nutr.* **2007**, *17*, 258–263. [CrossRef] [PubMed]
35. Fernandes, M.B.; Caldas, H.C.; Toloni, L.D.; Baptista, M.A.; Fernandes, I.M.; Abbud-Filho, M. Supplementation with omega-3 polyunsaturated fatty acids and experimental tacrolimus-induced nephrotoxicity. *Exp. Clin. Transplant.* **2014**, *12*, 522–527. [PubMed]
36. Devassy, J.G.; Yamaguchi, T.; Monirujjaman, M.; Gabbs, M.; Ravandi, A.; Zhou, J.; Aukema, H.M. Distinct effects of dietary flax compared to fish oil, soy protein compared to casein, and sex on the renal oxylipin profile in models of polycystic kidney disease. *Prostaglandins Leukot Essent Fatty Acids* **2017**, *123*, 1–13. [CrossRef] [PubMed]
37. Satoh, M.; Nagasu, H.; Morita, Y.; Yamaguchi, T.P.; Kanwar, Y.S.; Kashihara, N. Klotho protects against mouse renal fibrosis by inhibiting Wnt signaling. *Am. J. Physiol. Ren. Physiol.* **2012**, *303*, F1641–F1651. [CrossRef] [PubMed]
38. Sugiura, H.; Yoshida, T.; Shiohira, S.; Kohei, J.; Mitobe, M.; Kurosu, H.; Kuro-o, M.; Nitta, K.; Tsuchiya, K. Reduced klotho expression level in kidney aggravates renal interstitial fibrosis. *Am. J. Physiol. Ren. Physiol.* **2012**, *302*, F1252–F1264. [CrossRef] [PubMed]
39. Adema, A.Y.; van Ittersum, F.J.; Hoenderop, J.G.; de Borst, M.H.; Nanayakkara, P.W.; Ter Wee, P.M.; Heijboer, A.C.; Vervloet, M.G.; NIGRAM consortium. Reduction of oxidative stress in chronic kidney disease does not increase circulating α-klotho concentrations. *PLoS ONE* **2016**, *11*, e0144121. [CrossRef] [PubMed]
40. Yang, K.; Wang, C.; Nie, L.; Zhao, X.; Gu, J.; Guan, X.; Wang, S.; Xiao, T.; Xu, X.; He, T.; et al. Klotho protects against indoxyl sulphate-induced myocardial hypertrophy. *J. Am. Soc. Nephrol.* **2015**, *26*, 2434–2446. [CrossRef] [PubMed]
41. Dai, B.; David, V.; Martin, A.; Huang, J.; Li, H.; Jiao, Y.; Gu, W.; Quarles, L.D. A comparative transcriptome analysis identifying FGF23 regulated genes in the kidney of a mouse ckd model. *PLoS ONE* **2012**, *7*, e44161. [CrossRef] [PubMed]
42. Neyra, J.A.; Hu, M.C. Potential application of klotho in human chronic kidney disease. *Bone* **2017**, *100*, 41–49. [CrossRef] [PubMed]
43. Asai, O.; Nakatani, K.; Tanaka, T.; Sakan, H.; Imura, A.; Yoshimoto, S.; Samejima, K.; Yamaguchi, Y.; Matsui, M.; Akai, Y.; et al. Decreased renal α-klotho expression in early diabetic nephropathy in humans and mice and its possible role in urinary calcium excretion. *Kidney Int.* **2012**, *81*, 539–547. [CrossRef] [PubMed]
44. Chen, J.; Zhang, X.; Zhang, H.; Lin, J.; Zhang, C.; Wu, Q.; Ding, X. Elevated klotho promoter methylation is associated with severity of chronic kidney disease. *PLoS ONE* **2013**, *8*, e79856. [CrossRef] [PubMed]
45. Sun, C.Y.; Chang, S.C.; Wu, M.S. Suppression of klotho expression by protein-bound uremic toxins is associated with increased DNA methyltransferase expression and DNA hypermethylation. *Kidney Int.* **2012**, *81*, 640–650. [CrossRef] [PubMed]

46. Cardenas, H.; Vieth, E.; Lee, J.; Segar, M.; Liu, Y.; Nephew, K.P.; Matei, D. TGF-β induces global changes in DNA methylation during the epithelial-to-mesenchymal transition in ovarian cancer cells. *Epigenetics* **2014**, *9*, 1461–1472. [CrossRef] [PubMed]
47. Ruiz-Andres, O.; Sanchez-Nino, M.D.; Moreno, J.A.; Ruiz-Ortega, M.; Ramos, A.M.; Sanz, A.B.; Ortiz, A. Downregulation of kidney protective factors by inflammation: Role of transcription factors and epigenetic mechanisms. *Am. J. Physiol. Ren. Physiol.* **2016**, *311*, F1329–F1340. [CrossRef] [PubMed]
48. Okada, H.; Kaneko, Y.; Yawata, T.; Uyama, H.; Ozono, S.; Motomiya, Y.; Hirao, Y. Reversibility of adenine-induced renal failure in rats. *Clin. Exp. Nephrol.* **1999**, *3*, 82–88. [CrossRef]

8

Erythrocyte n-6 Fatty Acids and Risk for Cardiovascular Outcomes and Total Mortality in the Framingham Heart Study

William S. Harris [1,2,*], Nathan L. Tintle [3] and Vasan S. Ramachandran [4,5,6]

1 Department of Internal Medicine, Sanford School of Medicine, University of South Dakota, Vermillion, SD 57069, USA
2 OmegaQuant Analytics, LLC, Sioux Falls, SD 57106, USA
3 Department of Mathematics & Statistics, Dordt College, Sioux Center, IA 51250, USA; nathan.tintle@dordt.edu
4 National Heart Lung and Blood Institute's and Boston University's Framingham Heart Study, Framingham, MA 02118, USA; vasan@bu.edu
5 Departments of Cardiology and Preventive Medicine, Department of Medicine, Boston University School of Medicine, Boston, MA 02118, USA
6 Department of Biostatistics, Boston University School of Public Health, Boston, MA 02118, USA
* Correspondence: bill@omegaquant.com

Abstract: Background: The prognostic value of erythrocyte levels of n-6 fatty acids (FAs) for total mortality and cardiovascular disease (CVD) outcomes remains an open question. Methods: We examined cardiovascular (CV) outcomes and death in 2500 individuals in the Framingham Heart Study Offspring cohort without prevalent CVD (mean age 66 years, 57% women) as a function of baseline levels of different length n-6 FAs (18 carbon, 20 carbon, and 22 carbon) in the erythrocyte membranes. Clinical outcomes were monitored for up to 9.5 years (median follow up, 7.26 years). Cox proportional hazards models were adjusted for a variety of demographic characteristics, clinical status, and red blood cell (RBC) n-6 and long chain n-3 FA content. Results: There were 245 CV events, 119 coronary heart disease (CHD) events, 105 ischemic strokes, 58 CVD deaths, and 350 deaths from all causes. Few associations between either mortality or CVD outcomes were observed for n-6 FAs, with those that were observed becoming non-significant after adjusting for n-3 FA levels. Conclusions: Higher circulating levels of marine n-3 FA levels are associated with reduced risk for incident CVD and ischemic stroke and for death from CHD and all-causes; however, in the same sample little evidence exists for association with n-6 FAs. Further work is needed to identify a full profile of FAs associated with cardiovascular risk and mortality.

Keywords: epidemiology; prospective cohort study; n-6 fatty acids; n-3 fatty acids; linoleic acid; arachidonic acid

---

1. Introduction

The roles of n-3 and/or n-6 polyunsaturated fatty acids (PUFAs) in health and disease are controversial. Whereas most studies have reported that higher circulating levels of the long-chain n-3 PUFAs (i.e., eicosapentaenoic acid (EPA) and docosahexaenoic acid (DHA)) are protective against cardiovascular disease (CVD) and premature death [1], the story is not as clear for the n-6 PUFAs. Previous studies have reported that higher intakes of linoleic acid (LA) and higher circulating levels of arachidonic acid (AA) are associated with cardiovascular (CV) benefit [1,2]. In addition, LA blood levels are inversely associated with risk for type 2 diabetes mellitus [3]. Nevertheless, some warn that current intakes (and thus blood levels) of the n-6 PUFAs, especially these two major fatty acids (FAs) in the n-6 family, are dangerous [4,5]. The proposed mechanism of harm is via increased inflammation, driven by the conversion of AA into pro-inflammatory/pro-thrombotic eicosanoids such as prostaglandin E2, thromboxane A2, and leukotriene B4 [6]. Accordingly, ratios like n-6:n-3 [7] or AA:EPA [8] have been promoted as better summary metrics of PUFA status than either family alone. This perspective has, however, been criticized on both theoretical [9–12] and evidential [13–15] bases.

In a previous report from the Framingham Offspring cohort, we examined relations between red blood cell (RBC) n-3 FAs, specifically EPA and DHA (the sum of which is called the omega-3 index [16]) and risk for CVD and total mortality [17]. In this follow-up analyses, we focus on the n-6 FA family and their relations with these outcomes.

2. Materials and Methods

2.1. Methods

The Framingham Heart Study is a longitudinal community-based cohort study that was initiated in 1948. The selection criteria for the Framingham Offspring Cohort and the Framingham Omni Cohort have previously been described [18,19]. Briefly, adult children of the original cohort were recruited in 1971 into the Framingham Offspring Cohort. We evaluated Framingham Offspring participants (n = 3021) who attended their eighth examination cycle (2005–2008). Participants were excluded in hierarchical order if they were missing RBC fatty acid measurements or clinical covariates (n = 122), or having prevalent cardiovascular disease (e.g., nonfatal coronary heart disease (CHD) or stroke; n = 350), leaving n = 2500 for this analysis. The study protocol was approved by the Institutional Review Board of the Boston University Medical Center. Informed consent was provided by all participants.

2.2. Covariates and Mortality Outcomes

We considered seventeen primary baseline demographic and cardiovascular risk covariates: sex, age, body mass index (BMI), marital status, education level, employment status, health insurance status, regular aspirin use, prevalent hypertensive status, use of cholesterol medication, prevalent diabetes, alcohol consumption, smoking status, metabolic equivalent (METS), total to high-density lipoprotein (HDL) cholesterol ratio, systolic blood pressure and C-reactive protein. Seven endpoints were examined: four mortality-related outcomes ((1) any mortality, (2) CVD mortality (CHD death or sudden cardiac death), (3) cancer mortality, or (4) death from non-CVD or cancer causes) and three cardio-vascular related outcomes ((1) total stroke (any fatal or non-fatal ischemic stroke), (2) total CHD (fatal or non-fatal myocardial infarction (MI), or CHD death or sudden cardiac death), and (3) total CVD (any stroke, CHD or CHD mortality)). We focused our analyses on seven RBC FAs from the n-6 family: 18:2n6 (linoleic acid, LA), 18:3n6 (gamma-linolenic acid, GLA), 20:2n6 (eicosadienoic acid, EDA), 20:3n6 (dihomo-gamma linolenic acid, DGLA), 20:4n6 (arachidonic acid, AA), 22:4n6 (adrenic acid, ADA) and 22:5n6 (docosapentaenoic acid, DPA n-6). In some analyses, we adjusted for the omega-3 index (EPA + DHA).

2.3. RBC Fatty Acid Analysis

Blood was drawn after a 10–12 h fast into an EDTA tube, and RBCs were separated from plasma by centrifugation. The RBC fraction was frozen at −80 °C immediately after collection. RBC fatty acid composition was determined as described previously [20]. Briefly, RBCs were incubated at 100 °C with boron trifluoride-methanol and hexane to generate fatty acid methyl esters that were then analyzed by gas chromatography with flame ionization detection. The coefficients of variation for the seven n-6 FAs measured were <3% for 18:2n6, 20:3n6, 20:4n6, and 22:4n6; 7% for 22:5n6; 11% for 20:2n6 and 21% for 18:3n6.

2.4. Statistical Analysis

Description of sample characteristics was conducted using standard statistical metrics (e.g., means, SDs, correlations). Hazard ratios were estimated using the survival package in R [21]. Primary analyses predicted incident clinical outcomes (date of event (CVD or death) or date of censoring) by groups of n-6 FAs (the 18-carbon, 20-carbon, and 22-carbon moities), with follow-up analyses adjusting for a variety of demographic covariates, and finally for the omega-3 index. Secondary analyses explored the relationship between event risk and n-6 FA levels by quintiles, individual omega-6 FA levels, and the sum of all omega-6 FAs. All analyses used two-sided tests at the 0.05 significance level.

3. Results

3.1. Cohort Description

The Framingham Offspring study consists of 2500 individuals for whom FAs, clinical outcomes, and demographic covariates were available, and who also did not have prevalent CVD at baseline. At baseline, the average age was 66 and the sample contained slightly more females (57%) than males (43%). The sample was fairly well educated (over two-thirds of the sample had at least some college education), with approximately half of the sample employed and the majority of the remainder having retired. Most (88%) of the sample had insurance at baseline and the distribution of cardiometabolic traits followed expected distributions, with approximately 40% of the sample using aspirin regularly, with similar numbers with prevalent hypertension, and high cholesterol. Rates of prevalent diabetes was lower (13%). The majority of the sample periodically consumed alcohol, and the vast majority (over 90%) were nonsmokers. Table 1 provides a complete overview of the demographic profile of the sample. Supplemental Table S1 illustrates the correlation between and among the major n-3 and n-6 fatty acids in this sample. While correlations are generally higher within the n-3 or n-6 fatty acids than between, this is not always the case (e.g., moderate negative correlations between both 20:2n6, 20:3n6, and 20:4n6 levels). Supplemental Table S2 illustrates the number of events present in the sample with 350 of the participants having died from any cause during the course of the study, but only 58 of those deaths were attributable to CVD. The maximum time to follow-up was approximately 9 years.

3.2. Omega-6 Fatty Acids and Mortality and Cardiovascular Disease Risk

Across all three classes of n-6 FAs (18-carbon, 20-carbon and 22-carbon) little evidence of association with cardiovascular outcomes or mortality was observed. In unadjusted analyses, the 18-carbon n-6′s showed an association with reduced risk of CVD and other (non-CVD, non-cancer) mortality, however, these associations became non-significant after adjusting for demographic variables (Table 2a). No associations were detected before or after evaluating 20-carbon n-6s (Table 2b). While 22-carbon n-6′s showed some evidence of positive association with Total CVD, CHD, and stroke risk after adjusting for demographic covariates, all of these associations became non-significant after also adjusting for the omega-3 index (Table 2c). Notably, the omega-3 index remained significant in many of the models for CVD event risk and CVD, non-cancer/non-CVD and all-cause mortality (Table 2a–c; Figure 1).

Table 1. Demographic overview (n = 2500). METS: metabolic equivalent.

Variable	Died (n = 350)	Still Living (n = 2150)	Total	p-Value for Difference (Chi-Squared or t-Test)
	% (n) or Mean (SD)	% (n) or Mean (SD)	% (n) or Mean (SD)	
Sex				
Male	52.9% (185)	41.5% (893)	43.1% (1078)	<0.001
Female	47.1% (165)	58.5% (1257)	56.9% (1422)	
Age	72.9 (8.6)	64.4 (8.2)	65.56 (8.76)	<0.001
Body Mass Index (BMI)	27.9 (5.9)	28.3 (5.4)	28.2 (5.4)	<0.001
Marital Status				
Single/Never Married	4.3% (15)	6.7% (144)	6.4% (159)	<0.001
Married	63.7% (223)	70.7% (1519)	69.7% (1742)	
Separated/Divorced	12.0% (42)	12.7% (273)	12.6% (315)	
Widowed	18.3% (64)	9.4% (203)	10.7% (267)	
Education				
Some High School (HS) or less	6.0% (21)	2.4% (51)	2.9% (72)	<0.001
HS graduate	33.7% (118)	24.8% (533)	26.0% (651)	
Some college or vocational	22.9% (78)	21.9% (471)	22.0% (549)	
College graduate	36.6% (128)	50.5% (1086)	48.6% (1214)	
Employment				
Employed	31.1% (109)	56.3% (1210)	52.8% (1319)	<0.001
Disabled/unemployed	3.1% (11)	2.5% 53)	2.6% (64)	
Retired	64.3% (225)	40.8% (877)	44.1% (1102)	
Health insurance status				
No insurance	2.3% (8)	1.9% (40)	1.9% (48)	0.053
Insurance, but no prescription	11.4% (40)	8.4% (181)	8.8% (221)	
Full insurance	84.0% (294)	88.7% (1906)	88.0% (2200)	
Regular aspirin use	49.7% (174)	38.6% (830)	40.2% (1004)	<0.001
Prevalent hypertension	57.1% (200)	42.2% (908)	44.3% (1108)	<0.001
Cholesterol medication	41.4% (145)	36.9% (794)	37.6% (939)	0.06
Prevalent diabetes	22.3% (78)	11.6% (249)	13.1% (327)	<0.001
Alcohol consumption				
None	34.0% (119)	23.2% (499)	24.7% (618)	<0.001
<1 drink/day	36.0% (126)	50.7% (1089)	48.6% (1215)	
1–2 drinks/day	22.6% (79)	20.2% (434)	20.5% (513)	
>2 drinks/day	6.9% (24)	5.7% (123)	5.9% (147)	
Smoking				
Not current smoker	89.1% (312)	90.5% (1946)	90.3% (2258)	0.70
Current	10.6% (37)	9.3% (200)	9.5% (237)	
METS	4.7 (15.4)	3.3 (8.6)	3.5 (9.9)	<0.001
Total to High-Density Lipoprotein (HDL) cholesterol ratio	3.5 (1.1)	3.5 (1.0)	3.5 (1.1)	<0.001
Systolic Blood Pressure	133.6 (19.8)	128.2 (16.9)	129.0 (17.4)	<0.001
C-reactive protein	4.9 (12.7)	3.0 (6.1)	3.3 (7.4)	<0.001
Omega-3 index	0.054 (0.017)	0.056 (0.017)	0.0554 (0.0168)	<0.001

Table 2. Risk of events and mortality by n-6 fatty acid carbon chain length ($n = 2500$). (**a**) Eighteen-carbon n-6 fatty acids (18:2n6 + 18:3n6). (**b**) Twenty-carbon n-6 fatty acids (20:2n6 + 20:3n6 + 20:4n6). (**c**) Twenty-two-carbon n-6 fatty acids (22:4n6 + 22:5n6).

(a)

	Total Events			Mortality			
	CVD	CHD	Stroke	CVD	Cancer	Other	Total
	HR (95% CI)	HR (95% CI)	HR (95% CI)	HR (95% CI)	HR (95% CI)	HR (95% CI)	HR (95% CI)
A. Unadjusted							
<9.8% 18-carbon ($n = 433$)	1.0	1.0	1.0	1.0	1.0	1.0	1.0
9.8%–10.7% ($n = 488$)	1.07 (0.71, 1.61)	1.30 (0.72, 2.35)	1.28 (0.67, 2.43)	1.14 (0.45, 2.89)	0.96 (0.58, 1.58)	0.56 (0.31, 1.02)	0.92 (0.64, 1.31)
10.7%–11.5% ($n = 522$)	1.05 (0.71, 1.57)	1.08 (0.59, 1.98)	1.33 (0.72, 2.43)	0.86 (0.33, 2.19)	0.81 (0.48, 1.36)	*0.51 (0.29, 0.92)* *	0.77 (0.54, 1.11)
11.5%–12.5% ($n = 522$)	0.74 (0.48, 1.13)	0.80 (0.42, 1.52)	0.70 (0.35, 1.38)	1.74 (0.71, 4.25)	0.56 (0.32, 1.00)	0.86 (0.53, 1.39)	0.94 (0.67, 1.31)
>12.5% ($n = 535$)	0.73 (0.48, 1.13)	1.01 (0.56, 1.81)	0.80 (0.39, 1.63)	0.57 (0.22, 1.53)	0.74 (0.43, 1.25)	*0.52 (0.29, 0.93)* *	0.74 (0.52, 1.06)
p-value for linear trend	*0.032* *	0.45	0.15	0.26	0.08	0.17	0.14
B. Adjusted for demos							
<9.8% 18-carbon ($n = 433$)	1.0	1.0	1.0	1.0	1.0	1.0	1.0
9.8%–10.7% ($n = 488$)	1.28 (0.83, 1.95)	1.42 (0.76, 2.67)	1.46 (0.71, 3.00)	1.19 (0.48, 2.96)	1.09 (0.63, 1.88)	0.87 (0.47, 1.60)	1.21 (0.84, 1.73)
10.7%–11.5% ($n = 522$)	1.37 (0.90, 2.08)	1.38 (0.74, 2.56)	1.51 (0.77, 2.96)	1.12 (0.42, 2.97)	0.89 (0.49, 1.61)	0.83 (0.45, 1.56)	1.02 (0.69, 1.50)
11.5%–12.5% ($n = 522$)	0.78 (0.48, 1.27)	0.96 (0.46, 2.02)	0.72 (0.33, 1.61)	1.59 (0.67, 3.75)	0.65 (0.35, 1.20)	1.02 (0.58, 1.80)	0.99 (0.68, 1.44)
>12.5% ($n = 535$)	1.16 (0.72, 1.89)	1.53 (0.75, 3.13)	1.12 (0.52, 2.40)	0.96 (0.33, 2.80)	0.88 (0.47, 1.65)	0.62 (0.29, 1.33)	1.02 (0.68, 1.53)
p-value for linear trend	0.68	0.59	0.49	0.68	0.30	0.42	0.69
C. Adjusted for demos and O3I							
<9.8% 18-carbon ($n = 433$)	1.0	1.0	1.0	1.0	1.0	1.0	1.0
9.8%–10.7% ($n = 488$)	1.19 (0.78, 1.82)	1.32 (0.70, 2.49)	1.29 (0.62, 2.66)	1.08 (0.43, 2.73)	1.07 (0.62, 1.87)	0.74 (0.39, 1.41)	1.14 (0.79, 1.64)
10.7%–11.5% ($n = 522$)	1.28 (0.84, 1.95)	1.28 (0.69, 2.38)	1.34 (0.67, 2.65)	1.04 (0.38, 2.78)	0.87 (0.47, 1.61)	0.71 (0.38, 1.34)	0.95 (0.64, 1.41)
11.5%–12.5% ($n = 522$)	0.71 (0.44, 1.16)	0.86 (0.41, 1.79)	0.62 (0.28, 1.39)	1.49 (0.65, 3.44)	0.64 (0.34, 1.19)	0.83 (0.46, 1.50)	0.92 (0.63, 1.34)
>12.5% ($n = 535$)	1.03 (0.63, 1.67)	1.32 (0.64, 2.73)	0.93 (0.43, 2.03)	0.78 (0.26, 2.34)	0.86 (0.45, 1.63)	0.52 (0.24, 1.11)	0.92 (0.61, 1.40)
p-value for linear trend	0.34	0.92	0.23	0.87	0.28	0.18	0.38
p-value for omega-3	0.005 **	0.034 *	0.004 **	0.10	0.70	0.004 **	0.011

CVD, cardiovascular disease; CHD, coronary heart disease; CI, confidence interval; HR, hazard ratio; O3I, Omega-3 Index. * $p < 0.05$; ** $p < 0.01$. All significant hazard ratios/*p*-values are shown in bold italics. A. Unadjusted model, B. Adjusted for all variables in Table 1 except history of CVD, C. Adjusted for omega-3 index and all variables in Table 1 except history of CVD. Quintiles for 18-carbon n-6 fatty acids are shown in the left-most column. For example, 9.8%–10.7% means that the second quintile for RBC 18-carbon n-6 fatty acids are individuals for whom between 9.8 and 10.7% of all RBC fatty acids are 18-carbon n-6 fatty acids.

Table 2. *Cont.*

(b)

	Total Events			Mortality			
	CVD	CHD	Stroke	CVD	Cancer	Other	Total
	HR (95% CI)	HR (95% CI)	HR (95% CI)	HR (95% CI)	HR (95% CI)	HR (95% CI)	HR (95% CI)
A. Unadjusted							
<17.5% 20-carbon (n = 508)	1.0	1.0	1.0	1.0	1.0	1.0	1.0
17.5%–18.4% (n = 509)	1.03 (0.71, 1.50)	0.95 (0.53, 1.70)	0.96 (0.54, 1.70)	1.19 (0.54, 2.62)	0.80 (0.48, 1.32)	0.84 (0.49, 1.46)	0.89 (0.65, 1.22)
18.4%–19.1% (n = 502)	0.92 (0.61, 1.39)	0.95 (0.52, 1.71)	0.78 (0.41, 1.49)	0.83 (0.31, 2.20)	0.90 (0.53, 1.53)	1.59 (0.94, 2.67)	1.16 (0.83, 1.63)
19.1%–19.9% (n = 502)	0.88 (0.58, 1.33)	1.22 (0.71, 2.09)	0.63 (0.32, 1.24)	1.24 (0.55, 2.80)	0.87 (0.52, 1.46)	1.19 (0.67, 2.09)	1.02 (0.73, 1.42)
>19.9% (n = 479)	1.03 (0.70, 1.52)	0.99)0.55, 1.77)	1.04 (0.59, 1.82)	0.77 (0.37, 1.60)	0.92 (0.55, 1.53)	1.14 (0.65, 2.01)	0.95 (0.69, 1.33)
p-value for linear trend	0.82	0.71	0.68	0.54	0.83	0.32	0.90
B. Adjusted for demos							
<17.5% 20-carbon (n = 508)	1.0	1.0	1.0	1.0	1.0	1.0	1.0
17.5%–18.4% (n = 509)	1.10 (0.74, 1.65)	0.96 (0.52, 1.75)	1.19 (0.62, 2.30)	1.58 (0.61, 4.11)	0.84 (0.49, 1.42)	0.86 (0.45, 1.67)	1.01 (0.71, 1.44)
18.4%–19.1% (n = 502)	0.96 (0.61, 1.51)	0.93 (0.49, 1.79)	1.09 (0.54, 2.21)	1.23 (0.38, 4.02)	0.98 (0.53, 1.81)	1.91 (1.08, 3.36) *	1.33 (0.92, 1.92)
19.1%–19.9% (n = 502)	1.04 (0.67, 1.61)	1.29 (0.71, 2.36)	0.88 (0.43, 1.80)	1.98 (0.75, 5.19)	1.02 (0.58 1.78)	1.45 (0.77, 2.70)	1.27 (0.88, 1.81)
>19.9% (n = 479)	1.21 (0.78, 1.88)	1.06 (0.56, 2.02)	1.48 (0.75, 2.92)	1.19 (0.44, 3.21)	1.21 (0.69, 2.13)	1.40 (0.75, 2.61)	1.19 (0.82, 1.73)
p-value for linear trend	0.52	0.52	0.53	0.55	0.42	0.11	0.16
C. Adjusted for demos and O3I							
<17.5% 20-carbon (n = 508)	1.0	1.0	1.0	1.0	1.0	1.0	1.0
17.5%–18.4% (n = 509)	0.97 (0.65, 1.46)	0.84 (0.46, 1.51)	0.96 (0.50, 1.86)	1.30 (0.47, 3.61)	0.84 (0.49, 1.44)	0.77 (0.40, 1.51)	0.94 (0.65, 1.36)
18.4%–19.1% (n = 502)	0.81 (0.51, 1.30)	0.77 (0.39, 1.51)	0.82 (0.39, 1.72)	0.99 (0.28, 3.55)	0.99 (0.52, 1.88)	1.62 (0.92, 2.86)	1.19 (0.81, 1.75)
19.1%–19.9% (n = 502)	0.85 (0.53, 1.34)	1.03 (0.55, 1.91)	0.61 (0.28, 1.33)	1.55 (0.56, 4.30)	1.03 (0.57, 1.86)	1.17 (0.60, 2.27)	1.12 (0.76, 1.65)
>19.9% (n = 479)	0.97 (0.60, 1.56)	0.82 (0.41, 1.65)	1.03 (0.49, 2.15)	0.85 (0.27, 2.72)	1.23 (0.67, 2.26)	1.12 (0.58, 2.16)	1.04 (0.70, 1.56)
p-value for linear trend	0.72	0.87	0.91	0.89	0.42	0.44	0.58
p-value for omega-3	0.011 *	0.039 *	0.009 **	0.13	0.87	0.03 *	0.04 *

CVD, cardiovascular disease; CHD, coronary heart disease; CI, confidence interval; HR, hazard ratio; O3I, Omega-3 Index. * $p < 0.05$; ** $p < 0.01$. All significant hazard ratios/*p*-values are shown in bold italics. A. Unadjusted model, B. Adjusted for all variables in Table 1 except history of CVD, C. Adjusted for omega-3 index and all variables in Table 1 except history of CVD. Quintiles for 18-carbon n-6 fatty acids are shown in the left-most column. For example, 17.5%–18.4% means that the second quintile for RBC 20-carbon n-6 fatty acids are individuals for whom between 17.5 and 18.4% of all RBC fatty acids are 20-carbon n-6 fatty acids.

Table 2. *Cont.*

(c)

	Total Events		Mortality				
	CVD	**CHD**	**Stroke**	**CVD**	**Cancer**	**Other**	**Total**
	HR (95% CI)	**HR (95% CI)**	**HR (95% CI)**	**HR (95% CI)**	**HR (95% CI)**	**HR (95% CI)**	**HR (95% CI)**
A. Unadjusted							
<3.6% 22-carbon ($n = 508$)	1.0	1.0	1.0	1.0	1.0	1.0	1.0
3.6%–4.3% ($n = 508$)	1.37 (0.88, 2.12)	1.24 (0.63, 2.43)	1.25 (0.62, 2.53)	0.93 (0.42, 2.03)	0.86 (0.52, 1.42)	1.11 (0.64, 1.93)	0.96 (0.69, 1.31)
4.3%–4.7% ($n = 500$)	1.73 (1.14, 2.62) **	2.43 (1.34, 4.42) **	1.36 (0.71, 2.61)	0.81 (0.35, 1.83)	0.65 (0.38, 1.13)	0.96 (0.53, 1.73)	0.80 (0.57, 1.13)
4.7%–5.3% ($n = 509$)	1.46 (0.96, 2.22)	1.61 (0.86, 3.03)	1.58 (0.83, 2.98)	1.16 (0.54, 2.49)	0.78 (0.46, 1.31)	1.27 (0.72, 2.26)	1.04 (0.75, 1.45)
>5.3% ($n = 469$)	1.73 (1.12, 2.68) *	2.25 (1.22, 4.16) **	1.48 (0.74, 2.98)	0.63 (0.24, 1.67)	1.18 (0.71, 1.95)	1.43 (0.82, 2.50)	1.10 (0.77, 1.56)
p-value for linear trend	0.02 *	0.006 **	0.18	0.57	0.74	0.17	0.48
B. Adjusted for demos							
<3.6% 22-carbon ($n = 508$)	1.0	1.0	1.0	1.0	1.0	1.0	1.0
3.6%–4.3% ($n = 508$)	1.20 (0.75, 1.93)	1.05 (0.50, 2.20)	1.39 (0.62, 3.13)	0.83 (0.28, 2.41)	0.94 (0.56, 1.60)	1.06 (0.60, 1.88)	1.01 (0.71, 1.44)
4.3%–4.7% ($n = 500$)	1.74 (1.13, 2.67) *	2.38 (1.26,4.48) **	1.73 (0.85, 3.55)	0.65 (0.26, 1.62)	0.74 (0.41, 1.32)	0.85 (0.41, 1.76)	0.85 (0.58, 1.25)
4.7%–5.3% ($n = 509$)	1.36 (0.87, 2.13)	1.51 (0.76, 2.99)	1.89 (0.92, 3.87)	1.28 (0.62, 2.62)	0.74 (0.41, 1.31)	1.31 (0.68, 2.51)	1.11 (0.78, 1.59)
>5.3% ($n = 469$)	1.66 (1.02, 2.69) *	1.91 (0.95, 3.83)	2.01 (0.92, 4.42)	0.60 (0.18, 2.01)	1.21 (0.71, 2.07)	1.53 (0.85, 2.74)	1.17 (0.81, 1.71)
p-value for linear trend	0.031 *	0.04 *	0.04 *	0.80	0.91	0.10	0.32
C. Adjusted for demos and O3I							
<3.6% 22-carbon ($n = 508$)	1.0	1.0	1.0	1.0	1.0	1.0	1.0
3.6%–4.3% ($n = 508$)	1.11 (0.69, 1.79)	0.99 (0.48, 2.05)	1.20 (0.53, 2.69)	0.62 (0.20, 1.95)	0.93 (0.54, 1.60)	0.89 (0.48, 1.63)	0.89 (0.62, 1.29)
4.3%–4.7% ($n = 500$)	1.52 (0.96, 2.39)	2.09 (1.07, 4.06) *	1.35 (0.65, 2.80)	0.42 (0.17, 1.06)	0.72 (0.38, 1.36)	0.67 (0.32, 1.42)	0.69 (0.45, 1.05)
4.7%–5.3% ($n = 509$)	1.14 (0.70, 1.86)	1.25 (0.60, 2.62)	1.37 (0.64, 2.97)	0.69 (0.27, 1.76)	0.71 (0.38, 1.34)	0.97 (0.48, 1.94)	0.87 (0.58, 1.30)
>5.3% ($n = 469$)	1.33 (0.77, 2.28)	1.51 (0.69, 3.30)	1.38 (0.60, 3.18)	0.30 (0.07, 1.26)	1.15 (0.57, 2.33)	0.98 (0.48, 1.98)	0.85 (0.54, 1.34)
p-value for linear trend	0.42	0.34	0.44	0.14	0.97	0.88	0.57
p-value for omega-3	0.09	0.22	0.049 *	0.034 *	0.92	0.03 *	0.021 *

CVD, cardiovascular disease; CHD, coronary heart disease; CI, confidence interval; HR, hazard ratio; O3I, Omega-3 Index. * $p < 0.05$; ** $p < 0.01$. All significant hazard ratios/*p*-values are shown in bold italics. A. Unadjusted model, B. Adjusted for all variables in Table 1 except history of CVD, C. Adjusted for omega-3 index and all variables in Table 1 except history of CVD. Quintiles for 18-carbon n-6 fatty acids are shown in the left-most column. For example, 3.6%–4.3% means that the second quintile for RBC 22-carbon n-6 fatty acids are individuals for whom between 3.6 and 4.3% of all RBC fatty acids are 22-carbon n-6 fatty acids.

3.3. Additional Fatty Acid Analyses

Supplemental Table S3a–g illustrate parallel analyses for each of the seven individual n-6 FAs. In short, these analyses follow what was observed for the classes of FAs. Namely, few associations were observed between the individual FAs and either cardiovascular events or mortality and what few associations were observed in unadjusted models tended to become non-significant in models that adjusted for demographic covariates. One exception was the positive association between ESA (C20:2n6) and all-cause mortality, a relationship which remained even after adjusting for the omega-3 index (Table S3c). Other exceptions were the positive associations between DTA (C22:4n6) and stroke, and the positive associations between DPA (C22:5n6) and all-cause mortality and non-CVD/non-cancer mortality, though these associations all became non-significant after adjusting for the omega-3 index (Table S3f–g). An analysis on the sum of all seven omega-6 FAs identified no significant associations after adjusting for the omega-3 index.

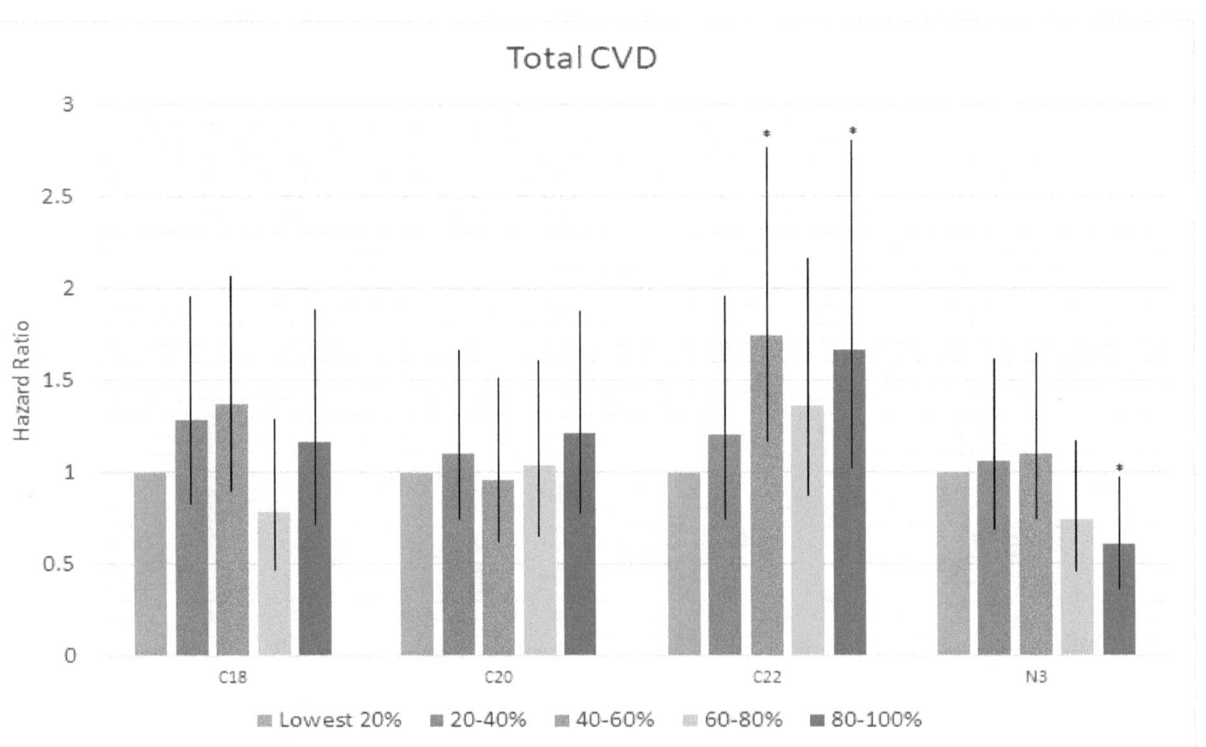

(a)

Figure 1. *Cont.*

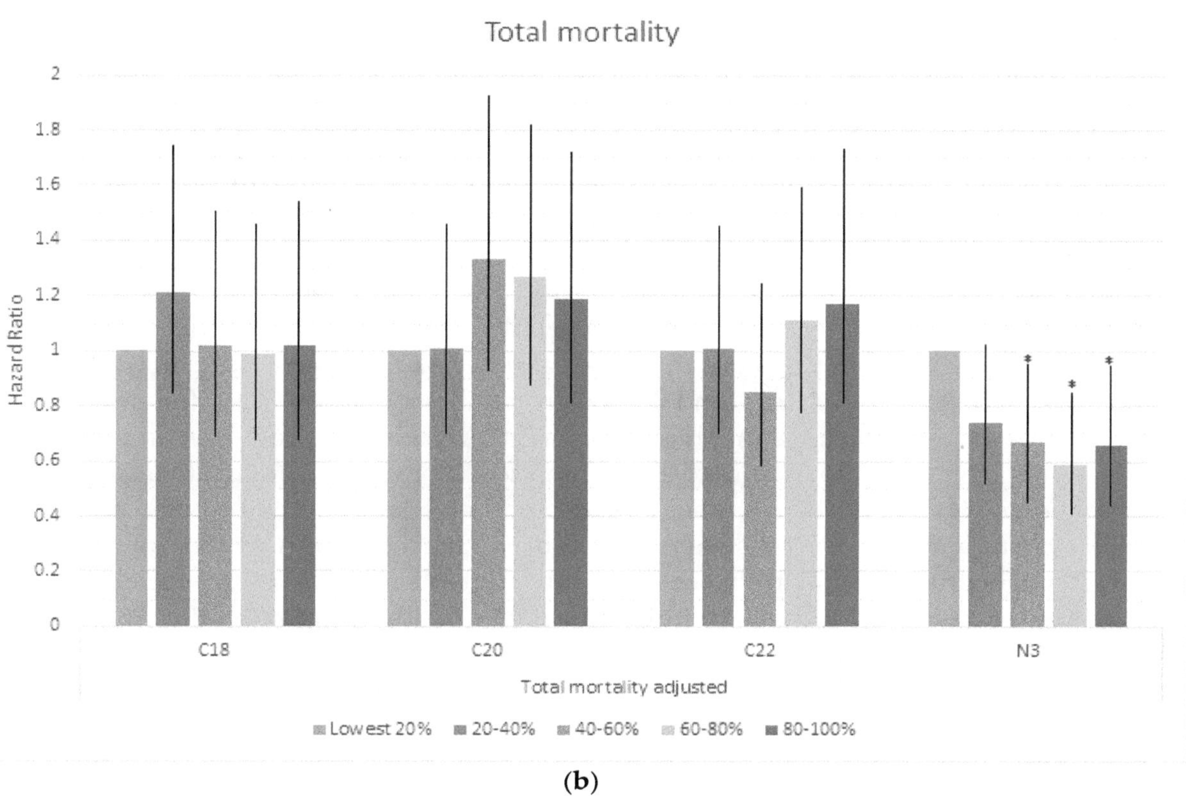

(b)

Figure 1. (**a**) Hazard ratios for total cardiovascular (CVD) risk by n-6 FAs and the omega-3 index. Figure 1a illustrates the associations between n-6 or n-3 fatty acids and total CVD risk. Bar heights are hazard ratios with 95% confidence intervals provided for each hazard ratio. Hazard ratios are provided for each quintile are all relative to the risk within the lowest quintile. Statistically significant HRs at the 0.05 level are denoted with asterisks. Hazard ratios depicted in this figure are from models adjusting for all demographic variables in Table 1, but do not adjust for the omega-3 index and/or other omega-6 FAs. There is no significant linear trend for the 18-carbon n-6 FAs ($p = 0.68$) or the 20-carbon n-6 FAs ($p = 0.52$), while the 22-carbon n-6 FAs ($p = 0.031$) and the omega-3 index ($p = 0.008$) both have significant linear trends across the 5 quintile groups (see Table 2a–c for additional details). Finally, we note that, as shown in Table 2c, both linear associations as well as all individual quintile group associations become non-significant ($p > 0.05$) for both the omega-3 index and 22 carbon n-6 FAs when both are simultaneously entered into the statistical model. (**b**) Hazard ratios for total mortality (CVD) risk by n-6 FAs and the omega-3 index. Figure 1b illustrates the associations between n-6 or n-3 fatty acids and Total mortality. Bar heights are hazard ratios with 95% confidence intervals provided for each hazard ratio. Hazard ratios are provided for each quintile are all relative to the risk within the lowest quintile. Statistically significant HRs at the 0.05 level are denoted with asterisks. Hazard ratios depicted in this figure are from models adjusting for all demographic variables in Table 1, but do not adjust for the omega-3 index and/or other omega-6 FAs. There is no significant linear trend for the 18 carbon n-6 FAs ($p = 0.69$), the 20 carbon n-6 FAs ($p = 0.16$) and the 22 carbon n-6 FAs ($p = 0.32$), while, the omega-3 index ($p = 0.02$) has a significant linear trend across the 5 quintile groups. Finally, we note that, as shown in Table 2c, linear associations as well as all individual quintile group associations become non-significant ($p > 0.05$) for all n-6 fatty acids when adjusting for the omega-3 index, while the omega-3 index remains significant ($p < 0.05$) in all models.

4. Discussion

In this study of participants in the Framingham Offspring study, the n-6 PUFAs were generally unrelated with vital status, especially in fully adjusted models accounting for subject characteristics and the omega-3 index. The only exception was for EDA which was directly related with risk all-cause mortality. The omega-3 index was inversely associated with most of the outcomes examined here even after adjustment for the n-6 FAs, whether in the full aggregate, the carbon-chain groups, or the individual n-6 FAs.

Delgado et al. recently reported the relations between red blood cell (RBC) n-6 FA levels and risk for death from all causes [22]. Using data from 3259 patients undergoing diagnostic coronary artery catheterization and followed for 10 years, these investigators found that RBC levels of n-6 FAs were inversely related with risk for death. However, a more granular examination revealed widely varying associations with n-6 FAs depending on chain length. The 18-carbon species (LA and GLA) were inversely associated with death, those with 20 carbons (AA and DGLA) were largely unrelated with risk, and those with 22 carbons (ADA and DPAn-6) were directly related with risk. A case-control study using RBC FA profiles from acute coronary syndrome patients found that a suite of 10 RBC FAs was able to predict case status better than the classical risk factors included in the Framingham Risk Score [23]. In that study, LA, AA, and GLA were predictors of lower risk for coronary disease, whereas EDA was associated with higher risk. In yet another study, RBC both EPA and DPAn-6 added independent predictive power to a standard algorithm used to predict risk for death in post myocardial infarction patients [24]. All of these studies suggest that n-6 FAs are not all created equal, and that to speak of them as a monolithic class of FAs with similar biochemical functions and physiological roles is probably incorrect. In this study, we further illustrated a widely varying correlation structure between n-3 FAs and n-6 FAs, as well as within the n-6 FAs, further supporting the argument that not each n-6 FA may have its own unique role to play in metabolism. However, one important trend worth noting is that, for 22 carbon FAs, associations with cardiovascular outcomes which were significant even after adjusting for demographic variables, became non-significant after adjusting for n-3 FAs. In these models (Table2c, fully adjusted model), n-3 FAs were significant, suggesting that the initial n-6 associations with cardiovascular outcomes were better explained by variation in n-3 FAs. Further work is needed to better understand the role of the full profile of fatty acids on disease risk.

The EDA finding in the present study was somewhat unexpected. EDA levels were adversely associated risk for acute coronary syndromes in a case-control study from Kansas City [23]. On the other hand, serum EDA levels were recently reported to be reduced in patients with inflammatory bowel disease [25], and in a large prospective study of plasma phospholipid FAs and risk for type 2 diabetes, EDA was inversely associated with incident disease [26]. These findings—along with those of the present study—would suggest that EDA participates in some manner in pathophysiology of these conditions. EDA is an elongation product of LA (C18 to C20, both with 2 double bonds), and on the biosynthetic path to DGLA and AA. These latter two n-6 FAs serve as substrates for the production of a wide variety of active metabolites called oxylipins [27], but whether the beneficial/harmful effects of EDA (if they indeed exist) are mediated by oxylipin metabolism is unknown. Complicating these inconsistent observations is the fact that levels of EDA in these subjects were very low, averaging only about 0.25% of total RBC FAs. Consequently, the ultimate meaning and impact of EDA in biology is unclear.

Strengths and Limitations

Strengths of this study include the large sample size and number of events, the unambiguous nature of the primary endpoint, the inclusion of community dwellers (instead of a patient population), and the use of an objective biomarker of PUFA exposure with low biological variability [28]. The previous detection of clear inverse relations between the omega-3 index and outcomes in this same cohort suggests that our failure to see associations with the n-6 FAs was not due to a lack of power, but a lack of effect. The assessment of PUFA exposure at only one time point cannot capture PUFA status changes throughout follow-up. Finally, the inability to rule out the possibility of residual or unmeasured confounding also precludes inferences about causality [29].

In conclusion, we found no meaningful relationship between RBC levels of n-6 PUFAs and risk for CVD or total mortality. Importantly, after adjustment for covariates, there was no increase in risk for adverse outcomes with higher n-6 PUFA levels, with the possible exception of EDA. These findings, in the context of the totality of available evidence on this subject, provide no support for a harmful role of n-6 PUFAs in these important clinical outcomes.

5. Conclusions

Higher circulating levels of marine n-3 FA levels are associated with reduced risk for incident CVD and ischemic stroke and for death from CHD and all-causes; however, in the same sample little evidence exists for association with n-6 FAs. Further work is needed to identify a full profile of FAs associated with cardiovascular risk and mortality.

Author Contributions: Conceptualization, W.S.H.; Formal analysis, N.L.T.; Funding acquisition, W.S.H. and V.S.R.; Writing—original draft, W.S.H., N.L.T., and V.S.R.; Writing—Review and editing, W.S.H. and N.L.T.

Abbreviations

ADA	adrenic acid
AA	arachidonic acid
CVD	cardiovascular disease
DGLA	dihomo-gamma linolenic acid
DHA	docosahexaenoic acid
DPA n-6	docosapentaenoic acid
EDA	eicosadienoic acid
EPA	eicosapentaenoic acid
FA	fatty acid
GLA	gamma-linolenic acid
HR	hazard ratio
LA	linoleic acid
MI	myocardial infarction
Omega-3 Index	erythrocyte EPA + DHA
PUFA	polyunsaturated FA
RBC	red blood cell
SD	standard deviation

References

1. Chowdhury, R.; Warnakula, S.; Kunutsor, S.; Crowe, F.; Ward, H.A.; Johnson, L.; Franco, O.H.; Butterworth, A.S.; Forouhi, N.G.; Thompson, S.G.; et al. Association of dietary, circulating, and supplement fatty acids with coronary risk: A systematic review and meta-analysis. *Ann. Int. Med.* **2014**, *160*, 398–406. [CrossRef]
2. Farvid, M.S.; Ding, M.; Pan, A.; Sun, Q.; Chiuve, S.E.; Steffen, L.M.; Willett, W.C.; Hu, F.B. Dietary linoleic acid and risk of coronary heart disease: A systematic review and meta-analysis of prospective cohort studies. *Circulation* **2014**, *130*, 1568–1578. [CrossRef] [PubMed]
3. Wu, J.H.Y.; Marklund, M.; Imamura, F.; Tintle, N.; Korat, A.V.A.; De Goede, J.; Zhou, X.; Yang, W.S.; de Oliveira Otto, M.C.; Kröger, J.; et al. Omega-6 fatty acid biomarkers and incident type 2 diabetes: Pooled

analysis of individual-level data for 39 740 adults from 20 prospective cohort studies. *Lancet Diabetes Endocrinol.* **2017**, *5*, 965–974. [CrossRef]

4. Ramsden, C.E.; Zamora, D.; Leelarthaepin, B.; Majchrzak-Hong, S.F.; Faurot, K.R.; Suchindran, C.M.; Ringel, A.; Davis, J.M.; Hibbein, J.R. Use of dietary linoleic acid for secondary prevention of coronary heart disease and death: Evaluation of recovered data from the Sydney Diet Heart Study and updated meta-analysis. *BMJ* **2013**, *346*, e8707. [CrossRef] [PubMed]
5. Blasbalg, T.L.; Hibbeln, J.R.; Ramsden, C.E.; Majchrzak, S.F.; Rawlings, R.R. Changes in consumption of omega-3 and omega-6 fatty acids in the United States during the 20th century. *Am. J. Clin. Nutr.* **2011**, *93*, 950–962. [CrossRef]
6. Lands, B. A critique of paradoxes in current advice on dietary lipids. *Prog. Lipid. Res.* **2008**, *47*, 77–106. [CrossRef] [PubMed]
7. Simopoulos, A.P. The importance of the omega-6/omega-3 fatty acid ratio in cardiovascular disease and other chronic diseases. *Exp. Biol. Med.* **2008**, *233*, 674–688. [CrossRef]
8. Yagi, S.; Aihara, K.I.; Fukuda, D.; Takashima, A.; Bando, M.; Hara, T.; Nishimoto, S.; Ise, T.; Kusunose, K.; Yamaguchi, K.; et al. Reduced ratio of eicosapentaenoic acid and docosahexaenoic acid to arachidonic acid is associated with early onset of acute coronary syndrome. *Nutr. J.* **2015**, *14*, 111. [CrossRef]
9. Harris, W.S. The omega-6/omega-3 ratio and cardiovascular disease risk: Uses and abuses. *Curr. Atheroscler. Rep.* **2006**, *8*, 453–459. [CrossRef]
10. Stanley, J.C.; Elsom, R.L.; Calder, P.C.; Griffin, B.A.; Harris, W.S.; Jebb, S.A.; Lovegrove, J.A.; Moore, C.S.; Riemersma, R.A.; Sanders, T.A.B. UK Food Standards Agency Workshop Report: The effects of the dietary n-6:n-3 fatty acid ratio on cardiovascular health. *Br. J. Nutr.* **2007**, *98*, 1305–1310. [CrossRef]
11. Harris, W.S.; Shearer, G.C. Omega-6 fatty acids and cardiovascular disease: Friend, not foe? *Circulation* **2014**, *130*, 1562–1564. [CrossRef] [PubMed]
12. Harris, W.S. The Omega-6:Omega-3 ratio: A critical appraisal and possible successor. *Prostaglandins Leukot. Essent. Fat. Acids* **2018**, *132*, 34–40. [CrossRef]
13. Mozaffarian, D.; Ascherio, A.; Hu, F.B.; Stampfer, M.J.; Willett, W.C.; Siscovick, D.S.; Rimm, E.B. Interplay Between Different Polyunsaturated Fatty Acids and Risk of Coronary Heart Disease in Men. *Circulation* **2005**, *111*, 157–164. [CrossRef] [PubMed]
14. Johnson, G.H.; Fritsche, K. Effect of dietary linoleic acid on markers of inflammation in healthy persons: A systematic review of randomized controlled trials. *J. Acad. Nutr. Diet.* **2012**, *112*, 1029–1041. [CrossRef] [PubMed]
15. Kakutani, S.; Ishikura, Y.; Tateishi, N.; Horikawa, C.; Tokuda, H.; Kontani, M.; Kawashima, H.; Sakakibara, Y.; Kiso, Y.; Shibata, H.; et al. Supplementation of arachidonic acid-enriched oil increases arachidonic acid contents in plasma phospholipids, but does not increase their metabolites and clinical parameters in Japanese healthy elderly individuals: A randomized controlled study. *Lipids Health Dis.* **2011**, *10*, 241. [CrossRef] [PubMed]
16. Harris, W.S.; von Schacky, C. The Omega-3 Index: A new risk factor for death from coronary heart disease? *Prev. Med.* **2004**, *39*, 212–220. [CrossRef] [PubMed]
17. Harris, W.S.; Tintle, N.L.; Etherton, M.R.; Vasan, R.S. Erythrocyte long-chain omega-3 fatty acid levels are inversely associated with mortality and with incident cardiovascular disease: The Framingham Heart Study. *J. Clin. Lipidol.* **2018**, *12*, 718–724. [CrossRef] [PubMed]
18. Kannel, W.B.; Feinleib, M.; McNamara, P.M.; Garrison, R.J.; Castelli, W.P. An investigation of coronary heart disease in families. The Framingham offspring study. *Am. J. Epidemiol.* **1979**, *110*, 281–290. [CrossRef] [PubMed]
19. Splansky, G.L.; Corey, D.; Yang, Q.; Atwood, L.D.; Cupples, L.A.; Benjamin, E.J.; D'Agostino, R.B., Sr.; Fox, S.C.; Larson, M.G.; Murabito, J.M.; et al. The Third Generation Cohort of the National Heart, Lung, and Blood Institute′s Framingham Heart Study: Design, recruitment, and initial examination. *Am. J. Epidemiol.* **2007**, *165*, 1328–1335. [CrossRef]
20. Harris, W.S.; Pottala, J.V.; Vasan, R.S.; Larson, M.G.; Robins, S.J. Changes in erythrocyte membrane trans and marine fatty acids between 1999 and 2006 in older Americans. *J. Nutr.* **2012**, *142*, 1297–1303. [CrossRef]
21. R. Version 3; Software for Statistical Analysis; the R-Project for Statistical Computing. Available online: www.r-project.org (accessed on 19 December 2018).

22. Delgado, G.E.; Marz, W.; Lorkowski, S.; von Schacky, C.; Kleber, M.E. Omega-6 fatty acids: Opposing associations with risk-The Ludwigshafen Risk and Cardiovascular Health Study. *J. Clin. Lipidol.* **2017**, *11*, 1082–1090. [CrossRef]
23. Shearer, G.C.; Pottala, J.V.; Spertus, J.A.; Harris, W.S. Red blood cell fatty acid patterns and acute coronary syndrome. *PLoS ONE*, **2009**, *4*, e5444. [CrossRef] [PubMed]
24. Harris, W.S.; Kennedy, K.F.; O'Keefe, J.H., Jr.; Spertus, J.A. Red blood cell fatty acid levels improve GRACE score prediction of 2-yr mortality in patients with myocardial infarction. *Int. J. Cardiol.* **2013**, *168*, 53–59. [CrossRef]
25. Sitkin, S.; Pokrotnieks, J. Alterations in Polyunsaturated Fatty Acid Metabolism and Reduced Serum Eicosadienoic Acid Level in Ulcerative Colitis: Is There a Place for Metabolomic Fatty Acid Biomarkers in IBD? *Dig. Dis. Sci.* **2018**, *63*, 2480–2481. [CrossRef] [PubMed]
26. Forouhi, N.G.; Imamura, F.; Sharp, S.J.; Koulman, A.; Schulze, M.B.; Zheng, J.; Ye, Z.; Sluijs, I.; Guevara, M.; Huerta, J.M.; et al. Association of Plasma Phospholipid n-3 and n-6 Polyunsaturated Fatty Acids with Type 2 Diabetes: The EPIC-InterAct Case-Cohort Study. *PLoS Med.* **2016**, *13*, e1002094. [CrossRef] [PubMed]
27. Shearer, G.C.; Walker, R.E. An overview of the biologic effects of omega-6 oxylipins in humans. Prostaglandins. *Leukot. Essent. Fat. Acids* **2018**, *137*, 26–38. [CrossRef] [PubMed]
28. Harris, W.S.; Thomas, R.M. Biological variability of blood omega-3 biomarkers. *Clin. Biochem.* **2010**, *43*, 338–340. [CrossRef] [PubMed]
29. Harris, W.S.; Kennedy, K.F.; Maddox, T.M.; Kutty, S.; Spertus, J.A. Multiple differences between patients who initiate fish oil supplementation post-myocardial infarction and those who do not: The TRIUMPH Study. *Nutr. Res.* **2016**, *36*, 65–71. [CrossRef]

9

10,12 Conjugated Linoleic Acid-Driven Weight Loss is Protective against Atherosclerosis in Mice and is Associated with Alternative Macrophage Enrichment in Perivascular Adipose Tissue

Jenny E. Kanter [1], Leela Goodspeed [1], Shari Wang [1], Farah Kramer [1], Tomasz Wietecha [1,2], Diego Gomes-Kjerulf [1], Savitha Subramanian [1], Kevin D. O'Brien [1,2] and Laura J. den Hartigh [1,*]

1 Department of Medicine, Division of Metabolism, Endocrinology and Nutrition, University of Washington Medicine Diabetes Institute, University of Washington, Box 358062, 750 Republican Street, Seattle, WA 98109, USA; jenka@u.washington.edu (J.E.K.); leelag@u.washington.edu (L.G.); sawang@u.washington.edu (S.W.); fkramer@u.washington.edu (F.K.); tomaszw@u.washington.edu (T.W.); gkjerulf@u.washington.edu (D.G.-K.); ssubrama@u.washington.edu (S.S.); cardiac@u.washington.edu (K.D.O.)

2 Department of Medicine, Cardiology, University of Washington, Box 356422, 1959 Pacific Ave NE, Seattle, WA 98195, USA

* Correspondence: lauradh@u.washington.edu

Abstract: The dietary fatty acid 10,12 conjugated linoleic acid (10,12 CLA) promotes weight loss by increasing fat oxidation, but its effects on atherosclerosis are less clear. We recently showed that weight loss induced by 10,12 CLA in an atherosclerosis-susceptible mouse model with characteristics similar to human metabolic syndrome is accompanied by accumulation of alternatively activated macrophages within subcutaneous adipose tissue. The objective of this study was to evaluate whether 10,12 CLA-mediated weight loss was associated with an atheroprotective phenotype. Male low-density lipoprotein receptor deficient ($Ldlr^{-/-}$) mice were made obese with 12 weeks of a high-fat, high-sucrose diet feeding (HFHS: 36% fat, 36% sucrose, 0.15% added cholesterol), then either continued on the HFHS diet with or without caloric restriction (CR), or switched to a diet with 1% of the lard replaced by either 9,11 CLA or 10,12 CLA for 8 weeks. Atherosclerosis and lipid levels were quantified at sacrifice. Weight loss in mice following 10,12 CLA supplementation or CR as a weight-matched control group had improved cholesterol and triglyceride levels, yet only the 10,12 CLA-treated mice had improved en face and aortic sinus atherosclerosis. 10,12 CLA-supplemented mice had increased lesion macrophage content, with enrichment of surrounding perivascular adipose tissue (PVAT) alternative macrophages, which may contribute to the anti-atherosclerotic effect of 10,12 CLA.

Keywords: alternatively activated macrophages; perivascular adipose tissue; type 2 cytokines

---

1. Introduction

Conjugated linoleic acids (CLAs), of which the major isomers are cis-9, trans-11 conjugated linoleic acid (9,11 CLA) and trans-10, cis-12 CLA (10,12 CLA), are microbial metabolites found naturally in ruminant animal food products and are major components of widely used CLA weight loss supplements [1–3]. Commercial CLA supplements differ significantly in the ratio of 9,11 CLA to 10,12 CLA (approximately 1:1) when compared to levels found in food (approximately 5:1). As such, CLA supplement users ingest significantly more 10,12 CLA than would be obtained from the diet.

Supplemental CLA promotes significant weight loss in animals and modest weight loss in humans, an effect now attributed to the 10,12 CLA isomer [4]. We have previously shown that 10,12 CLA reduces lipid accumulation by increasing fatty acid oxidation in a cell line derived from (mouse) 3T3 cells (3T3-L1) adipocytes [5]. Moreover, obese mice supplemented with 10,12 CLA lose body weight and fat mass due to enhanced fatty acid oxidation with increased energy expenditure and white adipose tissue browning [4]. These changes in energy expenditure are not the result of weight loss per se, as a control group undergoing caloric restriction to mirror weight loss by the 10,12 CLA-supplemented group did not exhibit these changes [4]. While the weight loss properties of 10,12 CLA are well established, if and how 10,12 CLA impacts atherosclerosis is less well-defined.

Studies of CLA supplementation in small animal models susceptible to the development of atherosclerosis have yielded mixed results. Initial studies in rabbits suggested that mixed CLA supplementation, an approximately equal mixture of the two most common isomers, 9,11 CLA and 10,12 CLA, was protective against atherosclerosis [6,7]. Subsequent studies have shown a similar effect in atherosclerosis-prone mice that lack the apolipoprotein-E gene (ApoE$^{-/-}$) when fed a diet containing mixed CLA [8,9], or a CLA diet containing 80% 9,11 CLA and 20% 10,12 CLA [10–12]. While these studies have shown atheroprotective effects of mixed CLA supplementation, there is also abundant evidence that CLA-containing diets do not provide protection from atherosclerosis, and may even contribute to its development [13–16]. Additional studies could clarify the impact of supplemental CLA on atherosclerosis.

Most previous CLA supplementation studies with the end point of atherosclerosis assessment utilized ApoE$^{-/-}$ mice. However, while these mice are an efficient model with which to study atherosclerosis, they poorly replicate human atherosclerotic lipoprotein profiles and co-morbidities such as obesity and insulin resistance. While ApoE$^{-/-}$ mice develop hypercholesterolemia due to elevated low-density lipoprotein (LDL) and very-low-density lipoprotein (VLDL), they also exhibit decreased high-density lipoprotein (HDL) [17]. Conversely, low-density lipoprotein receptor deficient (Ldlr$^{-/-}$) mice accumulate LDL and HDL cholesterol with more modest VLDL elevation, which more closely resembles dyslipidemic humans [18]. Humans inclined to take CLA supplements would likely be obese with characteristics of metabolic syndrome, including insulin resistance, hepatic steatosis, and systemic inflammation. As such, a better mouse model with which to study the effects of CLA supplementation on atherosclerosis would include these phenotypes, as well as the propensity to develop atherosclerosis. We therefore utilized Ldlr$^{-/-}$ mice consuming a diet high in saturated fat and refined carbohydrates, which has previously been shown to promote a phenotype closely resembling human metabolic syndrome [19], to study the effects of 10,12 CLA on atherosclerosis. In addition, and in contrast to previous studies, mice in this study were supplemented with individual isomers of CLA rather than mixed CLA in order to clearly identify effects due to 9,11 or 10,12 CLA alone.

2. Materials and Methods

2.1. Mouse Study Design

Ten-week-old adult male Ldlr$^{-/-}$ mice were randomized into treatment groups, and fed either normal chow or a high-fat, high-sucrose ((HFHS): 36% fat from lard, 36.2% sucrose diet with 0.15% added cholesterol) for 12 weeks (chow: n = 5; HFHS: n = 10–15). Mice were then switched to one of five test diets for an additional 8 weeks: (1) chow → chow diet; (2) HFHS → HFHS diet; (3) HFHS → HFHS + 1% 9,11 CLA; (4) HFHS → HFHS + 1% 10,12 CLA; (5) HFHS → HFHS + caloric restriction (CR). The study design is shown in Figure 1. CLA diets replaced 1% lard with 1% of either CLA isomer (>90%purity, Nu-Check Prep, Waterville, MN, USA). All test diets were prepared by BioServ (Flemington, NJ, USA) and have been previously described [4]. CR was begun at 85% total food intake per mouse and adjusted daily to mirror weight loss by 10,12 CLA, ending at an average of 74.4% CR after 8 weeks. HFHS, 9,11 CLA, and 10,12 CLA diets were fed ad libitum. Mice were individually housed for the duration of test diet feeding. Body weights were recorded weekly, and body composition, glucose and insulin tolerance, energy intake, and energy expenditure for these exact mice have been previously reported [4], with relevant phenotypes shown in Table S1. As such, this study adheres strongly to the "Reduction" component of the "Replacement, Reduction and Refinement (3Rs)" of animal research, as the same animals were utilized for multiple studies. At sacrifice, blood was collected and phosphate buffered saline (PBS)-perfused harvested tissues were snap-frozen in liquid nitrogen and stored at −70 °C or were fixed with 10% neutral-buffered formalin and embedded in paraffin wax. All experimental procedures were undertaken with approval from the Institution Animal Care and Use Committee of the University of Washington (#3104-01 03/15/13–02/28/19) and followed the guidelines of the National Institutes of Health guide for the care and use of laboratory animals (NIH Publications No. 8023, revised 1978).

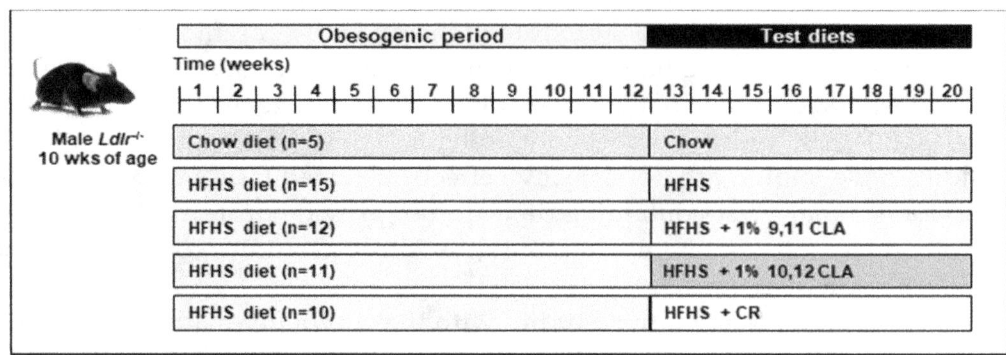

Figure 1. Study schematic. 10-week male low-density lipoprotein receptor deficiency (*Ldlr*$^{-/-}$) mice were fed either a chow or obesogenic high-fat, high-sucrose (HFHS) diet for 12 weeks, then either maintained on those diets or switched to a HFHS diet containing 1% 9,11 conjugated linoleic acid (9,11 CLA) (w/w), 1% 10,12 conjugated linoleic acid (10,12 CLA) (w/w), or calorically restricted (CR) on the HFHS diet to consume 85% of baseline food intake for an additional 8 weeks. wks: weeks.

2.2. *Plasma Analyses*

Triglycerides and cholesterol were measured from fasting plasma, and pooled plasma fast-phase liquid chromatography (FPLC) fractions using colorimetric assays as previously described [20]. Lipids were extracted from plasma using the Bligh and Dyer method [21], the fatty acid components were derivatized into methyl esters, and fatty acid compositions were quantified using gas chromatography as previously described [4]. Serum amyloid A (SAA) was quantified from plasma using enzyme-linked immunosorbent assay (ELISA) [22].

2.3. *Atherosclerosis*

Aortas were perfused with saline, the perivascular adipose tissue (PVAT) surrounding the thoracic aorta was completely removed and collected, and the thoracic aorta was excised down to the level of the diaphragm. PVAT samples were flash frozen and stored at −80 °C, and aortas were fixed in 4% formalin. Atherosclerosis from the aortic arch was quantified using the en face method using Sudan IV staining as described previously [23,24], and from the aortic sinus using Movat's pentachrome staining as described previously [25]. Quantification for total lesion size and necrotic core areas was performed blinded on digital images of stained tissue sections using Image Pro Plus analysis software Version 6 (Media Cybernetics, Inc., Rockville, MD, USA). Necrotic cores were identified and outlined for quantification using Image J software, as in shown in Figure S1.

2.4. *Immunohistochemistry*

Formalin-fixed, paraffin-embedded hearts were sectioned through the aortic sinus and stained with Movat's pentachrome for lesion quantification, Picro-Sirius Red for collagen quantification, and a rat monoclonal Galectin-3 (MAC2) antibody (1:3000 dilution, Cedarlane Laboratories, Burlington,

NC, USA) for relative quantification of atherosclerotic plaque macrophages. To further characterize plaque macrophage phenotypes, sequential sections were also stained with rabbit polyclonal antibodies against CD206 (Mannose receptor) to identify resident macrophages (1:100 dilution, AbCam, Cambridge, MA, USA). Area quantification for MAC2 and Cluster of Differentiation 206 (CD206) staining was performed on digital images of immunostained tissue sections using image analysis software Image Pro Plus software Version 6 (Media Cybernetics, Inc., Rockville, MD, USA).

2.5. Quantitative Real-Time PCR

Aortas were perfused through the left ventricle with RNA-later (Thermo Fisher Scientific, Waltham, MA, USA), excised from the heart to the diaphragm, snap frozen in liquid nitrogen and stored at −80 °C until processed. PVAT was completely removed from the aortas prior to freezing. Total RNA was extracted and purified using a commercially available kit (Qiagen RNeasy Mini Kit (Qiagen, Hilden, Nordrhein-Westfalen, Germany)). After spectroscopic quantification, 2 μg of RNA was reverse-transcribed, and the cDNA thus obtained was analyzed by real-time quantitative polymerase chain reaction (RT-PCR) by standard protocols using an ABI 7900HT instrument (Thermo Fisher Scientific, Waltham, MA, USA). Primer and probe set for individual genes (TaqMan system) were purchased from Thermo Fisher Scientific. Glyceraldehyde-3-Phosphate Dehydrogenase (GAPDH) was used as a housekeeping gene, levels of which did not change with the various treatments. Relative amounts of the target gene were calculated using the ΔΔCt formula and expressed as a fold change from HFHS-fed control mice. Accession numbers for Taqman primers used are shown in Table S2.

2.6. Bone Marrow-Derived Macrophage Culture

Bone marrow was isolated from donor C57Bl/6 male mice (n = 3) and differentiated into bone marrow-derived macrophages (BMDMs) in Roswell Park Memorial Institute (RPMI)-1640 medium (GE Life Sciences, Pittsburgh, PA, USA) that contained 30% L-cell conditioned medium over the course of 7 days. Non-polarized BMDMs were treated with media alone (control), lipopolysaccharides (LPS) (10 ng/mL for 4 h), interleukin-4 (IL-4) (10 ng/mL for 24 h), 9,11 CLA or 10,12 CLA (100 μM for 24 h, conjugated to bovine serum albumin (BSA, Sigma-Aldrich, St. Louis, MO, USA) as described previously [5]). In a separate experiment, BMDMs were treated for 24 h with 10% v/v serum that had been isolated from mice fed the HFHS diet with or without 1% 9,11 CLA or 1% 10,12 CLA. Total RNA was extracted from >1 × 10^6 macrophages and reverse transcribed for RT-PCR analysis as described above. To determine if CLA isomers influenced cholesterol loading, BMDMs were loaded with acetylated low-density lipoprotein (Ac-LDL, 50 μg/mL) in the presence or absence of 9,11 CLA or 10,12 CLA (100 μM) for 24 h. Intracellular cholesterol was quantified using an Amplex Red assay (Thermo Fisher Scientific), presented normalized to total protein content (bicinchoninic acid (BCA) assay, Thermo Fisher Scientific, Waltham, MA, USA).

2.7. Statistics

Data were analyzed using GraphPad Prism 6 software (GraphPad Software Inc., California, CA, USA) and are represented as means ± standard errors. One-way analysis of variance (ANOVA) was used to compare differences between mice receiving the different diets as indicated, and Bonferroni post-hoc testing was used to detect differences among mean values of the groups. A p value < 0.05 was considered statistically significant.

3. Results

3.1. Weight Loss by 10,12 CLA and CR Improves Plasma Triglycerides, Cholesterol, Fatty Acids, and Lipoprotein Profiles

We previously reported that mice supplemented with 10,12 CLA lost significant body weight and body fat, while mice calorically restricted to lose equivalent body weight lost mass equally from lean and fat compartments [4]. Control obese mice consuming the HFHS diet with or without 9,11 CLA remained obese [4]. Metabolic parameters such as glucose tolerance and energy expenditure have been reported previously [4]. Consistent with weight loss, 10,12 CLA supplementation improved plasma triglyceride (TG), cholesterol, and fatty acid (FA) levels when compared with obese HFHS-fed control mice with and without 9,11 CLA, as seen in Figure 2A–C. Circulating lipoprotein profiles measured using FPLC were similarly improved by 10,12 CLA, as seen in Figure 2D, with reduced cholesterol content of VLDL and LDL-containing fractions. While mice that had undergone CR lost equivalent body weight as 10,12 CLA-supplemented mice, they exhibited further improvements in plasma triglycerides (TG), cholesterol, fatty acids (FA), and lipoprotein profiles, as shown in Figure 2A–D. Moreover, plasma serum amyloid A (SAA), an acute phase reactant that becomes chronically elevated during obesity [26], was also improved by CR, as shown in Figure 2E, but not 10,12 CLA. Supplementation with 9,11 CLA had no effect on plasma lipids or SAA. Collectively, weight loss by both 10,12 CLA and CR resulted in improvements in plasma lipid levels, with significantly lower lipid levels and SAA seen following CR-mediated weight loss.

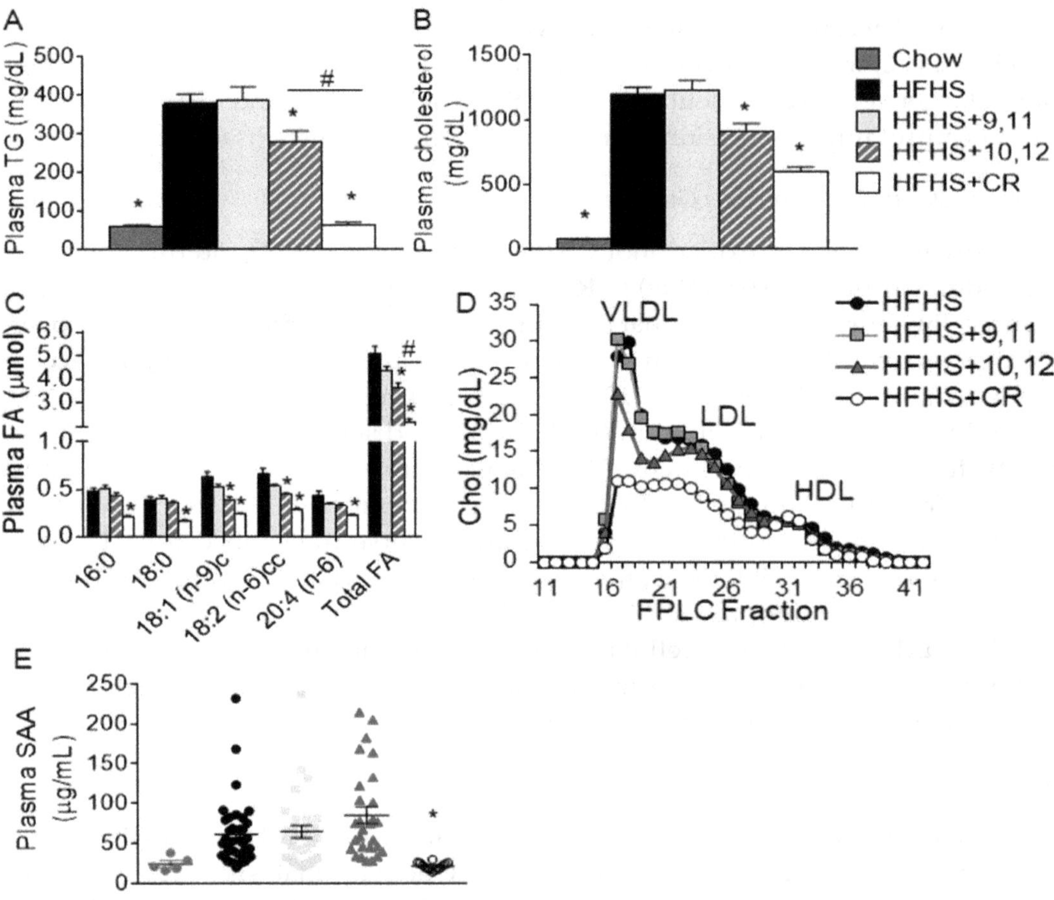

Figure 2. Fasting plasma lipid levels were decreased by 10,12 conjugated linoleic acid (CLA) and caloric restriction (CR). (**A**) Triglycerides (TG), (**B**) cholesterol, (**C**) fatty acids (FA), (**D**) fast phase liquid chromatography (FPLC)-fractionated cholesterol, and (**E**) serum amyloid A (SAA) were quantified from plasma following a 4-year. Fast in mice that had been fed chow or high-fat, high-sucrose (HFHS) diet for 12 weeks followed by 8 weeks of the indicated diets. Plasma samples were pooled prior to FPLC fractionation. Data are presented as mean ± standard error of mean (SEM), n = 5–15 mice/group. * $p < 0.05$ from HFHS control; # $p < 0.05$ from 10,12 CLA. LDL, low-density lipoprotein; VLDL, very-low-density lipoprotein; HDL, high-density lipoprotein.

3.2. Weight Loss Following 10,12 CLA Supplementation Improves Atherosclerosis

To determine if weight loss-mediated reductions in plasma lipids improved atherosclerosis, the extent of thoracic aortic atherosclerosis was evaluated using the en face technique. Obese mice consuming the HFHS diet with or without 9,11 CLA, shown in Figure 3A,B, displayed extensive atherosclerosis compared to chow-fed control mice, evident by increased Sudan IV staining. In contrast, mice supplemented with 10,12 CLA had significantly reduced levels of atherosclerosis, with no significant reductions following CR, despite having greater reductions in circulating lipid levels and systemic inflammation. To determine if the anti-atherogenic effect of 10,12 CLA was not an effect exclusive to the thoracic aorta, atherosclerotic lesions were quantified from the aortic sinus. Similarly, obese mice fed the HFHS diet with or without 9,11 CLA had extensive lesion development in the aortic sinus, as seen in Figure 3C,D. Also consistent with the en face analysis, 10,12 CLA supplementation significantly reduced aortic sinus lesion size, shown in Figure 3C,D, with no significant reductions following CR. Collagen levels were equivalent among treatment groups, shown in Figure 3E. Further, necrotic core areas represented a smaller proportion of atherosclerotic lesions in 10,12 CLA-treated mice as shown in Figure 3F,G. Taken together, 10,12 CLA supplementation significantly reduced atherosclerotic lesion area from both the aorta and the aortic sinus with reduced necrotic core size, with no significant differences evoked by CR-mediated weight loss or by 9,11 CLA. Thus, improved aortic atherosclerosis appears to be an effect specific to 10,12 CLA supplementation, and not weight loss or reduced circulating lipid levels per se.

3.3. Aortic Sinus Lesions Contain More Macrophages Following 10,12 CLA Supplementation

To further characterize the aortic sinus lesions in response to different diets, sections from the aortic sinus were stained for Mac2, a general macrophage-specific marker. As expected, obese mice fed the HFHS diet with or without 9,11 CLA or CR, shown in Figure 4A–C, exhibited higher Mac2-positive areas than lean chow-fed mice. However, mice supplemented with 10,12 CLA had significantly elevated Mac2 staining when expressed as total stained area or the percentage of total lesion area, as seen in Figure 4B,C. Gene expression from the aortic arches of a separate cohort of mice confirmed elevation of macrophage-specific genes Emr1 and Cd68 from mice given 10,12 CLA, as seen in Figure 4D. The lack of a corresponding increase in monocyte recruitment chemokines Ccl2 and Saa3 implies that the enrichment in lesion macrophages may not be due to increased monocyte recruitment, as shown in Figure 4F. These results suggest that while 10,12 CLA supplementation results in fewer atherosclerotic lesions, those lesions contain more macrophages.

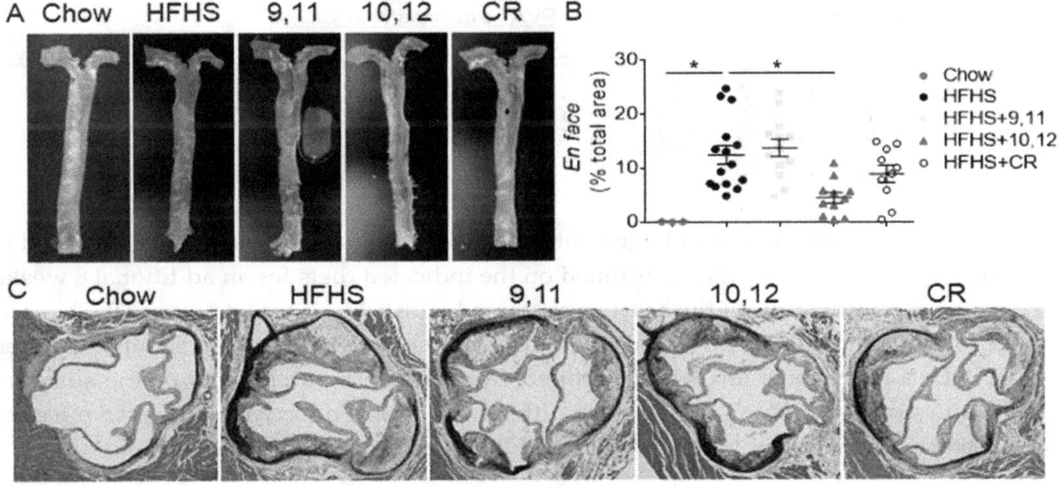

Figure 3. *Cont.*

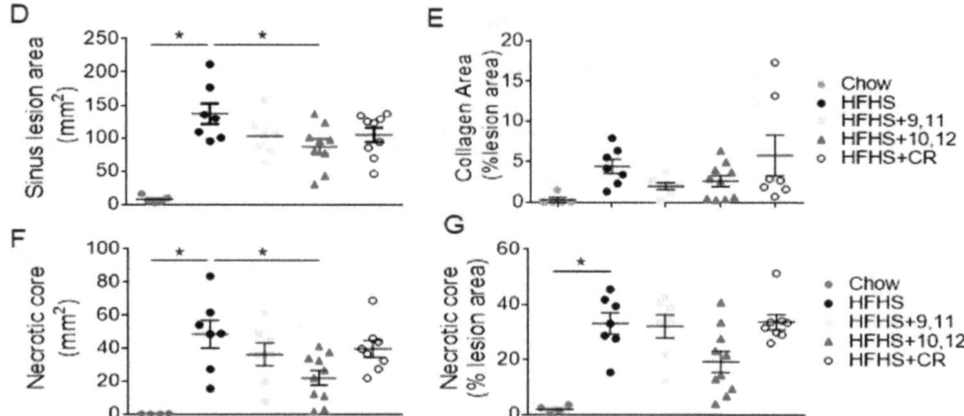

Figure 3. Atherosclerosis lesion size was decreased by 10,12 CLA, but not CR. Mice were fed either chow or HFHS diet for 12 weeks, then continued on the indicated diets for an additional 8 weeks. (**A**,**B**) Aortas were prepared en face (**A**), stained with Sudan IV, and lesions imaged and quantified using Image Pro Plus software (**B**). (**C–G**) Sections through the aortic sinus of the heart were stained with Movat's pentachrome, and lesion area (**C**), collagen (**D**), and necrotic core area (**F–G**) was quantified using Image Pro Plus software. Data are presented as mean ± SEM, n = 5–10 mice/group. * $p < 0.05$ from HFHS control.

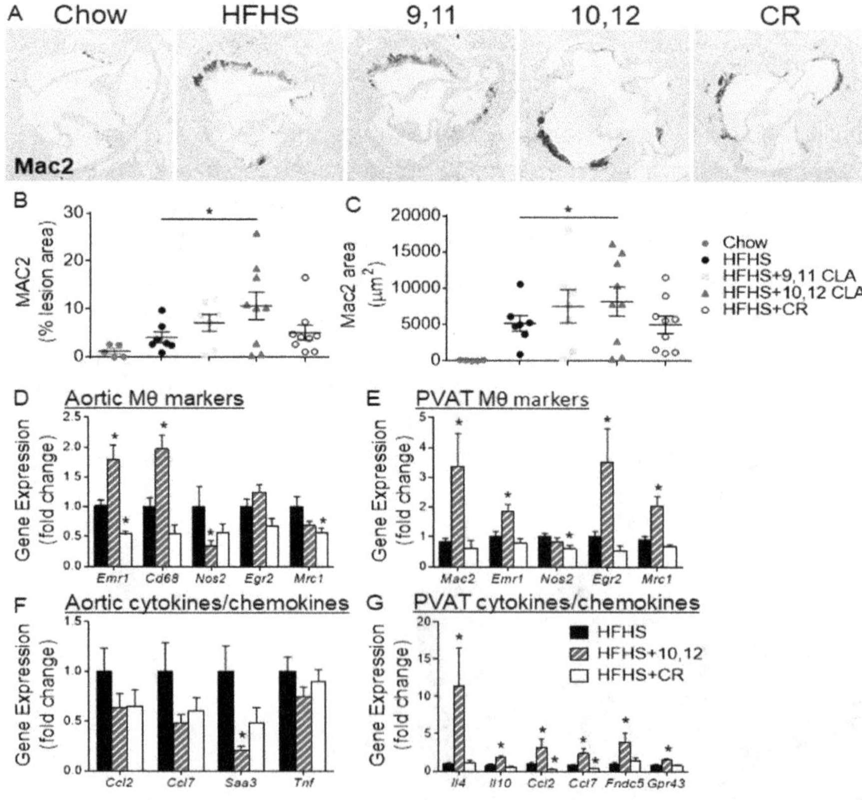

Figure 4. 10,12 CLA increases macrophage content of atherosclerotic lesions. Mice were fed either chow or HFHS diet for 12 weeks, then continued on the indicated diets for an additional 8 weeks. (**A**) Sections through the aortic sinus of the heart were stained with a Mac2 antibody, and (**B**,**C**) quantified using Image Pro Plus software. n = 5–10 mice/group. Different letters indicate a significant difference ($p < 0.05$). (**D–G**) Gene expression was quantified from the aortic arch (**D**,**F**) or the surrounding perivascular adipose tissue (PVAT, **E**,**G**) from a different cohort of different mice. n = 8 mice/group. Data are presented as mean ± SEM. * $p < 0.05$ from HFHS control.

Macrophages are generally classified based on their function, stratified as "classically", "alternatively", or "metabolically" activated [27]. Classically-activated macrophages will be defined herein as those that express Nos2 and secrete pro-inflammatory cytokines such as tumor necrosis factor (TNF), while alternatively-activated, or resident, macrophages express Egr2 and secrete type-2 cytokines such as IL-4 [27]. A previous study in the exact same mice presented herein showed that adipose tissue from 10,12 CLA-treated mice exhibited a significant elevation in gene expression for markers indicative of alternative activation, or resident M2 macrophages, including Arg1 and Egr2 [4]. To determine if the elevation of macrophages in sinus lesions was due to enrichment in M2 macrophages, sinus sections were stained for the mannose receptor, CD206. As shown in Figure S2A, there were no differences in CD206 staining between groups. Gene expression from aortic arches confirmed the lack of enrichment in resident macrophage markers *Egr2* and *Mrc1* (encodes CD206), with a significant reduction in the M1 marker *Nos2*, as seen in Figure 4D, promoting a reduction in the M1/M2 ratio shown in Figure S2B. This suggests that M2 macrophages may predominate in 10,12 CLA-supplemented mouse aortas. In contrast, perivascular adipose tissue (PVAT) surrounding the aortic arches was enriched in the general macrophage markers *Mac2* and *Emr1* as well as resident macrophage markers *Egr2* and *Mrc1* following 10,12 CLA supplementation as seen in Figure 4E. Moreover, PVAT from 10,12 CLA-supplemented mice was enriched with type-2 cytokine expression, including *Il4* and *Il10*, further supporting an M2 phenotype. Expression of chemokines *Ccl2* and *Ccl7* was increased in PVAT in response to 10,12 CLA, shown in Figure 4G, suggesting the recruitment of new macrophages. Finally, *Fndc5*, the gene encoding the browning marker irisin, and *Gpr43*, a major short-chain fatty acid (SCFA) receptor, were also enriched in PVAT from 10,12 CLA-treated mice, as seen in Figure 4G, supporting the known effects of 10,12 CLA to promote the browning of adipose tissue and increases in fecal and systemic SCFA [4,28]. In summary, while 10,12 CLA increased the macrophage content of aortic and sinus lesions and the surrounding PVAT, macrophage polarization towards a resident M2 phenotype was only observed in PVAT.

3.4. 10,12 CLA Induces a Resident Alternatively-Activated Macrophage Phenotype

To further examine what effect 10,12 CLA has on macrophage polarization in vitro, bone marrow-derived macrophages (BMDMs) were cultured with or without agents known to polarize macrophages towards classically- or alternatively-activated profiles. As shown in Figure 5A–F, BMDMs that have been classically-activated by treatment with lipopolysaccharide (LPS) express high levels of type-1 cytokines *Il1β* and *Tnf* and the classic marker of classically activated macrophages *Nos2*, while BMDMs that have been alternatively-activated by IL-4 treatment express *Il4*, *Arg1*, and *Egr2*, markers that have been previously associated with resident macrophage populations [29]. BMDMs treated with 10,12 CLA express a similar complement of markers as those treated with IL-4, as seen in Figure 5A–F, suggesting that 10,12 CLA promotes an alternative macrophage phenotype. Further, BMDMs treated with 10% serum collected from mice that had been fed a HFHS diet that contained 10,12 CLA, as in Figure 1, exhibited a similar gene expression profile as shown in Figure 5G–L, suggesting that a component of the serum in 10,12 CLA-supplemented mice promotes the alternative activation of macrophages. Co-treatment with 9,11 CLA or 10,12 CLA had no impact on acetylated LDL-mediated cholesterol loading of BMDMs as seen in Figure S3. Collectively, these results suggest that 10,12 CLA: (1) reduces plasma lipid levels and atherosclerotic lesion area, (2) increases atherosclerotic lesion macrophage content, and (3) polarizes the surrounding adipose tissue macrophages towards an alternative phenotype.

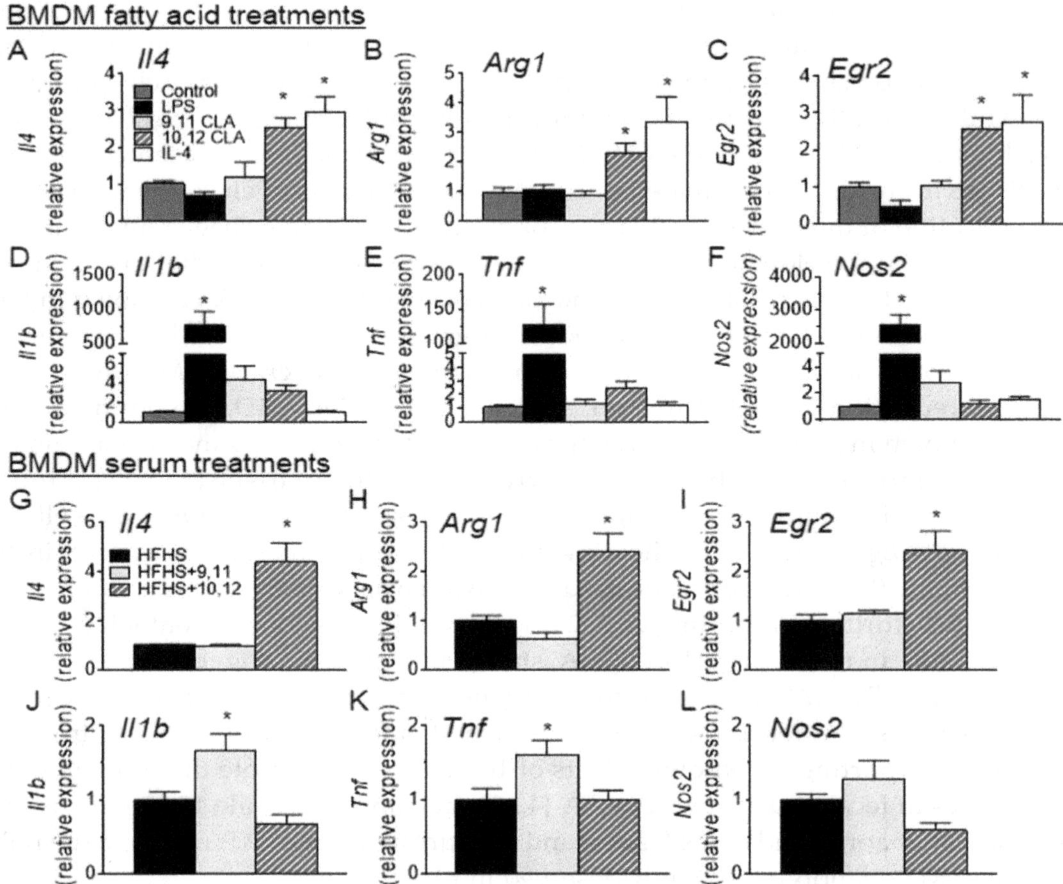

Figure 5. 10,12 CLA promotes the alternative polarization of macrophages in vitro. (**A–F**) bone marrow-derived macrophages (BMDMs) were treated with media alone (control), lipopolysaccharides (LPS) (10 ng/mL for 4 h), interleukin-4 (IL-4) (10 ng/mL for 24 h), or 10,12 CLA (100 µM for 24 h). (**G–L**) BMDMs were treated for 24 h with 10% serum isolated from mice fed a HFHS diet with or without 1% 9,11 or 10,12 CLA. Total RNA was extracted from $>1 \times 10^6$ macrophages and reverse transcribed for real-time quantitative polymerase chain reaction (RT-PCR) analysis. $n = 3$; data are presented as mean ± SEM. * $p < 0.05$ from media or HFHS control.

4. Discussion

While it has been suggested that mixed CLA supplementation may have anti-atherogenic properties in certain mouse models [8–12,30], we now show for the first time that obese HFHS diet-fed Ldlr$^{-/-}$ mice, which represent a more humanized model of metabolic syndrome, are protected from atherosclerosis following CLA supplementation, and that the 10,12 isomer of CLA is responsible for this protection. Further, the anti-atherosclerotic effects of 10,12 CLA may be independent from its weight loss and lipid-lowering effects, as a weight-matched control group undergoing CR-mediated weight loss does not exhibit equivalent atheroprotection. Moreover, a potential mechanism by which 10,12 CLA is atheroprotective may involve its effects on local macrophage populations.

It is well known that dramatic lipid-lowering therapies, such as statins or PCSK9 inhibitors, improve atherosclerosis in humans and mice [31,32], and that atherosclerosis has a strong inflammatory component [33]. It is therefore striking that 10,12 CLA supplementation resulted in reduced atherosclerotic lesion size while CR did not, despite profoundly improved systemic triglyceride, cholesterol, and SAA levels by CR. It is possible that CR-mediated improvements in lipids and SAA were insufficient to modulate atherosclerosis in the time frame of this study. It is also possible that the improvements in systemic lipids and inflammation by CR were trumped by a lack of improvement at the local tissue level.

The reduction of atherosclerosis by 10,12 CLA supplementation was also striking, given the increased macrophage content of those lesions. It has been previously reported that atherosclerosis regression in response to thiazolidinedione treatment occurs despite increased lesion macrophage content [34], which were identified as largely resident M2 macrophages. Moreover, it is becoming increasingly appreciated that M2 macrophages support lesion regression by resolving inflammation and promoting tissue remodeling [34–36]. Mice deficient in transcription factors that are required for M2 polarization have accelerated atherosclerosis [37], while administering type-2 cytokines such as IL-4 to mice protects against atherosclerosis [38]. Thus, it is tempting to speculate that the reduction in atherosclerosis in response to 10,12 CLA is due to enhanced M2 macrophage content. Indeed, we previously showed that these exact same mice supplemented with 10,12 CLA had increased markers of alternatively activated macrophages within adipose tissue as seen in Table S1 [4]. The polarization towards an M2 phenotype could explain the increased macrophage content, as IL-4 (which is secreted from M2 macrophages) is a strong stimulus for macrophage proliferation [39]. While we did not observe appreciable changes in alternative macrophage markers directly quantified from atherosclerotic lesions in these mice, it is possible that a more sensitive method such as analysis of laser capture microdissected macrophages would reveal a more robust effect. Nevertheless, the observed decrease in the M1/M2 ratio within the aortas of 10,12 CLA-treated mice suggest that M2 macrophages play a more dominant role, supporting previous observations that the M1/M2 ratio is positively correlated with the severity of coronary artery disease [40]. Notably, and in contrast to the current study, a growing body of work suggests that IL-4 may exert pro-atherogenic effects by accelerating endothelial cell apoptosis and/or enhancing vascular inflammation and oxidative stress [41–47]. While we did not observe enhanced inflammation (i.e., increased *Tnf*, *Saa3*, or *Ccl2*) in aortic or PVAT tissue from mice supplemented with 10,12 CLA, nor in macrophages treated with IL-4, whether the observed increase in IL-4 is causally associated with improved atherosclerosis in these mice remains to be explored.

The lesion microenvironment, which includes adjacent PVAT, is thought to be important for atherosclerotic progression and/or regression [48]. Mice deficient in PVAT exhibit endothelial dysfunction, and lose cold-mediated protection from atherosclerosis [49]. Our observation that resident macrophages and anti-inflammatory signals are enriched in the PVAT immediately adjacent to the aorta suggests that a signal from the PVAT may confer atheroprotection. It is possible that the "alternative" M2 milieu in the lesion microenvironment (in this case PVAT) promotes regression of atherosclerosis and/or plaque stabilization, as is evidenced by the reduced necrotic core size. Previous observations in humans support this notion, as epicardial adipose tissue M1:M2 macrophage ratios positively correlate with the severity of coronary artery disease [40]. PVAT is a plastic adipose tissue depot, and can possess a phenotype resembling brown adipose tissue [50]. As we have previously shown that 10,12 CLA supplementation promotes the browning and M2 macrophage enrichment of white adipose tissue [4], and we now show that PVAT in these mice expresses elevated levels of irisin and the M2 markers *Egr2* and *Mrc1*, it is plausible that M2 macrophage-containing PVAT secretes factors that promote atherosclerosis regression. Future PVAT transplantation studies could address whether this is the case.

In addition to changes in adipose tissue, 10,12 CLA consumption promotes significant alterations to the gut microbiota, characterized by increased abundance of species that produce SCFAs such as acetate and butyrate [28]. Metabolic diseases such as atherosclerosis are associated with decreased SCFA-producing bacteria such as the butyrate-producing genera *Butyrivibrio* and *Roseburia* [51]. In our previous study using the exact same mice presented herein, *Butyrivibrio* and *Roseburia* species were significantly enriched in the gut microbiota of mice given 10,12 CLA [28]. Atherosclerosis-prone $ApoE^{-/-}$ mice fed a butyrate-supplemented chow diet are protected from atherosclerosis [52,53], and mounting evidence shows that butyrate blunts macrophage inflammation [54–56], suggesting that butyrate has anti-atherogenic properties. Further, evidence suggests that butyrate promotes macrophage M2 polarization [57]. Thus, it is tempting to speculate that at least part of the atheroprotection incurred by 10,12 CLA may be related to its effects on the gut microbiota and gut-derived SCFA.

In conclusion, mice supplemented with 10,12 CLA experience reduced atherosclerosis and an anti-inflammatory, M2-like state in the aortic lesion microenvironment. Mice that are calorically restricted with markedly lowered cholesterol, triglyceride, and systemic inflammation do not experience such atheroprotection, suggesting that alterations to the aortic microenvironment may be more effective at impacting atherosclerosis. Future studies will evaluate a causal role for PVAT components and the gut microbiota in promoting atherosclerosis regression.

Author Contributions: Data curation, J.E.K., L.G., S.W., F.K., T.W., D.G.-K. and L.J.d.H.; Formal analysis, J.E.K., S.W., T.W., K.D.O. and L.J.d.H.; Funding acquisition, L.J.d.H.; Investigation, S.S. and L.J.d.H.; Methodology, J.E.K., S.W., F.K., T.W. and L.J.d.H.; Supervision, L.J.d.H.; Validation, J.E.K., S.W., T.W. and L.J.d.H.; Writing—original draft, L.J.d.H.; Writing—review & editing, J.E.K., L.G., S.W., F.K., T.W., D.G.-K., S.S. and K.D.O.

Acknowledgments: The authors utilized Metabolomics Core Services supported by the NIH Common Funds Project and the Nutrition Obesity Research Center, both from the University of Michigan. The authors acknowledge Alan Chait for critical review of the manuscript.

Abbreviations

CLA	conjugated linoleic acid
HFHS	high fat high sucrose
PVAT	perivascular adipose tissue
LDLR	low-density lipoprotein receptor
CR	caloric restriction
SAA	serum amyloid A
BMDM	bone marrow-derived macrophages
FPLC	fast phase liquid chromatography
TG	triglycerides
FA	fatty acids
SCFA	short-chain fatty acids

References

1. Ashwell, M.S.; Ceddia, R.P.; House, R.L.; Cassady, J.P.; Eisen, E.J.; Eling, T.E.; Collins, J.B.; Grissom, S.F.; Odle, J. Trans-10, cis-12-conjugated linoleic acid alters hepatic gene expression in a polygenic obese line of mice displaying hepatic lipidosis. *J. Nutr. Biochem.* **2010**, *21*, 848–855. [CrossRef] [PubMed]
2. Churruca, I.; Fernández-Quintela, A.; Zabala, A.; Macarulla, M.T.; Navarro, V.; Rodríguez, V.M.; Simón, E.; Milagro, F.; Portillo, M.P. The effect of trans-10, cis-12 conjugated linoleic acid on lipogenesis is tissue dependent in hamsters. *Genes Nutr.* **2007**, *2*, 121–123. [CrossRef] [PubMed]
3. Macarulla, M.T.; Fernández-Quintela, A.; Zabala, A.; Navarro, V.; Echevarría, E.; Churruca, I.; Rodríguez, V.M.; Portillo, M.P. Effects of conjugated linoleic acid on liver composition and fatty acid oxidation are isomer-dependent in hamster. *Nutrition* **2005**, *21*, 512–519. [CrossRef] [PubMed]
4. Den Hartigh, L.J.; Wang, S.; Goodspeed, L.; Wietecha, T.; Houston, B.; Omer, M.; Ogimoto, K.; Subramanian, S.; Gowda, G.A.; O'Brien, K.D.; et al. Metabolically distinct weight loss by 10,12 CLA and caloric restriction highlight the importance of subcutaneous white adipose tissue for glucose homeostasis in mice. *PLoS ONE* **2017**, *12*, e0172912. [CrossRef] [PubMed]
5. Den Hartigh, L.J.; Han, C.Y.; Wang, S.; Omer, M.; Chait, A. 10E,12Z-conjugated linoleic acid impairs adipocyte triglyceride storage by enhancing fatty acid oxidation, lipolysis, and mitochondrial reactive oxygen species. *J. Lipid Res.* **2013**, *54*, 2964–2978. [CrossRef] [PubMed]
6. Lee, K.N.; Kritchevsky, D.; Pariza, M.W. Conjugated linoleic acid and atherosclerosis in rabbits. *Atherosclerosis* **1994**, *108*, 19–25. [CrossRef]

7. Kritchevsky, D.; Tepper, S.A.; Wright, S.; Tso, P.; Czarnecki, S.K. Influence of conjugated linoleic acid (CLA) on establishment and progression of atherosclerosis in rabbits. *J. Am. Coll. Nutr.* **2000**, *19*, 472S–477S. [CrossRef] [PubMed]
8. Mitchell, P.L.; Karakach, T.K.; Currie, D.L.; McLeod, R.S. t-10, c-12 CLA Dietary Supplementation Inhibits Atherosclerotic Lesion Development Despite Adverse Cardiovascular and Hepatic Metabolic Marker Profiles. *PLoS ONE* **2012**, *7*, e52634. [CrossRef] [PubMed]
9. Franczyk-Zarów, M.; Kostogrys, R.B.; Szymczyk, B.; Jawień, J.; Gajda, M.; Cichocki, T.; Wojnar, L.; Chlopicki, S.; Pisulewski, P.M. Functional effects of eggs, naturally enriched with conjugated linoleic acid, on the blood lipid profile, development of atherosclerosis and composition of atherosclerotic plaque in apolipoprotein E and low-density lipoprotein receptor double-knockout mice (apoE/LDLR$^{-/-}$). *Br. J. Nutr.* **2008**, *99*, 49–58. [PubMed]
10. Toomey, S.; Harhen, B.; Roche, H.M.; Fitzgerald, D.; Belton, O. Profound resolution of early atherosclerosis with conjugated linoleic acid. *Atherosclerosis* **2006**, *187*, 40–49. [CrossRef] [PubMed]
11. McCarthy, C.; Duffy, M.M.; Mooney, D.; James, W.G.; Griffin, M.D.; Fitzgerald, D.J.; Belton, O. IL-10 mediates the immunoregulatory response in conjugated linoleic acid-induced regression of atherosclerosis. *FASEB J.* **2013**, *27*, 499–510. [CrossRef] [PubMed]
12. De Gaetano, M.; Alghamdi, K.; Marcone, S.; Belton, O. Conjugated linoleic acid induces an atheroprotective macrophage MΦ2 phenotype and limits foam cell formation. *J. Inflamm. (Lond.)* **2015**, *12*, 15. [CrossRef] [PubMed]
13. Kostogrys, R.B.; Franczyk-Żarów, M.; Maślak, E.; Gajda, M.; Mateuszuk, Ł.; Chłopicki, S. Effects of margarine supplemented with t10c12 and C9T11 CLA on atherosclerosis and steatosis in apoE/LDLR$^{-/-}$ mice. *J. Nutr. Health Aging* **2012**, *16*, 482–490. [CrossRef] [PubMed]
14. Cooper, M.H.; Miller, J.R.; Mitchell, P.L.; Currie, D.L.; McLeod, R.S. Conjugated linoleic acid isomers have no effect on atherosclerosis and adverse effects on lipoprotein and liver lipid metabolism in apoE$^{-/-}$ mice fed a high-cholesterol diet. *Atherosclerosis* **2008**, *200*, 294–302. [CrossRef] [PubMed]
15. Mitchell, P.L.; Langille, M.A.; Currie, D.L.; McLeod, R.S. Effect of conjugated linoleic acid isomers on lipoproteins and atherosclerosis in the Syrian Golden hamster. *Biochim. Biophys. Acta* **2005**, *1734*, 269–276. [CrossRef] [PubMed]
16. Arbonés-Mainar, J.M.; Navarro, M.A.; Guzmán, M.A.; Arnal, C.; Surra, J.C.; Acín, S.; Carnicer, R.; Osada, J.; Roche, H.M. Selective effect of conjugated linoleic acid isomers on atherosclerotic lesion development in apolipoprotein E knockout mice. *Atherosclerosis* **2006**, *189*, 318–327. [CrossRef] [PubMed]
17. Getz, G.S.; Reardon, C.A. Do the Apoe$^{-/-}$ and Ldlr$^{-/-}$ Mice Yield the Same Insight on Atherogenesis? *Arterioscler. Thromb. Vasc. Biol.* **2016**, *36*, 1734–1741. [CrossRef] [PubMed]
18. Getz, G.S.; Reardon, C.A. Diet and murine atherosclerosis. *Arterioscler. Thromb. Vasc. Biol.* **2006**, *26*, 242–249. [CrossRef] [PubMed]
19. Subramanian, S.; Han, C.; Chiba, T.; McMillen, T.; Wang, S.; Haw, A.R.; Kirk, E.; O'Brien, K.; Chait, A. Dietary cholesterol worsens adipose tissue macrophage accumulation and atherosclerosis in obese LDL receptor-deficient mice. *Arterioscler. Thromb. Vasc. Biol.* **2008**, *28*, 685–691. [CrossRef] [PubMed]
20. Lewis, K.E.; Kirk, E.A.; McDonald, T.O.; Wang, S.; Wight, T.N.; O'Brien, K.D.; Chait, A. Increase in serum amyloid a evoked by dietary cholesterol is associated with increased atherosclerosis in mice. *Circulation* **2004**, *110*, 540–545. [CrossRef] [PubMed]
21. Bligh, E.G.; Dyer, W.J. A rapid method of total lipid extraction and purification. *Can. J. Biochem. Physiol.* **1959**, *37*, 911–917. [CrossRef] [PubMed]
22. Den Hartigh, L.J.; Wang, S.; Goodspeed, L.; Ding, Y.; Averill, M.; Subramanian, S.; Wietecha, T.; O'Brien, K.D.; Chait, A. Deletion of serum amyloid A3 improves high fat high sucrose diet-induced adipose tissue inflammation and hyperlipidemia in female mice. *PLoS ONE* **2014**, *9*, e108564. [CrossRef] [PubMed]
23. Willecke, F.; Yuan, C.; Oka, K.; Chan, L.; Hu, Y.; Barnhart, S.; Bornfeldt, K.E.; Goldberg, I.J.; Fisher, E.A. Effects of High Fat Feeding and Diabetes on Regression of Atherosclerosis Induced by Low-Density Lipoprotein Receptor Gene Therapy in LDL Receptor-Deficient Mice. *PLoS ONE* **2015**, *10*, e0128996. [CrossRef] [PubMed]
24. Ding, Y.; Subramanian, S.; Montes, V.N.; Goodspeed, L.; Wang, S.; Han, C.; Teresa, A.S.; Kim, J.; O'Brien, K.D.; Chait, A. Toll-like receptor 4 deficiency decreases atherosclerosis but does not protect against inflammation in obese low-density lipoprotein receptor-deficient mice. *Arterioscler. Thromb. Vasc. Biol.* **2012**, *32*, 1596–1604. [CrossRef] [PubMed]

25. Umemoto, T.; Subramanian, S.; Ding, Y.; Goodspeed, L.; Wang, S.; Han, C.Y.; Teresa, A.S.; Kim, J.; O'Brien, K.D.; Chait, A. Inhibition of intestinal cholesterol absorption decreases atherosclerosis but not adipose tissue inflammation. *J. Lipid Res.* **2012**, *53*, 2380–2389. [CrossRef] [PubMed]
26. Zhao, Y.; He, X.; Shi, X.; Huang, C.; Liu, J.; Zhou, S.; Heng, C.K. Association between serum amyloid A and obesity: A meta-analysis and systematic review. *Inflamm. Res.* **2010**, *59*, 323–534. [CrossRef] [PubMed]
27. Chinetti-Gbaguidi, G.; Colin, S.; Staels, B. Macrophage subsets in atherosclerosis. *Nat. Rev. Cardiol.* **2015**, *12*, 10–17. [CrossRef] [PubMed]
28. Den Hartigh, L.J.; Gao, Z.; Goodspeed, L.; Wang, S.; Das, A.K.; Burant, C.F.; Chait, A.; Blaser, M.J. Obese Mice Losing Weight Due to trans-10,cis-12 Conjugated Linoleic Acid Supplementation or Food Restriction Harbor Distinct Gut Microbiota. *J. Nutr.* **2018**, *148*, 562–572. [CrossRef] [PubMed]
29. Martinez, F.O.; Sica, A.; Mantovani, A.; Locati, M. Macrophage activation and polarization. *Front. Biosci.* **2008**, *13*, 453–461. [CrossRef] [PubMed]
30. Toomey, S.; Roche, H.; Fitzgerald, D.; Belton, O. Regression of pre-established atherosclerosis in the apoE$^{-/-}$ mouse by conjugated linoleic acid. *Biochem. Soc. Trans.* **2003**, *31*, 1075–1079. [CrossRef] [PubMed]
31. Nissen, S.E. Halting the progression of atherosclerosis with intensive lipid lowering: Results from the Reversal of Atherosclerosis with Aggressive Lipid Lowering (REVERSAL) trial. *Am. J. Med.* **2005**, *118*, 22–27. [CrossRef] [PubMed]
32. Chapman, M.J.; Stock, J.K.; Ginsberg, H.N.; Forum, P. PCSK9 inhibitors and cardiovascular disease: Heralding a new therapeutic era. *Curr. Opin. Lipidol.* **2015**, *26*, 511–520. [CrossRef] [PubMed]
33. Ross, R. Atherosclerosis is an inflammatory disease. *Am. Heart J.* **1999**, *138*, S419–S420. [CrossRef]
34. Yamamoto, S.; Zhong, J.; Yancey, P.G.; Zuo, Y.; Linton, M.F.; Fazio, S.; Yang, H.; Narita, I.; Kon, V. Atherosclerosis following renal injury is ameliorated by pioglitazone and losartan via macrophage phenotype. *Atherosclerosis* **2015**, *242*, 56–64. [CrossRef] [PubMed]
35. Rahman, K.; Vengrenyuk, Y.; Ramsey, S.A.; Vila, N.R.; Girgis, N.M.; Liu, J.; Gusarova, V.; Gromada, J.; Weinstock, A.; Moore, K.J.; et al. Inflammatory Ly6Chi monocytes and their conversion to M2 macrophages drive atherosclerosis regression. *J. Clin. Investig.* **2017**, *127*, 2904–2915. [CrossRef] [PubMed]
36. Feig, J.E.; Vengrenyuk, Y.; Reiser, V.; Wu, C.; Statnikov, A.; Aliferis, C.F.; Garabedian, M.J.; Fisher, E.A.; Puig, O. Regression of atherosclerosis is characterized by broad changes in the plaque macrophage transcriptome. *PLoS ONE* **2012**, *7*, e39790. [CrossRef] [PubMed]
37. Hanna, R.N.; Shaked, I.; Hubbeling, H.G.; Punt, J.A.; Wu, R.; Herrley, E.; Zaugg, C.; Pei, H.; Geissmann, F.; Ley, K.; et al. NR4A1 (Nur77) deletion polarizes macrophages toward an inflammatory phenotype and increases atherosclerosis. *Circ. Res.* **2012**, *110*, 416–427. [CrossRef] [PubMed]
38. Cardilo-Reis, L.; Gruber, S.; Schreier, S.M.; Drechsler, M.; Papac-Milicevic, N.; Weber, C.; Wagner, O.; Stangl, H.; Soehnlein, O.; Binder, C.J. Interleukin-13 protects from atherosclerosis and modulates plaque composition by skewing the macrophage phenotype. *EMBO Mol. Med.* **2012**, *4*, 1072–1086. [CrossRef] [PubMed]
39. Jenkins, S.J.; Ruckerl, D.; Cook, P.C.; Jones, L.H.; Finkelman, F.D.; van Rooijen, N.; MacDonald, A.S.; Allen, J.E. Local macrophage proliferation, rather than recruitment from the blood, is a signature of TH2 inflammation. *Science* **2011**, *332*, 1284–1288. [CrossRef] [PubMed]
40. Hirata, Y.; Tabata, M.; Kurobe, H.; Motoki, T.; Akaike, M.; Nishio, C.; Higashida, M.; Mikasa, H.; Nakaya, Y.; Takanashi, S.; et al. Coronary atherosclerosis is associated with macrophage polarization in epicardial adipose tissue. *J. Am. Coll. Cardiol.* **2011**, *58*, 248–255. [CrossRef] [PubMed]
41. Rollins, B.J.; Pober, J.S. Interleukin-4 induces the synthesis and secretion of MCP-1/JE by human endothelial cells. *Am. J. Pathol.* **1991**, *138*, 1315–1319. [PubMed]
42. Lee, Y.W.; Kühn, H.; Hennig, B.; Toborek, M. IL-4 induces apoptosis of endothelial cells through the caspase-3-dependent pathway. *FEBS Lett.* **2000**, *485*, 122–126. [CrossRef]
43. Lee, Y.W.; Kühn, H.; Hennig, B.; Neish, A.S.; Toborek, M. IL-4-induced oxidative stress upregulates VCAM-1 gene expression in human endothelial cells. *J. Mol. Cell. Cardiol.* **2001**, *33*, 83–94. [CrossRef] [PubMed]
44. Walch, L.; Massade, L.; Dufilho, M.; Brunet, A.; Rendu, F. Pro-atherogenic effect of interleukin-4 in endothelial cells: Modulation of oxidative stress, nitric oxide and monocyte chemoattractant protein-1 expression. *Atherosclerosis* **2006**, *187*, 285–291. [CrossRef] [PubMed]

45. King, V.L.; Szilvassy, S.J.; Daugherty, A. Interleukin-4 deficiency decreases atherosclerotic lesion formation in a site-specific manner in female LDL receptor$^{-/-}$ mice. *Arterioscler. Thromb. Vasc. Biol.* **2002**, *22*, 456–461. [CrossRef] [PubMed]
46. Davenport, P.; Tipping, P.G. The role of interleukin-4 and interleukin-12 in the progression of atherosclerosis in apolipoprotein E-deficient mice. *Am. J. Pathol.* **2003**, *163*, 1117–1125. [CrossRef]
47. Lee, Y.W.; Lee, W.H.; Kim, P.H. Oxidative mechanisms of IL-4-induced IL-6 expression in vascular endothelium. *Cytokine* **2010**, *49*, 73–79. [CrossRef] [PubMed]
48. Tabas, I.; Bornfeldt, K.E. Macrophage Phenotype and Function in Different Stages of Atherosclerosis. *Circ. Res.* **2016**, *118*, 653–667. [CrossRef] [PubMed]
49. Chang, L.; Villacorta, L.; Li, R.; Hamblin, M.; Xu, W.; Dou, C.; Zhang, J.; Wu, J.; Zeng, R.; Chen, Y.E. Loss of perivascular adipose tissue on peroxisome proliferator-activated receptor-γ deletion in smooth muscle cells impairs intravascular thermoregulation and enhances atherosclerosis. *Circulation* **2012**, *126*, 1067–1078. [CrossRef] [PubMed]
50. Gil-Ortega, M.; Somoza, B.; Huang, Y.; Gollasch, M.; Fernández-Alfonso, M.S. Regional differences in perivascular adipose tissue impacting vascular homeostasis. *Trends Endocrinol. Metab.* **2015**, *26*, 367–375. [CrossRef] [PubMed]
51. Karlsson, F.H.; Fåk, F.; Nookaew, I.; Tremaroli, V.; Fagerberg, B.; Petranovic, D.; Bäckhed, F.; Nielsen, J. Symptomatic atherosclerosis is associated with an altered gut metagenome. *Nat. Commun.* **2012**, *3*, 1245. [CrossRef] [PubMed]
52. Aguilar, E.C.; Leonel, A.J.; Teixeira, L.G.; Silva, A.R.; Silva, J.F.; Pelaez, J.M.; Capettini, L.S.; Lemos, V.S.; Santos, R.A.; Alvarez-Leite, J.I. Butyrate impairs atherogenesis by reducing plaque inflammation and vulnerability and decreasing NFκB activation. *Nutr. Metab. Cardiovasc. Dis.* **2014**, *24*, 606–613. [CrossRef] [PubMed]
53. Aguilar, E.C.; Santos, L.C.; Leonel, A.J.; de Oliveira, J.S.; Santos, E.A.; Navia-Pelaez, J.M.; da Silva, J.F.; Mendes, B.P.; Capettini, L.S.; Teixeira, L.G.; et al. Oral butyrate reduces oxidative stress in atherosclerotic lesion sites by a mechanism involving NADPH oxidase down-regulation in endothelial cells. *J. Nutr. Biochem.* **2016**, *34*, 99–105. [CrossRef] [PubMed]
54. Cox, M.A.; Jackson, J.; Stanton, M.; Rojas-Triana, A.; Bober, L.; Laverty, M.; Yang, X.; Zhu, F.; Liu, J.; Wang, S.; et al. Short-chain fatty acids act as antiinflammatory mediators by regulating prostaglandin E(2) and cytokines. *World J. Gastroenterol.* **2009**, *15*, 5549–5557. [CrossRef] [PubMed]
55. Menzel, T.; Lührs, H.; Zirlik, S.; Schauber, J.; Kudlich, T.; Gerke, T.; Gostner, A.; Neumann, M.; Melcher, R.; Scheppach, W. Butyrate inhibits leukocyte adhesion to endothelial cells via modulation of VCAM-1. *Inflamm. Bowel Dis.* **2004**, *10*, 122–128. [CrossRef] [PubMed]
56. Lührs, H.; Gerke, T.; Müller, J.G.; Melcher, R.; Schauber, J.; Boxberge, F.; Scheppach, W.; Menzel, T. Butyrate inhibits NF-kappaB activation in lamina propria macrophages of patients with ulcerative colitis. *Scand. J. Gastroenterol.* **2002**, *37*, 458–466. [CrossRef] [PubMed]
57. Ji, J.; Shu, D.; Zheng, M.; Wang, J.; Luo, C.; Wang, Y.; Guo, F.; Zou, X.; Lv, X.; Li, Y.; et al. Microbial metabolite butyrate facilitates M2 macrophage polarization and function. *Sci. Rep.* **2016**, *6*, 24838. [CrossRef] [PubMed]

10

Medium-Chain Triglycerides Lower Blood Lipids and Body Weight in Streptozotocin-Induced Type 2 Diabetes Rats

Ming-Hua Sung [1], Fang-Hsuean Liao [1] and Yi-Wen Chien [1,2,3,*]

1 School of Nutrition and Health Sciences, Taipei Medical University, Taipei 11031, Taiwan; Glycine1016@hotmail.com (M.-H.S.); function0727@gmail.com (F.-H.L.)
2 Research Center of Geriatric Nutrition, College of Nutrition, Taipei Medical University, Taipei 11031, Taiwan
3 Graduate Institute of Metabolism and Obesity Sciences, Taipei Medical University, Taipei 11031, Taiwan
* Correspondence: ychien@tmu.edu.tw

Abstract: Medium-chain triglycerides (MCTs) are distinguished from other triglycerides in that each fat molecule consists of 6 to 12 carbons in length. MCTs and long-chain triglycerides (LCTs) are absorbed and utilized in different ways. The aim of this study was to assess the effects of replacing soybean oil with MCT oil, in a low- or high-fat diet, on lipid metabolism in rats with streptozotocin-induced type 2 diabetes mellitus (T2DM). There were, thirty-two T2DM Sprague-Dawley rats divided into low-fat-soybean oil (LS), low-fat-MCT oil (LM), high-fat-soybean oil (HS), and high-fat-MCT oil (HM) groups. After 8 weeks, blood sugar, serum lipids, liver lipids, and enzyme activities related to lipid metabolism were measured. Under a high-fat diet condition, replacement of soybean oil with MCT oil lowered serum low-density lipoprotein cholesterol (LDL-C), non-esterified fatty acids, and liver total cholesterol; whilst it increased serum high-density lipoprotein cholesterol (HDL-C) and the HDL-C/LDL-C ratio. A low-fat diet with MCT oil resulted in lower body weight and reproductive white adipose tissues compared to the HS groups, and higher hepatic acyl-CoA oxidase activities (the key enzyme in the peroxisomal beta-oxidation) compared to the LS group in T2DM rats. In conclusion, MCTs showed more protective effects on cardiovascular health in T2DM rats fed a high-fat diet, by improving serum lipid profiles and reducing hepatic total cholesterol.

Keywords: type 2 diabetes mellitus; medium-chain triglyceride; long-chain triglyceride; lipid metabolism

---

1. Introduction

Type 2 diabetes mellitus (T2DM) is the predominant form of diabetes worldwide and is accompanied with a heavy economic burden [1]. From a pathophysiological standpoint, persons with T2DM consistently show three cardinal abnormalities: (1) resistance to the action of insulin in peripheral tissues particularly muscles and fat; (2) defective insulin secretion, particularly in response to a glucose stimulus; and (3) increased glucose production by the liver. The pathogenesis of T2DM is complex and involves diet imbalances, life stresses, and obesity [2].

The prevalence rates of being overweight and obese in Taiwan, defined by the Taiwanese definition (body-mass index = 24~26.99 and $\geq$27 kg/m^2, respectively), were 22.9% and 10.5% for men and 20.3% and 13.2% for women, respectively [3]. Obesity reduces life expectancy and increases the risks of several non-communicable diseases (i.e., T2DM, hypertension, and dyslipidemia).

Medium-chain triglycerides (MCTs) are distinguished from other triglycerides in that each fat molecule is between 6 and 12 carbons in length. Medium-chain fatty acids (MCFAs) are transported in the portal blood directly to the liver, unlike low-chain fatty acids (LCFAs), which are incorporated into chylomicrons and transported through lymph [4]. Moreover, MCFAs do not require a carnitine shuttle system to penetrate mitochondria [5]. In β-oxidation, MCFAs cause the greatest induction of medium-chain acyl coenzyme A (CoA) dehydrogenase and increase the oxidation rate. Overall, the MCT transport pathway and the oxidation rate, differ from those of long-chain triglycerides (LCTs) [6]. The weight gain of rats fed an MCT-containing diet was 30% less than that of rats fed an LCT-containing diet [7]. MCTs have a reductive effect on body fat stores [8]. Body weight was significantly reduced (17%) in weanling rats fed high-MCT diets [9]. The decreased deposition of fat in MCT-overfed rats may result from obligatory oxidation of MCT-derived fatty acids in the liver [10]. MCT may decrease fat accumulation in adipocytes by increasing thermogenesis and satiety [11]. MCTs also improved plasma triglyceride and total cholesterol concentrations in rats [12].

Previous research, has verified that MCT oil has acceptable effects on body weight, fat, and blood lipids [7–10]. The aim of this study was to assess the effects of replacing soybean oil with MCT oil, in a low- or high-fat diet, on lipid metabolism and enzyme activities in rats with T2DM. The study had two hypotheses: (1) that MCTs improve cardiovascular health in T2DM, shown by loss of body weight and fat; and (2) that MCTs reduce serum and liver lipids accompanied by regulation of liver lipid metabolic enzyme activities.

2. Materials and Methods

MCT oil (lot no. 1959) was obtained from Kao Corporation (Tokyo, Japan). The fatty acid component percentages of the MCT and soybean oils were analyzed via gas chromatography [13]. The medium-chain fatty acid (MCFA) and long-chain fatty acid (LCFA) proportions of the MCT oil were 87.1% (containing 32.1 ± 0.5% caprylic acids, 37.9 ± 0.2% capric acids, and 17.2 ± 0.1% lauric acid) and 12.9%, respectively. There were no MCFAs in the soybean oil.

2.1. Animals and Diets

Male Sprague-Dawley rats (n = 60; aged 5 weeks with a body weight (BW) of 126~150 g) were obtained from Lasco (Taipei, Taiwan). Rats were housed individually in wire-bottomed stainless-steel cages, in an air-conditioned room (21 ± 2 °C and 50~70% relative humidity) with a 12-h light: dark cycle and free access to a basic diet and water for 1 week before diabetes was induced. Diabetes was induced via a high-fat diet (58% of calories as fat) for a period of 2 weeks, and an intraperitoneal injection of a low dose of streptozotocin (STZ) (35 mg/kg). After 2 weeks, a rat was considered diabetic when its fasting blood glucose concentration was ≥180 mg/dL [14]. At this point, baseline blood samples were collected from the tail vein of rats after anesthetization with ether gas. We then began to feed the rats with the experimental diets. Thirty-two T2DM Sprague-Dawley rats were divided into 4 groups, with similar average initial body weights. T2DM rats were divided into low-fat with soybean oil (LS), low-fat with MCT oil (LM), high-fat with soybean oil (HS), and high-fat with MCT oil (HM) groups. The LS diet per kilogram contained 70 g soybean oil (16% of calories as fat); the LM diet contained 35 g soybean oil (8% of calories as fat) and 38 g MCT oil (8% of calories as fat); the HS diet contained 254.4 g soybean oil (58% of calories as fat); and the HM diet contained 127.2 g soybean oil (29% of calories as fat) and 137.9 g MCT oil (29% of calories as fat). All diets contained 200 g casein and 50 g a-cellulose as fiber/kg of diet. Choline, cysteine, minerals, and vitamins were added as described in AIN-93 [15]. Calorie densities of low-fat diets and high-fat diets were 4 kcal/g and 5.1 kcal/g, respectively. The weight of animal diets was adjusted to fix total caloric intake and all rats received 109 kcal/day for 8 weeks. Calories from the daily food intake, during the experimental period did not differ among the groups (data not shown). After consuming the diets for 8 weeks, the rats were deprived of food overnight (~14 h); then they were anesthetized with ester. Blood was centrifuged at 3500 g at 4 °C for 10 min, and serum was collected. The livers and reproductive white adipose tissue (RDWAT) were removed. All samples were frozen at −80 °C until being analyzed. All animal experimental procedures followed published guidelines and were approved by the Institutional Animal Care and Use Committee of Taipei Medical University (Taipei, Taiwan).

2.2. Intraperitoneal Glucose Tolerance Test (IPGTT)

At 0 and 8 weeks, all rats were fasted for approximately 16 h and intraperitoneally injected with 50% glucose solution (0.1 mL/100 g), and venous blood samples were obtained at 0, 15, 30, 60, 90, 120 and 180 min to determine plasma glucose.

2.3. Assay of Serum and Hepatic Lipids

Blood glucose, triglyceride, total cholesterol (TC), high-density lipoprotein cholesterol (HDL-C), low-density lipoprotein cholesterol (LDL-C), and non-esterified fatty acid (NEFA) concentrations were determined spectrophotometrically using kits from Randox (Taipei, Taiwan). The serum insulin concentration was measured with a rat insulin enzyme-linked immunosorbent assay (ELISA) kit (Mercodia, Taipei, Taiwan). Triglycerides, cholesterol, and NEFAs in liver samples were extracted [16], and levels were measured using kits from Randox.

2.4. Enzyme Assay

The fatty acid synthase (FAS) activity assay, was based on measuring the initial rates of total NADP+ formation from NADPH, by cytosomes by an ELISA. The cytosomes in the medium were incubated with 2 M potassium phosphate, 20 mM dithiothreitol, 0.25 mM acetyl-CoA, 60 mM EDTA-2Na, and 0.39 mM malonyl-CoA, and the reaction was monitored at 340 nm [17,18].

The acyl-CoA oxidase (ACO) activity assay, was based on the method of Small et al. by an ELISA reader [19]. Liver postnuclear supernatant medium, were taken at 1% of total reaction volume and incubated with 11 mM potassium phosphate, 8 μg/μL horseradish peroxidase type II, and the 5% LAT mixture (contained 2.5 mM DCFH-DA, 4 M aminotriazole, and 20% Triton X-100). After 6 min (30 °C), 3 mM palmitoyl CoA was added. The reaction was monitored at 502 nm every minute for a total of 10 min, and the rate of H_2O_2 formation was calculated.

The acetyl-CoA carboxylase (ACC) activity assay [20], was based on measuring the initial rates of total NADP+ formation from NADPH, by cytosomes by an ELISA. Cytosomes in the medium, were incubated with 20 mM Tris-HCl, 10 mM $MgCl_2$, 10 mM potassium citrate, 3.75 mM glutathione, 12.5 mM KHCO3, 0.675 mM bovine serum albumin (BSA), 0.125 mM acetyl-CoA, and 3.75 mM ATP, and the reaction was monitored at 340 nm.

The carnitine palmitoyltransferase (CPT) activity assay [21], was based on measuring the initial rates of total free CoA (CoASH) formed by the 5,5′-dithio-bis-2-nitrobenzoic acid (DTNB) reaction from palmitoyl CoA by individual mitochondria with l(-) carnitine by an ELISA. Mitochondria in the medium, were incubated with 116 mM Tris-HCl buffer, 0.09% Triton X-100, 1.1 mM EDTA-2Na, 0.035 mM palmitoyl CoA (Sigma, Darmstadt, Germany), 0.12 mM DTNB, and 1.1 mM 1(-) carnitine. The reaction was monitored at 412 nm.

The assay of 3-hydroxy-3-methylglutaryl coenzyme A (HMG-CoA) reductase activity was based on measuring the initial rates of total NADP+ formed from NADPH, by microsomes by an ELISA. Microsomes in the medium, were incubated with 0.2 M KCl, 0.16 M potassium phosphate, 0.004 M EDTA, 0.01 M DL-dithiothreitol, 0.1 mM HMG-CoA, and 0.2 mM NADPH, and the reaction was monitored at 340 nm [22–24].

2.5. Histology

Livers and RDWATs were steeped in 10% formalin, dehydrated, and packed in wax. After 2 days, the specimens were stained with a hematoxylin and eosin solution.

2.6. Statistical Analysis

All data are expressed as the mean ± SEM. Data from multiple groups were compared by two-way ANOVA, and each group was compared with the others by Fisher's protected least significant difference (LSD) test. Statistical significance was defined as $p < 0.05$.

3. Results

3.1. Weight Gain and Organ Weights

Calories in the daily food intake during the experimental period did not differ among the groups. After 8 weeks of treatment, the average body weight in the HS group was higher than in the other three groups, and it was significantly higher than that of the LM group ($p < 0.05$, see Table 1). The average RDWAT (%) in the HS group was significantly higher than that of the LM group ($p < 0.05$). The average liver weight (w/w) in the HS group was lower than in the other three groups, and it was significantly lower than that of the LM group ($p < 0.05$). The average brown fat and kidney weights of rats did not differ among the groups (Table 1).

Table 1. Body and organ weights of type 2 diabetes mellitus rats fed the different diets for 8 weeks.

	LS	LM	HS	HM
0 week-Weight (g)	353.8 ± 11.5	354.1 ± 8.0	357.4 ± 18.7	350.6 ± 12.81
8 week-Weight (g)	373.1 ± 18.4 ^{ab}	340.3 ± 14.3 ^{b}	435.4 ± 12.0 ^{a}	392.8 ± 19.2 ^{ab}
RDWAT (g)	5.1 ± 1.0	4.9 ± 0.9	9.3 ± 0.9	8.4 ± 1.2
RDWAT %	1.2 ± 0.2 ^{ab}	1.2 ± 0.2 ^{b}	2.1 ± 0.2 ^{a}	1.9 ± 0.2 ^{ab}
BAT (g)	0.3 ± 0.1	0.3 ± 0.0	0.33 ± 0.0	0.34 ± 0.0
BAT %	0.1 ± 0.0	0.1 ± 0.0	0.1 ± 0.0	0.1 ± 0.0
Liver (g)	11.5 ± 0.6	12.5 ± 0.6	12.6 ± 0.4	12.1 ± 0.4
Liver %	3.2 ± 0.1 ^{ab}	3.4 ± 0.1 ^{a}	3.0 ± 0.1 ^{b}	3.1 ± 0.1 ^{ab}
Kidney (g)	3.0 ± 0.1	3.2 ± 0.1	3.7 ± 0.2	3.1 ± 0.1

Data are expressed as mean ± SEM ($n = 8$ in each group). LS, diet contained 16% soybean oil; LM, diet contained 8% soybean oil and 8% medium-chain triglyceride oil; HS, diet contained 58% soybean oil; HM, diet contained 29% soybean oil and 29% medium-chain triglyceride oil. RDWAT, reproductive white adipose tissue; BAT, brown adipose tissue. Values with different superscripts significantly differ at $p < 0.05$.

3.2. Blood Glucose, Insulin Concentrations, Intraperitoneal Glucose Tolerance Test (IPGTT) and Lipid Levels

After 8 weeks of treatment, blood glucose and serum insulin concentrations of T2DM rats did not differ among the four groups (Table 2). The LM group had the least area under the curve (AUC) of IPGTT, and the HS group had the greatest AUC of IPGTT (Figure 1). The LM group had a lower TG concentration than the HS group ($p = 0.07$) (Table 2). The blood TC concentration did not differ among the groups. The serum LDL-C concentration of the HS group was significantly higher than in the other three groups ($p < 0.05$), and that in the HS group was higher than that of the HM group alone ($p < 0.05$). The HS group had a lower HDL-C concentration than the HM group. Also, the MCT oil groups had significantly higher HDL-C values than the soybean oil groups, with both the low- and high-fat diets. The serum HDL-C/LDL-C ratio of the HM group was significantly higher than that in the HS group ($p < 0.05$), and the NEFA concentration of the HS group was significantly higher than that of the HM group ($p < 0.05$) (Figure 2).

3.3. Liver Lipid Levels

After 8 weeks of treatment, the low-fat diet groups had significantly lower hepatic TG levels, than the high-fat diet groups ($p < 0.05$, Figure 3). The HS group had the highest levels of the hepatic TG, TC, and NEFA. In groups with a low-fat diet, the hepatic TG, TC, and NEFA levels of the MCT oil and soybean oil groups did not significantly differ. However, the hepatic TC levels of the HM group, were significantly lower than those of the HS group ($p < 0.05$, Figure 3).

Table 2. Blood glucose, insulin, triglyceride, and total cholesterol concentrations of type 2 diabetes mellitus rats fed the different diets for 8 weeks.

	LS	LM	HS	HM
Blood glucose (mg/dL)	302.5 ± 15.4	287.9 ± 22.7	368.2 ± 32.8	297.9 ± 22.1
Insulin (ug/L)	0.4 ± 0.1	0.4 ± 0.1	0.5 ± 0.1	0.4 ± 0.1
Triglyceride (mg/dL)	55.9 ± 2.0	52.2 ± 1.8	69.2 ± 5.0	57.4 ± 3.6
Total cholesterol (mg/dL)	63.8 ± 3.3	63.3 ± 3.6	70.6 ± 1.6	64.2 ± 2.7

Data are expressed as the mean ± SEM (n = 8 in each group). LS, diet contained 16% soybean oil; LM, diet contained 8% soybean oil and 8% medium-chain triglyceride oil; HS, diet contained 58% soybean oil; HM, diet contained 29% soybean oil and 29% medium-chain triglyceride oil.

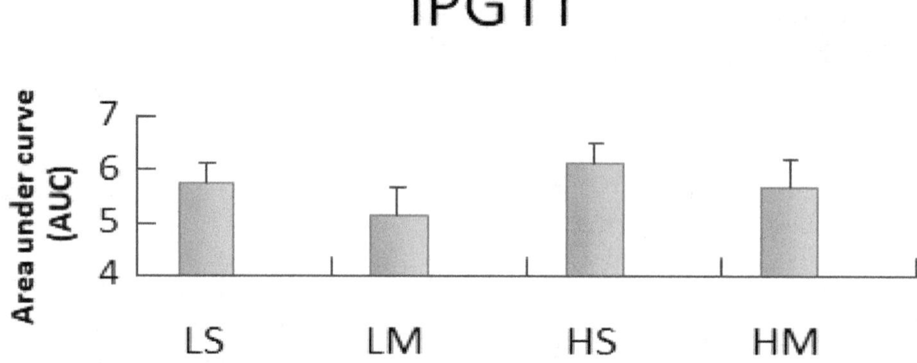

Figure 1. Area under the curve (AUC) of intraperitoneal glucose tolerance test (IPGTT) of type 2 diabetes mellitus rats fed the different diets for 8 weeks. Data are expressed as mean ± SEM (n = 8). LS: diet contains 16% soybean oil, LM: diet contains 8% soybean oil and 8% medium-chain triglyceride oil, HS: diet contains 58% soybean oil, HM: diet contains 29% soybean oil and 29% medium-chain triglyceride oil. All values are multiplied by 10^{-4}.

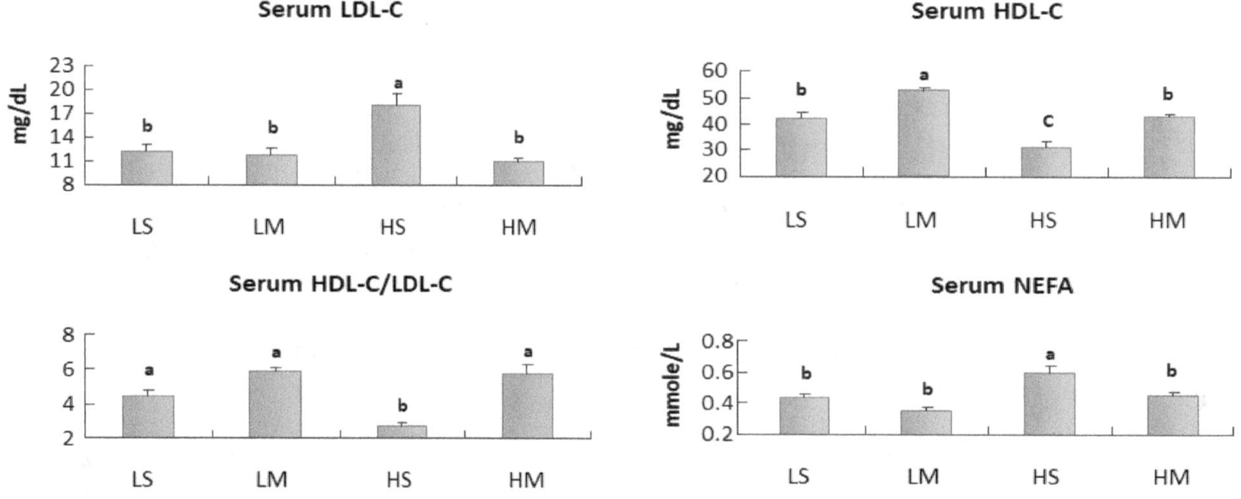

Figure 2. Serum low-density lipoprotein cholesterol (LDL-C), high-density lipoprotein cholesterol (HDL-C), the HDL-C/LDL-C ratio, and non-esterified fatty acid (NEFA) concentrations of type 2 diabetes mellitus rats fed the different diets for 8 weeks. Data are expressed as the mean ± SEM (n = 8). LS, diet contained 16% soybean oil; LM, diet contained 8% soybean oil and 8% medium-chain triglyceride oil; HS, diet contained 58% soybean oil; HM, diet contained 29% soybean oil and 29% medium-chain triglyceride oil. Values with different superscripts significantly differ at $p < 0.05$.

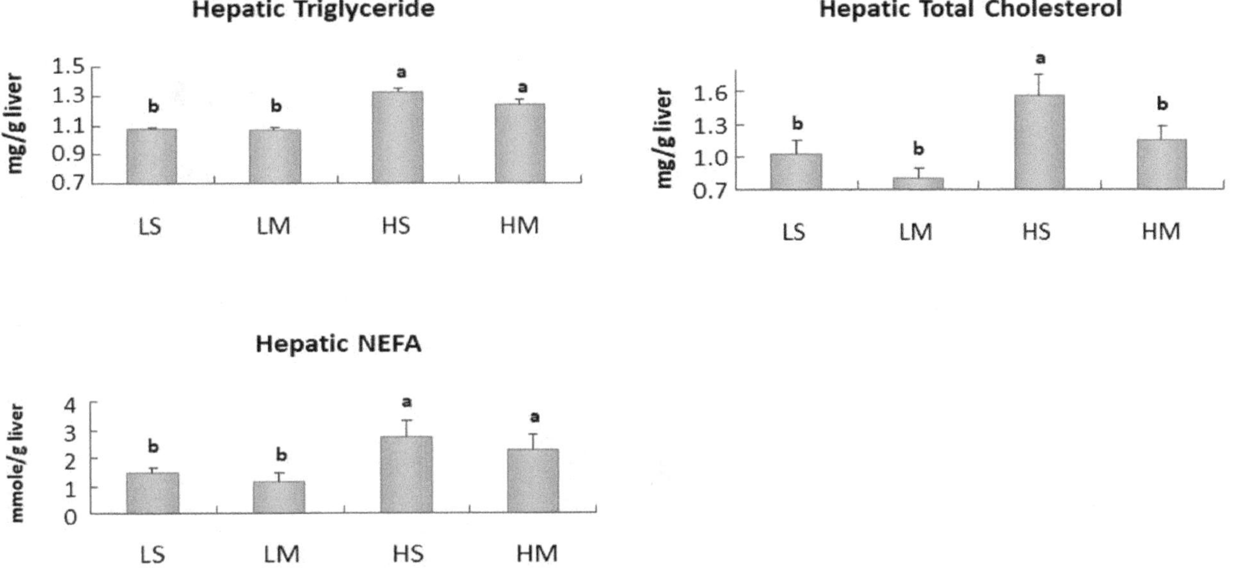

Figure 3. Hepatic triglyceride, total cholesterol, and non-esterified fatty acid concentrations of type 2 diabetes mellitus rats fed the different diets for 8 weeks. Data are expressed as the mean ± SEM ($n = 8$ in each group). LS, diet contained 16% soybean oil; LM, diet contained 8% soybean oil and 8% medium-chain triglyceride oil; HS, diet contained 58% soybean oil; HM, diet contained 29% soybean oil and 29% medium-chain triglyceride oil. Values with different superscripts significantly differ at $p < 0.05$.

3.4. Liver Enzyme Activity Assay

Hepatic FAS is the enzyme involved in de novo lipogenesis pathway, leading to the accumulation of fatty acids in tissues. After 8 weeks of treatment, no difference in hepatic FAS activity was found among the four groups (Figure 4). The formation of malonyl-CoA from acetyl-CoA was an irreversible process, catalyzed by ACC. T2DM rats, fed both low-fat diet groups had significantly lower hepatic ACC activities than those fed the HS group ($p < 0.05$). There were no differences in hepatic ACC activity between the HM group and the LM group. ACO is the key enzyme in the peroxisomal β-oxidation pathway. When the activity of ACO increases, β-oxidation increases. In T2DM rats fed low-fat diets, the MCT oil group had higher activity of hepatic ACO increases than the soybean oil group ($p < 0.05$). Liver carnitine palmitoyltransferase (CPT), is the key step in mitochondrial β-oxidation for long-chain fatty acid, binding to carnitine from cytosol to the matrix. T2DM rats fed a low-fat diet had significantly lower hepatic CPT activities than the high-fat diet groups ($p < 0.05$). HMG-CoA reductase, is the key enzyme for endogenous cholesterol synthesis in the liver. In groups with a low-fat diet, the MCT group had slightly less activity than the soybean oil group; the same result was found for the high-fat diet (Figure 4).

3.5. Histology

Examination of RDWAT slices showed that the HS group had the largest adipocytes, and the LM group had the smallest (Figure 5). The LM group had smaller adipocytes than the LS group; the same result was found in high-fat diet groups. The HM group had smaller adipocytes than the HS group. The liver tissue slice results showed that the two high-fat diet groups had more lipid droplets than the two low-fat diet groups, corresponding to the hepatic TG concentrations (Figure 5).

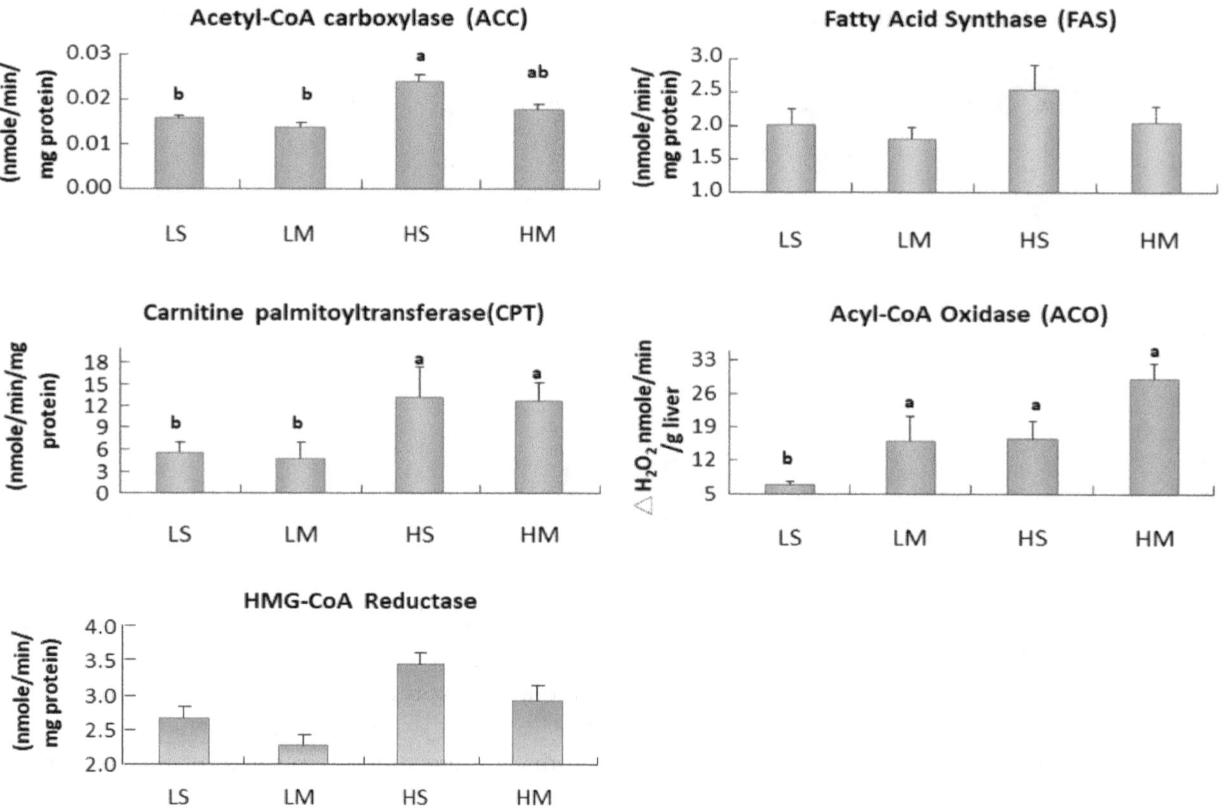

Figure 4. Liver acetyl-CoA carboxylase, fatty acid synthase, acyl-CoA oxidase, carnitine palmityltransferase, and HMG-CoA reductase activities of type 2 diabetes mellitus rats fed the different diets for 8 weeks. Data are expressed as the mean ± SEM ($n = 8$ in each group). LS, diet contained 16% soybean oil; LM, diet contained 8% soybean oil and 8% medium-chain triglyceride oil; HS, diet contained 58% soybean oil; HM, diet contained 29% soybean oil and 29% medium-chain triglyceride oil. Values with different superscripts significantly differ at $p < 0.05$.

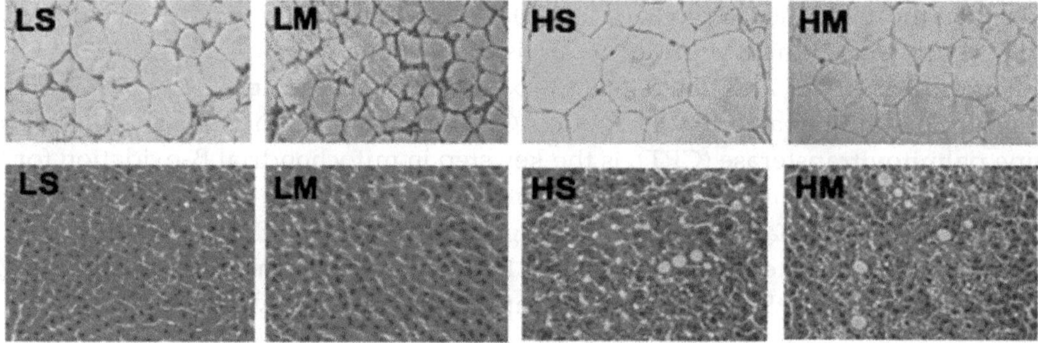

Figure 5. Reproductive white adipose tissues (upper row) and liver tissues (lower row) of type 2 diabetes mellitus rats fed the different diets for 8 weeks, shown with hematoxylin and eosin staining (10×). LS, diet contained 16% soybean oil; LM, diet contained 8% soybean oil and 8% medium-chain triglyceride oil; HS, diet contained 58% soybean oil; HM, diet contained 29% soybean oil and 29% medium-chain triglyceride oil.

4. Discussion

After 8 weeks of treatment, the body weight of diabetic rats consuming a high-fat diet with soybean oil was significantly higher than that of rats consuming a low-fat diet with MCT oil ($p < 0.05$). MCT undergoes faster and more-complete hydrolysis to MCFA than LCT to LCFA [25,26], and MCFAs are absorbed and oxidized more quickly than LCFAs, reducing body weight by decreasing fat accumulation [4–6]. However, the daily calories from food intake during the experimental period did not differ among the groups. Additionally, the body weight of the LS group was approximately 18% less than that of the HS group. Thus, the LM group compared with the HS group, not only had MCT oil, but also had a lower percentage of oil in the diet. The LM group had a significant decrease in RDWAT compared to the HS group. MCT reduces the percentage of body fat by increasing the activity of hepatic lipolytic enzymes (ACO) [6]. Thus, feeding a low-fat with MCTs-rich diet, caused a much greater reduction of body weight and adipose tissues in T2DM rats.

In the low-fat diet, the MCT oil group had a slightly smaller AUC (glucose) than the soybean oil groups; the same was found for the high-fat diet. Insulin resistance in mice is reduced by a low-fat diet [27]. Also, the area under the curve can be an index of the body's insulin resistance [28]. MCT oil consumption might have benefits to blood glucose levels and insulin resistance [27], although our results did not have statistical significance. In our study, the serum TG of the LM group was less than that of the HS group, and the serum NEFA concentration in the HM group was significantly lower than that of the HS group. MCT oil reduced hepatic TG synthesis by decreasing hepatic lipogenic enzyme (ACC) activity, increasing hepatic lipolytic enzyme (ACO) activity, and lowering serum TG [6]. Reducing the percentage of oil in the diet may have the same effect [29]. Thus, MCT reduced body fat more effectively with a low-fat diet. The serum LDL-C concentration of the HS group was significantly higher than that of the HM group. The number of hepatic LDL receptors is reduced significantly by high insulin concentrations [30,31]. High hepatic TC also diminishes hepatic LDL receptors [32]. Thus, MCT oil might increase the recovery of serum LDL-C, accompanied with the reduction in serum NEFA concentrations, by increasing hepatic LDL receptors, not hepatic HMG-CoA reductase activity. The most common form of atherosclerosis in diabetes, is induced by abnormal LDL-C metabolism [33]; rats in the HS group were most likely at risk of atherosclerosis. In addition, subjects with higher plasma small-dense LDL levels have up to a 3-fold increased risk of myocardial infarction [34]. Future research, may need to investigate the effect of MCT oil on advanced lipoprotein particles. The serum HDL-C concentrations of the MCT oil groups were significantly higher than those of the soybean oil groups, in both the low- and high-fat diets. Defective ABCA1 mediating the efflux of cellular free cholesterol, defective LCAT activity, or increased selective delivery of HDL cholesteryl ester to hepatocytes may be involved in the low HDL levels present with severe insulin resistance [35]. The serum HDL-C/LDL-C ratio of the HM group was significantly higher than that of the HS group. The HDL-C/LDL-C ratio can be a predictor of the risk of coronary heart disease [36]. Thus, the HS group might have the highest risk of coronary heart disease. Additionally, MCTs enhanced serum HDL-C concentrations, and may have achieved more efficient protection of cardiovascular health in T2DM rats fed a high-fat diet.

After 8 weeks of treatment, the low-fat diet groups had significantly lower hepatic TG and NEFA levels than the high-fat diet groups. A high-fat diet induced TG accumulation in adipose tissues. In T2DM, resistance to the action of insulin in adipose tissues increased NEFAs from TG hydrolysis and released them to the blood, and seriously high NEFAs in the blood were carried into the liver where the de novo synthesis of TGs occurred [37]. Hepatic TC levels in the HM group were significantly lower than those of the HS group; but hepatic HMG-CoA reductase activity in the HM group did not differ compared to that of the HS group. Takase et al. reported that hepatic HMG-CoA reductase activity was significantly lower in MCT-fed rats [38]. The reason why a high-fat with MCT oil diet reduced hepatic TC levels, accompanied with higher serum HDL-C levels, might be associated with hepatic LDL receptors [32] and other proteins, such as the hepatic scavenger receptor (SR-B1) and hepatic cholesterol 7-hydroxylase (CYP7A1), involved in liver cholesterol metabolism [39,40].

White adipose tissue is an energy storage and is related with insulin resistance of T2DM and cardiovascular complications of obesity. With a low-fat diet, replacement of soybean oil with MCT oil may improve fat oxidation by increasing hepatic ACO activities to reduce reproductive white adipocyte size. In some animal studies, the mean adipocyte size was smaller in MCT- than in LCT-fed rats [10]; those of the LM group were smallest. In obese and diabetic B6 mice that were switched from a high- to a low-fat diet, obesity was completely reversed [41]. Thus, the small adipocyte size of our LM group was related to consumption of MCT, accompanied with a reduction in the percentage of oil. Rats fed a higher-fat diet had higher ACC and FAS activities, and a faster hepatic lipogenetic pathway to accumulate TGs in the liver. The liver tissue slice results corresponded to hepatic TG levels.

5. Conclusions

Consequently, we concluded that MCTs can achieve more efficient protection of cardiovascular health in T2DM rats fed a high-fat diet, by improving serum lipid profiles and reducing hepatic total cholesterol. Moreover, T2DM rats fed a low-fat and MCTs-rich diet, had much greater losses of body weight and adipose tissues, compared with those fed a high-fat with soybean oil diet.

Author Contributions: M.-H.S. and Y.-W.C. were responsible for study design. M.-H.S. was responsible for data collection and analysis. All authors were responsible for writing the manuscript. None of the authors had a conflict of interest, either financial or personal, with this study.

Acknowledgments: This study was supported by a grant from the National Science Council of Taiwan (NSC95-2320-B-038-039). The authors gratefully acknowledge Hsing-Hsien Cheng for assistance with the Stabilwax-DA capillary column and G-3000 chromatograph detection system. The results/data/figures in this manuscript have not been published elsewhere, nor are they under consideration (from all our contributing authors) by another publisher.

References

1. Bommer, C.; Sagalova, V.; Heesemann, E.; Manne-Goehler, J.; Atun, R.; Bärnighausen, T.; Davies, J.; Vollmer, S. Global Economic Burden of Diabetes in Adults: Projections from 2015 to 2030. *Diabetes Care* **2018**, *41*, 963–970. [CrossRef] [PubMed]
2. Wu, Y.; Ding, D.; Tanaka, Y.; Zhang, W. Risk Factors Contributing to Type 2 Diabetes and Recent Advances in the Treatment and Prevention. *Int. J. Med. Sci.* **2014**, *11*, 1185–1200. [CrossRef] [PubMed]
3. Chang, H.C.; Yang, H.C.; Chang, H.Y.; Yeh, C.J.; Chen, H.H.; Huang, K.C.; Pan, W.H. Morbid obesity in Taiwan: Prevalence, trends, associated social demographics, and lifestyle factors. *PLoS ONE* **2017**, *12*, e0169577. [CrossRef] [PubMed]
4. Bach, A.C.; Babayan, V.K. Medium-chain triglycerides: An update. *Am. J. Clin. Nutr.* **1982**, *36*, 950–962. [CrossRef] [PubMed]
5. Johnson, R.C.; Young, S.K.; Cotter, R.; Lin, L.; Rowe, W.B. Medium-chain-triglyceride lipid emulsion: Metabolism and tissue distribution. *Am. J. Clin. Nutr.* **1990**, *52*, 502–508. [CrossRef] [PubMed]
6. Schönfeld, P.; Wojtczak, L. Short- and medium-chain fatty acids in energy metabolism: The cellular perspective. *J. Lipid Res.* **2016**, *57*, 943–954. [CrossRef] [PubMed]
7. Crozier, G.; Bois-Joyeux, B.; Chanez, M.; Girard, J.; Peret, J. Metabolic effects induced by long-term feeding of medium-chain triglycerides in the rat. *Metabolism* **1987**, *36*, 807–814. [CrossRef]
8. Lavau, M.M.; Hashim, S.A. Effect of medium chain triglyceride on lipogenesis and body fat in the rat. *J. Nutr.* **1978**, *108*, 613–620. [CrossRef] [PubMed]
9. Birk, R.Z.; Brannon, P.M. Regulation of pancreatic lipase by dietary medium chain triglycerides in the weanling rat. *Pediatr. Res.* **2004**, *55*, 921–926. [CrossRef] [PubMed]
10. Geliebter, A.; Torbay, N.; Bracco, E.F.; Hashim, S.A.; Van Itallie, T.B. Overfeeding with medium-chain triglyceride diet results in diminished deposition of fat. *Am. J. Clin. Nutr.* **1983**, *37*, 1–4. [CrossRef] [PubMed]
11. Hill, J.O.; Peters, J.C.; Yang, D.; Sharp, T.; Kaler, M.; Abumrad, N.N.; Greene, H.L. Thermogenesis in humans during overfeeding with medium-chain triglycerides. *Metabolism* **1989**, *38*, 641–648. [CrossRef]
12. Geelen, M.J.; Schoots, W.J.; Bijleveld, C.; Beynen, A.C. Dietary medium-chain fatty acids raise and (*n*-3) polyunsaturated fatty acids lower hepatic triacylglycerol synthesis in rats. *J. Nutr.* **1995**, *125*, 2449–2456. [PubMed]
13. Lepage, G.; Roy, C.C. Direct transesterification of all classes of lipids in a one-step reaction. *J. Lipid Res.* **1986**, *27*, 114–120. [PubMed]

14. Srinivasan, K.; Viswanad, B.; Asrat, L.; Kaul, C.L.; Ramarao, P. Combination of high-fat diet-fed and low-dose streptozotocin-treated rat: A model for type 2 diabetes and pharmacological screening. *Pharmacol. Res.* **2005**, *52*, 313–320. [CrossRef] [PubMed]
15. Reeves, P.G.; Nielsen, F.H.; Fahey, G.C., Jr. AIN-93 purified diets for laboratory rodents: Final report of the American Institute of Nutrition ad hoc writing committee on the reformulation of the AIN-76A rodent diet. *J. Nutr.* **1993**, *123*, 1939–1951. [CrossRef] [PubMed]
16. Folch, J.; Lees, M.; Sloane Stanley, G.H. A simple method for the isolation and purification of total lipides from animal tissues. *J. Biol. Chem.* **1957**, *226*, 497–509. [PubMed]
17. Erickson, R.H.; Zakim, D.; Vessey, D.A. Preparation and properties of a phospholipid-free form of microsomal UDP-glucuronyltransferase. *Biochemistry* **1978**, *17*, 3706–3711. [CrossRef] [PubMed]
18. Nepokroeff, C.M.; Lakshmanan, M.R.; Porter, J.W. Fatty-acid synthase from rat liver. *Methods Enzymol.* **1975**, *35*, 37–44. [PubMed]
19. Small, G.M.; Burdett, K.; Connock, M.J. A sensitive spectrophotometric assay for peroxisomal acyl-CoA oxidase. *Biochem. J.* **1985**, *227*, 205–210. [CrossRef] [PubMed]
20. Numa, S.; Ringelmann, E.; Lynen, F. On inhibition of acetyl-CoA-carboxylase by fatty acid-coenzyme A compounds. *Biochem. Z.* **1965**, *343*, 243–257. [PubMed]
21. Bieber, L.L.; Abraham, T.; Helmrath, T. A rapid spectrophotometric assay for carnitine palmitoyltransferase. *Anal. Biochem.* **1972**, *50*, 509–518. [CrossRef]
22. Edwards, P.A.; Gould, R.G. Turnover rate of hepatic 3-hydroxy-3-methylglutaryl coenzyme A reductase as determined by use of cycloheximide. *J. Biol. Chem.* **1972**, *247*, 1520–1524. [PubMed]
23. Edwards, P.A.; Lemongello, D.; Fogelman, A.M. Improved methods for the solubilization and assay of hepatic 3-hydroxy-3-methylglutaryl coenzyme A reductase. *J. Lipid Res.* **1979**, *20*, 40–46. [PubMed]
24. Heller, R.A.; Gould, R.G. Solubilization and partial purification of hepatic 3-hydroxy-3-methylglutaryl coenzyme A reductase. *Biochem. Biophys. Res. Commun.* **1973**, *50*, 859–865. [CrossRef]
25. Fernando-Warnakulasuriya, G.J.; Staggers, J.E.; Frost, S.C.; Wells, M.A. Studies on fat digestion, absorption, and transport in the suckling rat. I. Fatty acid composition and concentrations of major lipid components. *J. Lipid Res.* **1981**, *22*, 668–674. [PubMed]
26. Mascioli, E.A.; Lopes, S.; Randall, S.; Porter, K.A.; Kater, G.; Hirschberg, Y.; Babayan, V.K.; Bistrian, B.R.; Blackburn, G.L. Serum fatty acid profiles after intravenous medium chain triglyceride administration. *Lipids* **1989**, *24*, 793–798. [CrossRef] [PubMed]
27. Muurling, M.; Jong, M.C.; Mensink, R.P.; Hornstra, G.; Dahlmans, V.E.; Pijl, H.; Voshol, P.J.; Havekes, L.M. A low-fat diet has a higher potential than energy restriction to improve high-fat diet-induced insulin resistance in mice. *Metabolism* **2002**, *51*, 695–701. [CrossRef] [PubMed]
28. Monzillo, L.U.; Hamdy, O. Evaluation of insulin sensitivity in clinical practice and in research settings. *Nutr. Rev.* **2003**, *61*, 397–412. [CrossRef] [PubMed]
29. Gerhard, G.T.; Ahmann, A.; Meeuws, K.; McMurry, M.P.; Duell, P.B.; Connor, W.E. Effects of a low-fat diet compared with those of a high-monounsaturated fat diet on body weight, plasma lipids and lipoproteins, and glycemic control in type 2 diabetes. *Am. J. Clin. Nutr.* **2004**, *80*, 668–673. [CrossRef] [PubMed]
30. Kissebah, A.H. Low density lipoprotein metabolism in non-insulin-dependent diabetes mellitus. *Diabetes Metab. Rev.* **1987**, *3*, 619–651. [CrossRef] [PubMed]
31. Streicher, R.; Kotzka, J.; Müller-Wieland, D.; Siemeister, G.; Munck, M.; Avci, H.; Krone, W. SREBP-1 mediates activation of the low density lipoprotein receptor promoter by insulin and insulin-like growth factor-I. *J. Biol. Chem.* **1996**, *271*, 7128–7133. [CrossRef] [PubMed]
32. Fernandez, M.L.; West, K.L. Mechanisms by which dietary fatty acids modulate plasma lipids. *J. Nutr.* **2005**, *135*, 2075–2078. [CrossRef] [PubMed]
33. Betteridge, D.J. Diabetes, lipoprotein metabolism and atherosclerosis. *Br. Med. Bull.* **1989**, *45*, 285–311. [CrossRef] [PubMed]
34. Austin, M.A.; Breslow, J.L.; Hennekens, C.H.; Buring, J.E.; Willett, W.C.; Krauss, R.M. Low-density lipoprotein subclass patterns and risk of myocardial infarction. *JAMA* **1988**, *260*, 1917–1921. [CrossRef] [PubMed]
35. Ginsberg, H.N.; Zhang, Y.L.; Hernandez-Ono, A. Regulation of plasma triglycerides in insulin resistance and diabetes. *Arch. Med. Res.* **2005**, *36*, 232–240. [CrossRef] [PubMed]
36. Baliarsingh, S.; Beg, Z.H.; Ahmad, J. The therapeutic impacts of tocotrienols in type 2 diabetic patients with hyperlipidemia. *Atherosclerosis* **2005**, *182*, 367–374. [CrossRef] [PubMed]

37. Raz, I.; Eldor, R.; Cernea, S.; Shafrir, E. Diabetes: Insulin resistance and derangements in lipid metabolism. Cure through intervention in fat transport and storage. *Diabetes Metab. Res. Rev.* **2005**, *21*, 3–14. [CrossRef] [PubMed]
38. Takase, S.; Morimoto, A.; Nakanishi, M.; Muto, Y. Long-term effect of medium-chain triglyceride on hepatic enzymes catalyzing lipogenesis and cholesterogenesis in rats. *J. Nutr. Sci. Vitaminol.* **1977**, *23*, 43–51. [CrossRef] [PubMed]
39. Trapani, L.; Segatto, M.; Pallottini, V. Regulation and deregulation of cholesterol homeostasis: The liver as a metabolic "power station". *World J. Hepatol.* **2012**, *4*, 184–190. [CrossRef] [PubMed]
40. Xu, Q.; Xue, C.; Zhang, Y.; Liu, Y.; Wang, J.; Yu, X.; Zhang, X.; Zhang, R.; Yang, X.; Guo, C. Medium-chain fatty acids enhanced the excretion of fecal cholesterol and cholic acid in C57BL/6J mice fed a cholesterol-rich diet. *Biosci. Biotechnol. Biochem.* **2013**, *77*, 1390–1396. [CrossRef] [PubMed]
41. Parekh, P.I.; Petro, A.E.; Tiller, J.M.; Feinglos, M.N.; Surwit, R.S. Reversal of diet-induced obesity and diabetes in C57BL/6J mice. *Metabolism* **1998**, *47*, 1089–1096. [CrossRef]

11

Dietary Fats and Chronic Noncommunicable Diseases

Hayley E. Billingsley [1], Salvatore Carbone [1,*] and Carl J. Lavie [2]

1 Pauley Heart Center, Virginia Commonwealth University, Richmond, VA, 23298, USA; hayley.billingsley@vcuhealth.org
2 John Ochsner Heart and Vascular Institute, Ochsner Clinical School, University of Queensland School of Medicine, New Orleans, LA 70121, USA; clavie@ochsner.org
* Correspondence: salvatore.carbone@vcuhealth.org

Abstract: The role of dietary fat has been long studied as a modifiable variable in the prevention and treatment of noncommunicable cardiometabolic disease. Once heavily promoted to the public, the low-fat diet has been demonstrated to be non-effective in preventing cardiometabolic disease, and an increasing body of literature has focused on the effects of a relatively higher-fat diet. More recent evidence suggests that a diet high in healthy fat, rich in unsaturated fatty acids, such as the Mediterranean dietary pattern, may, in fact, prevent the development of metabolic diseases such as type 2 diabetes mellitus, but also reduce cardiovascular events. This review will specifically focus on clinical trials which collected data on dietary fatty acid intake, and the association of these fatty acids over time with measured cardiometabolic health outcomes, specifically focusing on morbidity and mortality outcomes. We will also describe mechanistic studies investigating the role of dietary fatty acids on cardiovascular risk factors to describe the potential mechanisms of action through which unsaturated fatty acids may exert their beneficial effects. The state of current knowledge on the associations between dietary fatty acids and cardiometabolic morbidity and mortality outcomes will be summarized and directions for future work will be discussed.

Keywords: cardiometabolic disease; unsaturated fat; Mediterranean diet; low-fat diet

---

1. Introduction

Cardiometabolic diseases are estimated to cause over 700,000 deaths per year in the United States (US) and nearly 50% of these deaths are directly related to diet [1,2], although this could be questioned due to so much data being based on potentially flawed food frequency questionnaires (FFQs) [3,4]. Numerous foods, dietary patterns, and individual nutrient consumption have been studied for associations with cardiometabolic disease and its risk factors, but few have received scrutiny as intense and lengthy as dietary fat. As early as 1953, Ancel Keys published a proposed link between dietary fat and cardiovascular diseases (CVD), and five years later, his Seven Countries study began collecting data in an effort to establish a relationship between diet and CVD [5,6]. During the same period, controlled-feeding studies demonstrated a link between increasing saturated fatty acids (SFA) in the diet and increased levels of total cholesterol and, more importantly, of low-density lipoprotein cholesterol (LDL-C), which were known to be associated with incidence of coronary heart disease (CHD) [7]. These controlled-feeding studies, in addition to observational evidence, were relied on as sufficient evidence that a higher total fat and SFA intake leads to an increased incidence of CHD by increasing plasma total cholesterol and LDL-C—the "diet-heart hypothesis" [7–9]. In response to this accruing evidence, the very first Dietary Guidelines for Americans in 1980 recommended lowering total fat and SFA [10], which was updated in 1990 to recommend Americans select a low-fat diet, specifically one that consisted of $\leq$30% total fat and $\leq$10% SFA of total daily energy [11].

In the decades following these recommendations, total dietary fat decreased in the American diet [12], refined grain intake increased [13], prevalence of type 2 diabetes mellitus (T2DM) continued to rise, and CVD remained the most common cause of death in US adults [14,15]. It is evident that perhaps the most important finding from the Seven Countries Study, that unsaturated fatty acids (UFA) were correlated with a lower risk of CVD in the context of a Mediterranean-style dietary pattern, was not properly communicated and implemented [16]. Evidence in favor of higher UFA consumption within a healthy dietary pattern has continued to accumulate and in 2015, the Dietary Guidelines for Americans was published for the first time in 35 years without a recommended limit on total dietary fat consumption while continuing to promote UFA consumption [17].

This review will discuss the evidence behind the recommendation of the low-fat diet for the past few decades as well as the evidence of UFA intake for cardiometabolic health by first reviewing morbidity and mortality outcomes. Finally, we will discuss the potential underlying mechanisms through which fatty acids may affect overall cardiometabolic health.

2. Methodology

To identify the works used in this critical review, the comprehensive electronic literature search using PubMed and Google Scholar included the use of the following key words and their combination: "Low-fat diet", "high-fat diet", "Mediterranean diet", "fatty acids", "mortality", "cardiovascular disease", "weight gain", "weight loss", "type II diabetes", "insulin resistance", "blood pressure", "heart failure", "dyslipidemia", and "cancer". All works meeting the subject matter were considered including observational cohort studies, randomized controlled trials, reviews, meta-analyses, and editorials, in animals and adult humans. Preference was placed on the most recent papers with the exception of those providing historical context to subject matter.

3. Introduction to Dietary Fat Nomenclature

Dietary fat can be broadly broken down into 3 broad subtypes—UFA, SFA and trans fat. UFA can be further divided into monounsaturated fat (MUFA) and polyunsaturated fats (PUFA). Numerous unique fatty acid molecules belong to each subtype of fat, sometimes with divergent effects due to their unique properties as well as the foods they exist within. Additionally, complex mechanisms exist within the body to process consumed nutrients and knowledge continues to accrue regarding the metabolism of dietary fat. A recent example is the recognition of the skeleton and particularly bone marrow as major contributors to fatty acid metabolism [18]. SFA exist in small amounts in many diverse sources of dietary fat, but animal products such as dairy (milk, butter, cheese) and meat are higher in SFA than most plant oils. Notable exceptions are tropical plant oils such as palm and coconut oil, which are also rich sources of SFA. Major sources of SFA include lauric acid (C12:0), myristic acid (C14:0), and palmitic acid (PA) (C16:0) which all increase LDL-C, and stearic acid (C18:0), which does not [19]. There has been some suggestion that PA (C16:0) found in both animal products and palm oil has particularly deleterious effects on cardiometabolic health, such as increased inflammation, oxidative stress, and impaired nitric oxide and insulin signaling, but due to food sources being high in multiple SFAs and endogenous production of PA by the body it is somewhat difficult to distinguish divergent effects [20,21]. Different sources of SFA may have slightly different risk profiles—recent data has suggested that dairy fat in particular may be neutral or even beneficial on cardiovascular (CV) outcomes [22,23]. This, however, seems to be related to the relative risk compared to refined carbohydrate: animal meat sources of SFA and dairy fat still increases atherosclerotic lipoproteins and replacement with UFA results in a decreased risk of CHD [24]. MUFA are also found in meat and dairy, but rich plant sources of MUFA include extra-virgin olive oil, canola oil, and some other plant oils such as rapeseed and high-oleic sunflower and safflower. The major MUFA present in Western diets and referenced in this review is oleic acid (C18:1*n*-9), however, some populations have a high intake of rapeseed oil, and therefore a high intake of erucic acid (c22:1*n*-9) [19]. PUFA are found in nuts and seeds, cold-water fish, and plant oils such as soybean and flaxseed. PUFA are divided in two categories, n-6 and n-3, based on the position of the first double bond from the omega end of the fatty acid. The primary source of PUFA in the diet is linoleic acid (LA) (C18:2n-6), an n-6 fatty acid [19]. Plant sourced n-3 alpha linolenic acid (ALA) (C18:3n-3) is present to a lesser degree, and even less prevalent are the marine n-3 fatty acids eicosapentaenoic acid (EPA) (C22:5n-3) and docosahexaenoic acid (DHA) (C22:6n-3) [19]. Though n-3 and n-6 PUFAs will be discussed separately in this review, both have been shown to be beneficial to human health when consumed in food sources and n-6 PUFAs are no longer considered to be inflammatory [25]. Trans fats occur to a very small degree naturally but mostly exist in the form of engineered fats in highly-processed convenience foods or fast food. Engineered trans fats have been established as harmful to human health and widespread efforts to remove sources of trans fat from the global food supply are ongoing [19,26].

3.1. Low-Fat Diet and CVD

In spite of the decades of guidelines recommending a low-fat diet, few trials have explored the long-term implementation of a low-fat diet and the resulting morbidity and mortality outcomes. The largest trial examining the cardiometabolic effects of the low-fat diet was the Women's Health Initiative Dietary Modification Trial (WHI) which tested the effects of a low-fat diet targeted at reducing the percentage of daily calories from dietary fat to 20%, while increasing servings of grains, fruits, and vegetables [27]. Over 48,000 postmenopausal women were randomized to either a low-fat intervention (40% of participants) or a control arm with minimal dietary interference (60% of participants) [28]. The women in the intervention arm received 18 group counseling sessions focused on dietary modification in the first year and then quarterly for the reminder of the trial [28]. A prescription for grams of daily dietary fat was given to each participant but no weight loss or physical activity goal was specified or encouraged [29]. Subjects in the control group received no dietary guidance but regular clinic visits [28]. After an average of 8.1 years follow up, the intervention group successfully decreased dietary fat intake by an absolute 8.2% from a baseline of 32%. No difference in the rate of CHD, stroke, or CVD was found between the intervention group and the control group, as recorded in Table 1. Although the women decreased total fat by 8.2%, SFA intake only decreased by an absolute 2.9% to a mean of 9.5% calories from SFA in the intervention group, which was significantly above the indicated target of 7% defined at the begin of the study. Although this aligns with the World Health Organization and American Dietary Guidelines 2015–2020 recommendations to reduce SFA to below 10% of total calorie intake in the general population, this recommendation did not result in improved clinical outcomes in the WHI study. Of note, the women enrolled in the WHI trial were post-menopausal and overweight with a mean body-mass index (BMI) of 29 kg/m^2, and were perhaps at a greater CVD risk compared to the general population [17,27,30]. The American Heart Association recommends that individuals with a high LDL-C reduce SFA to 5–6% of daily calories, which may have applied to many of the individuals who developed CVD events during the trial [31].

A recent analysis explored deeper into the neutral CVD outcomes of the WHI trial, examining the difference in CVD disease risk modification for those in the low-fat intervention group [32]. This analysis divided the women into three strata: subjects with baseline CVD, normotensive subjects without baseline CVD, and hypertensive subjects without baseline CVD [32]. Interestingly, the results diverged: in subjects with a prior history of CVD randomized to the low-fat intervention, risk was significantly increased for composite CHD as well as all causes of death [32]. In contrast, normotensive women without a history of CVD had a significantly reduced risk of CHD, which was overshadowed by an increase in stroke risk, particularly ischemic stroke risk [32]. No difference in disease risk was seen in hypertensive women without a history of CVD [32]. It is important to note that CHD was a secondary outcome for the WHI trial, while stroke risk was not a designated primary or secondary trial outcome. The authors of the analysis attribute the adverse CHD outcomes in the subjects with prior CVD to alterations in statin use and the increased stroke risk seen in normotensive women without baseline CVD to possible multiple-testing bias [32]. The findings of this analysis are inconclusive but do bring up a disturbing possibility that the low-fat diet is not just neutral on cardiometabolic outcomes, but could potentially be harmful.

3.2. *Low-Fat Diet and Metabolic Diseases*

The WHI investigators also tracked the incidence of T2DM throughout the length of the trial [29]. They hypothesized that a low-fat dietary pattern, even in the absence of weight loss or exercise, would reduce T2DM incidence [29]. Type I diabetes mellitus was an exclusion factor for the trial and subjects with T2DM at baseline were excluded from this analysis [29]. Incidence of T2DM was self-reported and based on medication reconciliation at regular 6-month visits throughout the trial as only around 5% of the over 45,000 women included in this analysis had regular lab work drawn as part of the trial for a confirmative diagnosis [29]. Participants did not differ in risk factors for T2DM at baseline [29]. After 8.1 years, as shown in Table 1, there was no difference in incidence of self-reported T2DM between subjects in the low-fat intervention and control groups [29,33]. Greater reduction of dietary fat from baseline was initially associated with reduced T2DM but this was no longer significant after controlling for weight loss [29].

Low-fat diets were once considered to be superior weight loss tools as fat, at 9 calories per gram, is more energy-dense than carbohydrate and protein, so reducing fat intake appeared to be an effective way to cut calories from a person' diet [34]. In contrast, evidence suggests that low-fat diets are equivalent, at best, to other diets for weight loss, not superior [35–39]. A recent meta-analysis that included randomized controlled trials (RCTs) with over one year of follow up concluded that low-fat dietary trials did not result in greater weight loss when compared to higher fat interventions of similar intensity as measured by the time, individual attention, and program materials given by the investigative team to participants [37]. When weight loss was the goal, higher fat, lower-carbohydrate diets actually resulted in greater weight loss over time [37]. A lack of difference between the two diets in terms of weight loss was recently demonstrated in the high-profile Diet Intervention Examining the Factors Interacting with Treatment Success (DIETFITS) trial, which examined the effects of genotyping and insulin response on weight loss in 609 overweight and obese individuals randomized to a low-fat or low-carbohydrate diet [38]. The DIETFITS intervention employed intensive counseling and education over a 12 months period to both groups, but at the conclusion of the trial, no difference in weight loss was seen between individuals randomized to a low-fat or low-carbohydrate diet, regardless of genotype or insulin-response at baseline [38].

In summary, low-fat dietary patterns do not seem to aid in the prevention of CVD or T2DM, and are not superior to other diets in terms of weight loss. Continued promotion of the low-fat diet is ineffective at preventing cardiometabolic disease at best, and exploratory findings cannot exclude harms.

3.3. *High-Fat Diet and CVD*

In the last decades, strong evidence has emerged to suggest a diet higher in UFA in the context of a healthy dietary pattern holds strong promise in the prevention and treatment of cardiometabolic disease. This is exemplified in a traditional Mediterranean diet (MedDiet) which is best known as the traditional dietary pattern consumed in Greece, southern Italy and the island of Crete, first brought to the attention of the nutrition scientific community by Ancel Key's Seven Countries Study [16,40]. Briefly, the MedDiet is a diet rich in fruits, vegetables, whole grains, legumes and UFA, principally from extra-virgin olive oil (EVOO) and nuts. Other features of the MedDiet include the consumption of fish and poultry in moderate amounts, red wine with meals, and low consumption of red meat and refined carbohydrates compared to other Western societies. The Prevención con Dieta Mediterránea (PREDIMED) trial, first published in 2013 [41] and retracted and subsequently republished with corrections in 2018 with similar results [42,43], tested a Mediterranean diet (MedDiet) supplemented with nuts or EVOO against a low-fat control diet in nearly 7500 individuals at high CVD risk to assess prevention on a primary composite endpoint of nonfatal myocardial infarction (MI), stroke, and death from CVD [41–43]. This multicenter randomized controlled trial performed in Spain assigned patients 1:1:1 to a MedDiet plus at least 4 tablespoons of EVOO, a MedDiet with 30 g of mixed nuts per day, or a low-fat control diet [42,44]. Notably, no caloric restriction was recommended, and at conclusion of the trial after an average of 4.8 years follow-up the MedDiet groups were consuming 42% total daily energy from fat while individuals in the relatively low-fat control group were consuming around 37% [45]. Patients in the MedDiet groups received group and individual counseling by a dietitian at baseline and then quarterly for the remaining duration of the study [42]. The subjects assigned to the low-fat diet group were initially only given a leaflet with advice on adopting a low-fat diet, but midway through the trial were transitioned to quarterly dietary counseling as well [42].

Adherence to a MedDiet using a 14-point dietary questionnaire was assessed at baseline in all subjects and quarterly thereafter in the MedDiet groups [42]. Control subjects filled out a 9-point dietary questionnaire at dietary counseling sessions assessing their adherence to a low-fat diet [42]. The planned duration of the trial was 6 years but an interim analysis at 4.8 years demonstrated sufficient evidence for benefit to terminate the trial early [46]. In fact, both MedDiet groups demonstrated a 30% relative risk reduction for the primary endpoint compared to their control counterparts [42], as shown in Table 1. This may have been largely driven by a reduction in stroke risk—the combined MedDiet groups demonstrated an impressive 42% relative risk reduction, as seen in Table 1, while death from CVD and nonfatal MI were non-significant independently [42].

The benefit of the relatively high fat MedDiet was not limited to CVD. Although fear of weight gain exists with a higher-fat diet, after 5 years of follow up all three groups showed a weight reduction from baseline and the MedDiet group supplemented with EVOO demonstrated greater weight reduction compared to control participants [47]. Furthermore, both MedDiet groups exhibited a lower increase in waist circumference during the trial than the control group [47,48]. Another analysis of the PREDIMED examined development and reversal of metabolic syndrome (MetS), defined under the integrated International Diabetes Federation/American Heart Association/National Heart, Lung and Blood Institute standards, and found that while there was not a difference between groups in risk of developing MetS, reversal from baseline MetS was more likely in the MedDiet groups compared to control [49]. Additionally, participants in the EVOO group were more likely to have developed a decrease in fasting plasma glucose from baseline [49]. Remarkably, after a median follow-up of 4 years, incidence of new-onset T2DM was reduced by 53% in the two MedDiet groups compared to the control [50,51] (Table 1).

Table 1. Cardiometabolic outcomes comparison of the Prevención con Dieta Mediterránea (PREDIMED) and Women's Health Initiative Dietary Modification Trial (WHI) trials.

Outcome of Interest [1]	WHI (Low-Fat Diet)	PREDIMED (High-Unsaturated Fat Diet)
Composite Cardiovascular Outcome [2]	0.94 (0.86–1.02)	0.70 (0.55–0.89)
Non-fatal myocardial infarction	0.91 (0.80–1.04)	0.80 (0.53–1.21)
Nonfatal Stroke	1.02 (0.90–1.17)	0.58 (0.42–0.82)
Type 2 Diabetes Mellitus Incidence	0.96 (0.90–1.03)	0.47 (0.26–0.87)
Breast Cancer incidence	0.91 (0.83–1.01)	0.49 (0.25–0.94)

[1] Data are presented as hazard ratio and 95% confidence interval. [2] For WHI: myocardial infarction, coronary heart disease, death or revascularization. For PREDIMED: non-fatal myocardial infarction, cardiovascular death or non-fatal stroke. Hazard ratios and confidence intervals for the WHI versus the PREDIMED on primary prevention of cardiovascular, metabolic and cancer-related endpoints [27,29,42,50–53].

Prevention of heart failure (HF) was also explored in the PREDIMED, but while levels of HF prognostic biomarkers (i.e., NT-proBNP) were reduced in the MedDiet groups in one analysis [54], incidence of new-onset HF was not lower in the MedDiet groups than the control group, perhaps due to a small number of events making the study likely underpowered to investigate the effects on new-incident HF [55]. A recent prospective cohort study, Mediterranean Diet in Acute Heart Failure (MEDIT-AHF), explored secondary prevention potential of the MedDiet for patients who had already experienced acute HF (AHF) [56]. Individuals were enrolled in this study in the emergency department (ED) setting and were administered the 14-point dietary questionnaire used in PREDIMED to assess adherence to the MedDiet [56]. The primary outcome of the MEDIT-AHF trial was all-cause mortality at the end of the trial, secondary outcomes consisted of ED visits for HF, hospitalization due to HF, all-cause mortality, and a composite of the three secondary outcomes if one was present [56]. After an average follow up of 2.1 years, ED visits, all-cause mortality, and the combined variable were not different between adherent and non-adherent individuals, however hospitalization was significantly lower in individuals adhering to the MedDiet [56]. It should be noted that both individuals with HF with a preserved ejection fraction (HFpEF) and HF with a reduced ejection fraction (HFrEF) were enrolled in this study. HFpEF is a condition that currently lacks effective clinical therapies and therefore the reduction in hospitalization seen in this study has important implications for future work [57]. Recently, higher consumption of UFA was correlated with greater cardiorespiratory fitness (CRF) as well as better cardiac diastolic function and body composition in a cohort of obese HFpEF patients [58]. The investigators have initiated a novel pilot study in obese HFpEF patients (NCT03310099) exploring the capabilities of UFA supplementation to improve CRF, metabolic flexibility and glucose tolerance.

3.4. High-Fat Diet and Metabolic Diseases

Recently, the results of the Prospective Urban Rural Epidemiological (PURE) study, a prospective cohort of over 135,000 individuals from 18 different countries, called into question whether the type of fatty acid consumed matters in the human diet [59]. Briefly, PURE collected dietary intake through FFQs and followed participants for an average of 7.4 years. Primary outcomes were designated as major CVD events and total mortality. At analysis, high carbohydrate intake was associated with an increased risk of total mortality but was not associated with CVD events or mortality [59]. Total fat and each category of fats (SFA, MUFA and PUFA) were associated with lower risk of total morality but not MI or overall CVD mortality [59]. The investigators stated they were unable to analyze trans fatty acids [59]. SFA alone were associated with lower risk of stroke [59]. The findings of PURE are in direct opposition to current guidelines, which recommend that SFA should be limited in the diet to help prevent CVD [17,60,61]. It is possible in the PURE cohort that FFQs estimated UFA mostly from food sources not deriving from vegetable oils and missed or underestimated vegetable oils [62]. Vegetable oils are major sources of UFA that mostly lack SFA, while animal sources of UFA are also rich sources of SFA [62,63]. It is possible that analyses of the trial, which take different dietary sources into account, could show divergent results between the consumption of different fatty acids.

A recent analysis of the Nurse's Health Study (NHS) and Health Professional's Follow Up Study (HPFS) in a cohort of similar size to PURE (>126,000), which also utilized FFQs in a prospective cohort design, illustrated careful comparison of the effects of different fatty acids consumption on clinical outcomes [64]. Similar to what was found in PURE, total dietary fat consumption was inversely associated with total mortality when substituted for total dietary carbohydrates [64]. The authors then performed substitution analysis of different macronutrients [64]. When SFA and trans fatty acids were substituted for total carbohydrate, a higher risk of mortality ensued, but when PUFA and MUFA were substituted for carbohydrate, as seen in Figure 1, a significant reduction in mortality was observed. Likewise, when PUFA and MUFA were substituted for 5% of energy from SFA, a 27% and 13% reduction in mortality was observed [64]. When trans fatty acids were substituted for 2% of energy from SFA, a 16% mortality increase followed [64].

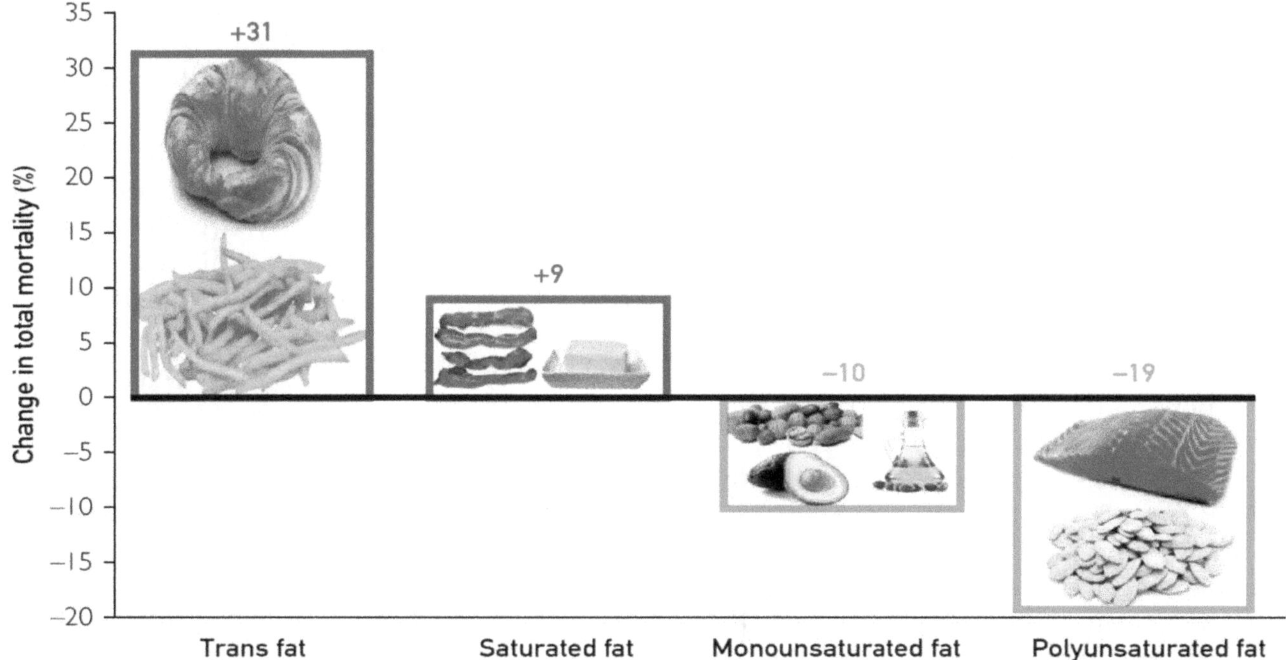

Figure 1. Substitution of different fatty acids for carbohydrate in the Nurse's Health Study (NHS) and Health Professional's Follow Up Study (HPFS). Hazard ratios for total mortality by replacing carbohydrates with specific dietary fats. Used with permission from O'Keefe et al. [65].

The results of the PURE study also called into question the ideal percentage of calories from carbohydrates vs. protein and fat, as high carbohydrate intake was associated with increased risk of total mortality [59]. The composition of a very low-carbohydrate diet or "ketogenic diet" varies in the literature, making up from <30–130 g of carbohydrate per day [66]. In a true ketogenic state, reserves of glycogen are depleted over the course of a few days on extremely low carbohydrate intake, and the liver begins producing ketone bodies as an alternate fuel source for the central nervous system [66]. In human subjects, positive cardiometabolic effects have been seen, including improved lipid panels and glucose metabolism, but concerns have been raised over the lack of long-term data, high intakes of saturated fat and/or protein, and maintaining adherence to a strict dietary pattern [66]. Additionally, a recent analysis suggested that both low (<40% daily calories from carbohydrate) and high (>70%) carbohydrate diets were associated with a greater risk for all-cause mortality [67]. The lowest mortality occurred with a diet composed of 50–55% of calories from carbohydrate [67]. Importantly, low-carbohydrate diets varied in risk profile—when carbohydrate was replaced by a diet high in plant-based protein and fat, a lower mortality risk was observed, but when calories from carbohydrate were replaced by animal fat and protein, an increased risk of all-cause mortality was observed [67]. Notably, participants in the PREDIMED consumed around 42% of their energy from carbohydrate at baseline, and MedDiet groups slightly decreased intake, while control participants slightly increased. Future work should focus on the effects of a plant-based ketogenic diet (KD) vs. animal-based KD as well as modulating carbohydrates (low vs. moderate) in a high-UFA Mediterranean dietary pattern.

4. Potential Mechanisms of Action of Fatty Acids on Cardiometabolic Disease Risk Factors

The cardiometabolic risk reduction observed with a diet higher in UFA is likely multifaceted. Evidence suggests that a diet higher in UFA may affect multiple related risk factors for cardiometabolic disease, including blood pressure (BP), weight maintenance, blood-glucose levels, blood lipids, and inflammation [68]. Though the discussion below focuses on independent mechanisms of improvement for each risk factor, these improvements may also be achieved by the nature of their relation to other risk factors (i.e., weight loss and blood pressure improvement).

Hypertension is responsible for more deaths from CVD in the US than any other modifiable risk factor. Consuming a diet rich in UFA may help lowering BP modestly, by less than 5 mmHg each in systolic and diastolic pressure [69,70], while SFA have an unclear relationship with BP [25]. The mechanism for this reduction is not fully established and may differ between different sources of UFA. Particularly for EVOO, the BP reduction induced may be mediated by OA (C18:1*n*-9) [71], the main fatty acid of EVOO. In pre-clinical studies, administration of EVOO actually altered membrane lipid structure by increasing the amount of OA (C18:1*n*-9) in the cell membrane, which altered G-protein mediated signaling and reduced BP in rats [72].

Nuts may also contribute to the BP-lowering effects of UFA, however, the effects seem to differ, perhaps due to the varying nutrient profile of different nuts. In a meta-analysis including 21 randomized-controlled trials with BP as the primary or secondary outcome, pistachios, but not other nuts, were significantly associated with a significant reduction in systolic BP (SBP) and diastolic BP(DBP) [73]. The authors postulated this could be due to their higher amount of MUFA (particularly OA (C18:1*n*-9)), antioxidants, and the amino acid arginine—a precursor to nitric oxide (NO), a potent vasodilator [74]. A meta-analysis of *n*-3 fatty acids, EPA (C22:5*n*-3) and DHA (C22:6*n*-3) and from food sources and supplementation found that SBP and DBP was lowered in both hypertensive and non-hypertensive subjects [75]. Multiple mechanisms have been suggested for this effect, predominantly relating to endothelial improvements. A recent retrospective analysis of a double-blind, placebo-controlled crossover study supplementing EPA (C22:5*n*-3) and DHA (C22:6*n*-3) in adult subjects attempted to isolate the hypotensive mechanisms of these fatty acids. Though there were no changes in endothelial function or BP in the overall group, SBP was lowered in individuals found to have systolic hypertension [76]. As for the mechanism of action, results demonstrated no effect of adhesion molecule expression in the endothelium or improvement in microvascular function [76]. The investigators also examined the effect of the eNOSrs1799983 gene, associated with lower circulating NO and CVD incidence, and found no treatment x genotype effect leading to speculation that the hypotensive response is independent of the effects of NO [76]. Overall, the effects of different sources of UFA on BP appear to be modest. However, a diet rich in UFA from multiple sources may produce a greater additive effect and subsequent protection against CVD.

Diverging effects on lipid panels are perhaps the one of the earliest and most often cited properties of dietary fats on cardiometabolic health. The National Lipid Association recommends that UFA should be substituted for SFA in lieu of carbohydrates for greater lowering of atherogenic cholesterol levels [77]. The expert consensus was that oils rich in *n*-6 PUFA lower atherogenic cholesterol levels more effectively than MUFA based on controlled feeding trials [77]. However, fatty acids exist within different food sources creating complex effects on lipoproteins. MUFA, especially as part of EVOO, has protective effects against oxidation of LDL-C and high-density lipoprotein cholesterol (HDL-C) as well as promoting an increase in HDL-C [78]. Nuts have varying nutrient profiles and therefore a likely variable effect on lipoproteins [79]. A pooled analysis of 25 intervention trials demonstrated that dietary interventions consisting of nuts alone reduced total cholesterol, LDL-C, and the ratio of LDL-C to HDL-C, but had no effect on HDL-C [80]. The investigators found that this was dose-responsive with higher nut consumption leading to a greater reduction in TC and LDL-C [80]. In addition to UFA, nuts are a source of dietary fiber and plant sterols, which may help reduce cholesterol absorption at the gut level. Lastly, the *n*-3 fatty acids EPA (C22:5*n*-3) and DHA (C22:6*n*-3) have a well-recognized lowering effect on triglycerides (TGs) [81,82]. This reduction in TGs is possibly mediated by multiple mechanisms, including a reduction in circulating fatty acids by increased beta oxidation/decreased lipogenesis, decreased TG synthesizing enzymes, and increased phospholipid synthesis [82]. Again, sources of UFA provide varying effects and mechanisms by which they improve lipid panels and therefore reduce cardiometabolic risk. It is likely the best result is achieved by consuming a diet rich in multiple different sources of UFA.

Weight gain in adulthood is a major risk factor for cardiometabolic disease and some evidence has demonstrated that low-fat diets are not superior to higher-fat diets in terms of weight maintenance or loss [35,37,38,47]. Results from the PREDIMED discussed above suggest that a diet relatively high in UFA may be protective against weight gain [47]. A recent analysis of the European Prospective Investigation into Cancer and Nutrition (EPIC) cohort of over 375,000 European participants corroborated an association between nut consumption and protection against weight gain [83]. The investigators demonstrated that for every 15 g of additional nut consumption per day, participants gained slightly less weight, average of −0.04 kg over 5 years compared to their counterparts, which corresponded to a small but significant 2.5% reduction in body weight increase [83]. Additionally, individuals in the highest quartile of nut consumption who were of a normal weight or overweight at baseline had a 5% lower chance of moving up a body-mass index (BMI) category [83]. Strong evidence is available to indicate that nuts, which contain 50% calories from fat, at the very least do not contribute to increased adiposity [84] and may aid in weight maintenance [47,83]. Nuts likely exert their protective effects against weight gain through several different mechanisms including the effects of the dietary fiber, protein, and fat on satiety, and incomplete absorption of fat at the intestinal level from physical structure [84]. EVOO also demonstrated a protective effect against weight gain and central adiposity during the PREDIMED trial [47]. This was previously demonstrated in the 7368-subject SUN prospective cohort in Spain [85]. In this cohort, participants with the lowest EVOO consumption at baseline who did not increase consumption during the 28.5-month follow-up period gained the most weight [85]. The lowest weight gain was demonstrated in individuals with moderate baseline consumption who increased EVOO during follow up [85]. The mechanisms behind the protective effects of EVOO on weight maintenance are not well established but could be due in part to lowered action of stearoyl-CoA desaturase 1 (SCD1), an obesogenic enzyme that catalyzes the production of MUFA from SFA [86]. Moreover, MUFA can slightly increase resting metabolic rate [87] and physical activity [88], which are, in turn, associated with weight loss in absence of major changes in food intake. Pre-clinical studies also support the beneficial effects on body weight of high-UFA diet, independent of caloric intake [58]. Overall, the evidence shows that nutrient-rich foods high in UFA do not increase the risk of weight gain and may be even protective against increased adiposity. Since 1980, prevalence of T2DM worldwide has doubled in men and increased by 60% in women [89]. Around 8–9% of the world's adult population now suffers from diabetes, and 8–95% from T2DM, which is heavily associated with lifestyle factors [89]. The scale of this epidemic underlines the importance of the PREDIMED sub-analysis that demonstrated new-onset T2DM was reduced over 50% in the higher-fat MedDiet groups compared to the low-fat control [50,51]. The authors suggested this may be due to the effects of lowered chronic systemic low-grade inflammation—an early sub-analysis showed significantly lowered markers of inflammation including Interleukin-6 (IL-6), soluble intercellular adhesion molecule-1 (ICAM-1), and vascular cell adhesion molecule (VCAM-1) in the MedDiet groups [90]. Additionally, C-Reactive Protein (CRP) was reduced in the EVOO MedDiet group [90]. The anti-inflammatory effects of EVOO and nuts are multi-factorial and may include enhancement of the body's endogenous antioxidant defenses, protection against weight gain for individuals in the MedDiet groups and the rich source of polyphenols EVOO provides [91]. Additionally, intake of EVOO with a meal has been shown to affect glycemia by improving insulin sensitivity and increasing glucagon like peptide-1 [92].

However, despite the impressive findings of the PREDIMED, evidence associating total dietary fat and subtypes of dietary fat has been inconsistent, which may be due to the differing food sources of fatty acids [93]. For example, *n*-3 FA supplementation is not recommended by the American Diabetes Association due to lack of demonstrated benefit, but the organization continues to recommend the intake of marine fish rich in *n*-3 for more general health benefits [94]. A meta-analysis and systematic review of 102 trials and over 4200 subjects enrolled in controlled feeding trials demonstrated overall beneficial effects of UFA on glucose-insulin homeostasis [95]. In a replacement analysis of 5% of calories, PUFA and MUFA were associated with improved HOMA-IR and HbA1c when replacing carbohydrate or SFA [95]. PUFA improved insulin secretion capacity whether the PUFA replaced carbohydrate or SFA or MUFA [95]. Only the replacement of SFA with PUFA reduced fasting glucose levels [95]. When SFA or PUFA was substituted for carbohydrate, fasting insulin was reduced but substitution of SFA for carbohydrate resulted in a significantly increased c-peptide in several trials [95]. Longer-term randomized-controlled trials supplementing UFA in individuals at risk for T2DM are needed.

5. Discussion and Conclusions

Preventing cardiometabolic disease with targeted lifestyle therapy such as evidence-based nutrition interventions must be made a global health priority [96]. There is a lack of evidence demonstrating that a low-fat diet is protective against the development of cardiometabolic disease [27,29,32,33]. Evidence continues to accrue that a diet higher in fat, particularly of UFA, especially in the context of a Mediterranean style dietary pattern may be protective against multiple risk factors for cardiometabolic disease [47,49,90,97]. Most importantly, evidence indicates that improvement in these intermediate markers does translate to prevention of CVD and T2DM in individuals consuming a higher UFA diet [42,50].

It should be noted that while a low-fat diet is not effective in the prevention of cardiometabolic disease, the WHI did demonstrate a reduction in death after breast cancer in the low-fat intervention group versus the control during the trial and throughout the 16.1-year follow up period [52]. No significant reduction in breast cancer incidence was observed [52], as seen in Table 1. Breast cancer incidence was also analyzed in the PREDIMED [53]. During the 4.8 years of follow up, as shown in Table 1, incidence of breast cancer was significantly reduced in both MedDiet groups—the released analysis did not include mortality outcomes [53]. Further research is needed to directly compare a healthy low-fat dietary pattern with a higher-fat MedDiet pattern to determine which pattern is superior in preventing breast cancer as well as mortality during and after treatment.

The PREDIMED was conducted in Spain, a country where a Mediterranean dietary pattern rich in UFA is commonly consumed—EVOO is the main dietary fat source in the Spanish population studied [98]. Interest in replicating the PREDIMED in a non-Mediterranean country is substantial. An expert working group has thoroughly explored the necessary resources, accommodations, and anticipated problems investigators may face in attempting to replicate the PREDIMED in the US [98]. Compared to the PREDIMED participants at baseline, the Mediterranean diet adherence score (MEDAS) of US participants estimated from the National Health and Nutrition Examination Survey is substantially lower [98], as seen in Table 2. Importantly, whether the supplementation of nuts and EVOO works in the context of a non-Mediterranean dietary pattern such as in United States is unknown [99]. The working group suggested that a goal of the trial would be to increase the MEDAS score of the US modestly and not to the level of Spanish participants which they felt would be very difficult to achieve and perhaps maintain [98], as seen in Table 2.

Table 2. Dietary pattern comparison of PREDIMED MedDiet groups and U.S. average intake.

	Mediterranean Diet + Extra-Virgin Olive Oil	Mediterranean Diet + Nuts	NHANES 2011–2012	Change Needed
Nutrient intake				
Energy, kcal/day	2172	2229	2141	
Carbohydrate, % Energy	40	40	48	Decrease (type matters)
Protein, % Energy	16	16	16	
Total fat, % Energy	41	42	34	Increase (type matters)
Saturated fat, % Energy	9	9	11	Decrease
Monounsaturated Fatty Acids, % E	22	21	12	Increase
Polyunsaturated Fatty Acids, % Energy	6	8	8	None
α-Linolenic acid, g/day	1.3	1.9	Not Available	Not Available
Marine *n*-3 fatty-acids, g/day	0.9	0.8	0.1	Increase

Table 2. *Cont.*

	Mediterranean Diet + Extra-Virgin Olive Oil	Mediterranean Diet + Nuts	NHANES 2011–2012	Change Needed
Fiber, g/day	25	27	17	Increase
Cholesterol, g/day	339	338	293	None
Food intake				
Virgin olive oil, g/day	50	32	Not Available	Increase
Refined olive oil, g/day	0.9	10.3	Not Available	
Nuts, g/day	10	40	11	Increase
Fruit, g/day	401	406	149	Increase
Vegetables, g/day	340	336	246	Increase
Legumes, g/day	22	22	6	Increase
Whole grains, g/day	27	28	28	None
Refined grains, g/day	181	178	165	None
Pastry, sweets, g/day	17	16	Not Available	Decrease
Meat, g/day	119	119	118	None
Fish/seafood, g/day	101	103	17	Increase
Dairy, g/day	366	370	399	None

Characteristics of average US diet gathered from NHANES 2011–2012 data as compared to PREDIMED MedDiet participant's diets. Used with permission from Jacobs Jr. et al. [98].

In summary, a relatively high-UFA diet, especially in the context of the MedDiet, decreases risk factors as well as morbidity and mortality related to CVD. In contrast, there is no evidence that a low-fat diet leads to lower morbidity or mortality related to cardiometabolic disease. Randomized controlled trials are warranted to test the effects of UFA-supplemented MedDiet in diverse global populations on risk factors and outcomes of T2DM and CVD.

Author Contributions: H.E.B. writing-original draft preparation. S.C. and C.J.L. writing-review and editing.

Acknowledgments: Salvatore Carbone is supported by the VCU DOIM Pilot Project Grant Program 2017 and by the VCU Pauley Heart Center Pilot Project Grant Program 2017. We would like to thank Stefano Canepa, BS for his help with formatting the tables and figures for the manuscript.

References

1. Micha, R.; Peñalvo, J.L.; Cudhea, F.; Imamura, F.; Rehm, C.D.; Mozaffarian, D. Association between dietary factors and mortality from heart disease, stroke, and type 2 diabetes in the United States. *JAMA* **2017**, *317*, 912. [CrossRef] [PubMed]
2. Yu, E.; Malik, V.S.; Hu, F.B. Cardiovascular disease prevention by diet modification. *J. Am. Coll. Cardiol.* **2018**, *72*, 914–926. [CrossRef] [PubMed]
3. Archer, E.; Hand, G.A.; Blair, S.N. Validity of U.S. nutritional surveillance: National health and nutrition examination survey caloric energy intake data, 1971–2010. *PLoS ONE* **2013**, *8*, e76632. [CrossRef] [PubMed]
4. Ioannidis, J.P.A. Implausible results in human nutrition research. *BMJ* **2013**, *347*, f6698. [CrossRef] [PubMed]
5. Keys, A. Prediction and possible prevention of coronary disease. *Am. J. Public Heal. Nations Heal.* **1953**, *43*, 1399–1407. [CrossRef]
6. Pett, K.D.; Willett, W.C.; Vartiainen, E.; Katz, D.L. The seven countries study. *Eur. Heart J.* **2017**, *38*, 3119–3121. [CrossRef] [PubMed]
7. Hu, F.B. Optimal diets for prevention of coronary heart disease. *JAMA* **2002**, *288*, 2569–2578. [CrossRef] [PubMed]
8. Keys, A.; Menotti, A.; Aravanis, C.; Blackburn, H.; Djordevič, B.S.; Buzina, R.; Dontas, A.S.; Fidanza, F.; Karvonen, M.J.; Kimura, N.; et al. The seven countries study: 2289 deaths in 15 years. *Prev. Med.* **1984**, *13*, 141–154. [CrossRef]
9. Kato, H.; Tillotson, J.; Nichaman, M.Z.; Rhoads, G.G.; Hamilton, H.B. Epidemiologic studies of coronary heart disease and stroke in japenese men living in Japan, Hawaii and California- Serum lipids and diet. *Am. J. Epidemiol.* **1973**, *97*, 372–385. [CrossRef] [PubMed]

10. U.S. Department of Agriculture: U.S. Department of Health and Human Services. *Nutrition and Your Health: Dietary Guidelines for Americans*; Government Printing Office: Washington, DC, USA, 1980.
11. U.S. Department of Agriculture: U.S. Department of Health and Human Services. *Nutrition and Your Health: Dietary guidelines for Americans*; Government Printing Office: Washington, DC, USA, 1990.
12. Austin, G.L.; Ogden, L.G.; Hill, J.O. Trends in carbohydrate, fat, and protein intakes and association with energy intake in normal-weight, overweight, and obese individuals: 1971–2006. *Am. J. Clin. Nutr.* **2011**, *93*, 836–843. [CrossRef] [PubMed]
13. Gross, L.S.; Li, L.; Ford, E.S.; Liu, S. Increased consumption of refined carbohydrates and the epidemic of type 2 diabetes in the United States: An ecologic assessment. *Am. J. Clin. Nutr.* **2004**, *79*, 774–779. [CrossRef] [PubMed]
14. Benjamin, E.J.; Virani, S.S.; Callaway, C.W.; Chang, A.R.; Cheng, S.; Chiuve, S.E.; Cushman, M.; Delling, F.N.; Deo, R.; de Ferranti, S.D.; et al. Heart disease and stroke statistics—2018 update: A report from the American heart association. *Circulation* **2018**. [CrossRef] [PubMed]
15. Menke, A.; Casagrande, S.; Geiss, L. Prevalence of and trends in diabetes among adults in the United States, 1988–2012. *JAMA* **2015**, *314*, 1021–1029. [CrossRef] [PubMed]
16. Keys, A.; Mienotti, A.; Karvonen, M.J.; Aravanis, C.; Blackburn, H.; Buzina, R.; Djordjevic, B.S.; Dontas, A.S.; Fidanza, F.; Keys, M.H.; et al. The diet and 15-year death rate in the seven countries study. *Am. J. Epidemiol.* **1986**, *124*, 903–915. [CrossRef] [PubMed]
17. U.S. Department of Health and Human Services. *2015–2020 Dietary Guidelines for Americans*, 8th ed.; U.S. Department of Agriculture: Washington, DC, USA, 2015. Available online: http://health.gov/dietaryguidelines/2015/guidelines/ (assessed on 27 September 2018).
18. Bartelt, A.; Koehne, T.; Tödter, K.; Reimer, R.; Müller, B.; Behler-Janbeck, F.; Heeren, J.; Scheja, L.; Niemeier, A. Quantification of bone fatty acid metabolism and its regulation by adipocyte lipoprotein lipase. *Int. J. Mol. Sci.* **2017**, *18*, 1264. [CrossRef] [PubMed]
19. FAO. Fats and fatty acids in human nutrition: Report of an expert consultation. *FAO Food Nutr. Pap.* **2010**, *91*, 1–166.
20. Risérus, U.; Willett, W.C.; Hu, F.B. Dietary fats and prevention of type 2 diabetes. *Prog. Lipid Res.* **2009**, *48*, 44–51. [CrossRef] [PubMed]
21. Mancini, A.; Imperlini, E.; Nigro, E.; Montagnese, C.; Daniele, A.; Orrù, S.; Buono, P. Biological and nutritional properties of palm oil and palmitic acid: Effects on health. *Molecules* **2015**, *20*, 17339–17361. [CrossRef] [PubMed]
22. Guo, J.; Astrup, A.; Lovegrove, J.A.; Gijsbers, L.; Givens, D.I.; Soedamah-Muthu, S.S. Milk and dairy consumption and risk of cardiovascular diseases and all-cause mortality: Dose–response meta-analysis of prospective cohort studies. *Eur. J. Epidemiol.* **2017**, *32*, 269–287. [CrossRef] [PubMed]
23. Dehghan, M.; Mente, A.; Rangarajan, S.; Sheridan, P.; Mohan, V.; Iqbal, R.; Gupta, R.; Lear, S.; Wentzel-Viljoen, E.; Avezum, A.; et al. Association of dairy intake with cardiovascular disease and mortality in 21 countries from five continents (PURE): A prospective cohort study. *Lancet* **2018**. [CrossRef]
24. Briggs, M.; Petersen, K.; Kris-Etherton, P. Saturated fatty acids and cardiovascular disease: Replacements for saturated fat to reduce cardiovascular risk. *Healthcare* **2017**, *5*, 29. [CrossRef] [PubMed]
25. Wang, D.D.; Hu, F.B. Dietary fat and risk of cardiovascular disease: Recent controversies and advances. *Annu. Rev. Nutr.* **2017**, *37*, 423–446. [CrossRef] [PubMed]
26. Ghebreyesus, T.A.; Frieden, T.R. REPLACE: A roadmap to make the world trans fat free by 2023. *Lancet* **2018**, *391*, 1978–1980. [CrossRef]
27. Howard, B.V.; Van Horn, L.; Hsia, J.; Manson, J.E.; Stefanick, M.L.; Wassertheil-Smoller, S.; Kuller, L.H.; LaCroix, A.Z.; Langer, R.D.; Lasser, N.L.; et al. Low-fat dietary pattern and risk of cardiovascular disease: The women's health initiative randomized controlled dietary modification trial. *JAMA* **2006**, *295*, 655–666. [CrossRef] [PubMed]
28. Group, W.H.I.S. Dietary adherence in the women's health initiative dietary modification trial. *J. Am. Diet. Assoc.* **2004**, *104*, 654–658.
29. Tinker, L.; DE, B.; Margolis, K.L.; Manson, J.E.; Howard, B.; Larson, J.; Perri, M.; Beresford, S.; Robinson, J.G.; Rodríguez, B.; et al. Low-fat dietary pattern and risk of treated diabetes mellitus in postmenopausal women: The women's health initiative randomized controlled dietary modification trial. *Arch. Intern. Med.* **2008**, *168*, 1500–1511. [CrossRef] [PubMed]

30. Collins, P.; Rosano, G.; Casey, C.; Daly, C.; Gambacciani, M.; Hadji, P.; Kaaja, R.; Mikkola, T.; Palacios, S.; Preston, R.; et al. Management of cardiovascular risk in the peri-menopausal woman: A consensus statement of European cardiologists and gynaecologists. *Eur. Heart J.* **2007**, *28*, 2028–2040. [CrossRef] [PubMed]
31. Eckel, R.H.; Jakicic, J.M.; Ard, J.D.; de Jesus, J.M.; Houston Miller, N.; Hubbard, V.S.; Lee, I.-M.; Lichtenstein, A.H.; Loria, C.M.; Millen, B.E.; et al. 2013 AHA/ACC guideline on lifestyle management to reduce cardiovascular risk: A report of the American college of cardiology/American heart association task force on practice guidelines. *Circulation* **2014**, *129*. [CrossRef] [PubMed]
32. Prentice, R.L.; Aragaki, A.K.; Horn, L.; Thomson, C.A.; Beresford, S.A.A.; Robinson, J.; Snetselaar, L.; Anderson, G.L.; Manson, J.E.; Allison, M.A.; et al. V Low-fat dietary pattern and cardiovascular disease: Results from the women's health initiative randomized controlled trial. **2017**, *106*, 25–43. [CrossRef] [PubMed]
33. Howard, B.V.; Aragaki, A.K.; Tinker, L.F.; Allison, M.; Hingle, M.D.; Johnson, K.C.; Manson, J.E.; Shadyab, A.H.; Shikany, J.M.; Snetselaar, L.G.; et al. A low-fat dietary pattern and diabetes: A secondary analysis from the women's health initiative dietary modification trial. *Diabetes Care* **2018**, *41*, 680–687. [CrossRef] [PubMed]
34. Hill, J.O.; Melanson, E.L.; Wyatt, H.T. Dietary fat intake and regulation of energy balance: Implications for obesity. *J. Nutr.* **2000**, *130*, S284–S288. [CrossRef]
35. Nordmann, A.J.; Nordmann, A.; Briel, M. Effects of low-carbohydrate vs low-fat diets on weight loss and cardiovascular risk factors: A meta-analysis of randomized controlled trials. *Arch. Intern. Med.* **2006**, *166*, 285–293. [CrossRef] [PubMed]
36. Shai, I.; Schwarzfuchs, D.; Henkin, Y.; Shahar, D.R.; Witkow, S.; Greenberg, I.; Golan, R.; Fraser, D.; Bolotin, A.; Vardi, H.; et al. Weight loss with a low-carbohydrate, Mediterranean, or low-fat diet. *N. Engl. J. Med.* **2008**, *359*, 229–241. [CrossRef] [PubMed]
37. Tobias, D.K.; Chen, M.; Manson, J.E.; Ludwig, D.S.; Willett, W.; Hu, F.B. Effect of low-fat diet interventions versus other diet interventions on long-term weight change in adults: A systematic review and meta-analysis. *Lancet. Diabetes Endocrinol.* **2015**, *3*, 968–979. [CrossRef]
38. Gardner, C.D.; Trepanowski, J.F.; Del Gobbo, L.C.; Hauser, M.E.; Rigdon, J.; Ioannidis, J.P.A.; Desai, M.; King, A.C. Effect of low-fat vs. low-carbohydrate diet on 12-month weight loss in overweight adults and the association with genotype pattern or insulin secretion: The DIETFITS randomized clinical trial. *JAMA* **2018**, *319*, 667–679. [CrossRef] [PubMed]
39. McManus, K.; Antinoro, L.; Sacks, F. A randomized controlled trial of a moderate-fat, low-energy diet compared with a low fat, low-energy diet for weight loss in overweight adults. *Int. J. Obes.* **2001**, *25*, 1503. [CrossRef] [PubMed]
40. Hu, F.B. The Mediterranean diet and mortality—Olive oil and beyond. *N. Engl. J. Med.* **2003**, *348*, 2595–2596. [CrossRef] [PubMed]
41. Estruch, R.; Ros, E.; Salas-Salvadó, J.; Covas, M.-I.; Corella, D.; Arós, F.; Gómez-Gracia, E.; Ruiz-Gutiérrez, V.; Fiol, M.; Lapetra, J.; et al. Primary prevention of cardiovascular disease with a Mediterranean diet. *N. Engl. J. Med.* **2013**, *368*, 1279–1290. [CrossRef] [PubMed]
42. Estruch, R.; Ros, E.; Salas-Salvadó, J.; Covas, M.-I.; Corella, D.; Arós, F.; Gómez-Gracia, E.; Ruiz-Gutiérrez, V.; Fiol, M.; Lapetra, J.; et al. Primary prevention of cardiovascular disease with a Mediterranean diet supplemented with extra-virgin olive oil or nuts. *N. Engl. J. Med.* **2018**, *378*, e34. [CrossRef] [PubMed]
43. Mayor, S. Sixty seconds on the Mediterranean diet. *BMJ* **2018**, *361*. [CrossRef] [PubMed]
44. Martínez-González, M.Á.; Corella, D.; Salas-salvadó, J.; Ros, E.; Covas, M.I.; Fiol, M.; Wärnberg, J.; Arós, F.; Ruíz-Gutiérrez, V.; Lamuela-Raventós, R.M.; et al. Cohort profile: Design and methods of the PREDIMED study. *Int. J. Epidemiol.* **2012**, *41*, 377–385. [CrossRef] [PubMed]
45. Mozaffarian, D. Food and weight gain: Time to end our fear of fat. *Lancet Diabetes Endocrinol.* **2017**, *4*, 633–635. [CrossRef]
46. Guasch-Ferré, M.; Salas-Salvadó, J.; Ros, E.; Estruch, R.; Corella, D.; Fitó, M.; Martínez-González, M.A.; Arós, F.; Gómez-Gracia, E.; Fiol, M.; et al. The PREDIMED trial, Mediterranean diet and health outcomes: How strong is the evidence? *Nutr. Metab. Cardiovasc. Dis.* **2017**, *27*, 624–632. [CrossRef] [PubMed]

47. Estruch, R.; Martínez-González, M.A.; Corella, D.; Salas-Salvadó, J.; Fitó, M.; Chiva-Blanch, G.; Fiol, M.; Gómez-Gracia, E.; Arós, F.; Lapetra, J.; et al. PREDIMED Study Investigators Effect of a high-fat Mediterranean diet on bodyweight and waist circumference: A prespecified secondary outcomes analysis of the PREDIMED randomised controlled trial. *Lancet Diabetes Endocrinol.* **2016**, *4*, 666–676. [CrossRef]
48. The editors of the lancet diabetes & endocrinology expression of concern. Effect of a high-fat Mediterranean diet on bodyweight and waist circumference: A prespecified secondary outcomes analysis of the PREDIMED randomised controlled trial. *Lancet Diabetes Endocrinol.* **2018**. [CrossRef]
49. Babio, N.; Toledo, E.; Estruch, R.; Ros, E.; Martínez-González, M.A.; Castañer, O.; Bulló, M.; Corella, D.; Arós, F.; Gómez-Gracia, E.; et al. Mediterranean diets and metabolic syndrome status in the PREDIMED randomized trial. *C. Can. Med. Assoc. J.* **2014**, *186*, E649–E657. [CrossRef] [PubMed]
50. Salas-Salvadó, J.; Bullo, M.; Babió, N.; Martínez-González, M.Á.; Ibarrola-Jurado, N.; Basora, J.; Estruch, R.; Covas, M.I.; Corella, D.; Arós, F.; et al. Reduction in the incidence of type 2 diabetes with the Mediterranean diet: Results of the PREDIMED-Reus nutrition intervention randomized trial. *Diabetes Care* **2011**, *34*, 14–19, Erratum in **2011**. [CrossRef] [PubMed]
51. Salas-Salvadó, J.; Bullo, M.; Babió, N.; Martínez-González, M.Á.; Ibarrola-Jurado, N.; Basora, J.; Estruch, R.; Covas, M.I.; Corella, D.; Arós, F.; et al. Reduction in the Incidence of Type 2 Diabetes with the Mediterranean Diet. *Diabetes Care* **2011**, *34*, 14–19. [CrossRef] [PubMed]
52. Chlebowski, R.T.; Aragaki, A.K.; Anderson, G.L.; Thomson, C.A.; Manson, J.E.; Simon, M.S.; Howard, B.V.; Rohan, T.E.; Snetselar, L.; Lane, D.; et al. Low-fat dietary pattern and breast cancer mortality in the women's health initiative randomized controlled trial. *J. Clin. Oncol.* **2017**, *35*, 2919–2926. [CrossRef] [PubMed]
53. Toledo, E.; Salas-Salvado, J.; Donat-Vargas, C.; Buil-Cosiales, P.; Estruch, R.; Ros, E.; Corella, D.; Fito, M.; Hu, F.B.; Aros, F.; et al. Mediterranean diet and invasive breast cancer risk among women at high cardiovascular risk in the PREDIMED trial: A randomized clinical trial. *JAMA Intern. Med.* **2015**, *175*, 1752–1760. [CrossRef] [PubMed]
54. Fitó, M.; Estruch, R.; Salas-Salvadó, J.; Martínez-Gonzalez, M.A.; Arós, F.; Vila, J.; Corella, D.; Díaz, O.; Sáez, G. Effect of the Mediterranean diet on heart failure biomarkers: A randomized sample from the PREDIMED trial. *Eur. J. Heart Fail.* **2014**, *16*, 543–550. [CrossRef] [PubMed]
55. Papadaki, A.; Martinez-Gonzalez, M.A.; Alonso-Gomez, A.; Rekondo, J.; Salas-Salvado, J.; Corella, D.; Ros, E.; Fito, M.; Estruch, R.; Lapetra, J.; et al. Mediterranean diet and risk of heart failure: Results from the PREDIMED randomized controlled trial. *Eur. J. Heart Fail.* **2017**, *19*, 1179–1185. [CrossRef] [PubMed]
56. Miró, Ò.; Estruch, R.; Martín-Sánchez, F.J.; Gil, V.; Jacob, J.; Herrero-Puente, P.; Herrera Mateo, S.; Aguirre, A.; Andueza, J.A.; Llorens, P.; et al. Adherence to Mediterranean diet and all-cause mortality after an episode of acute heart failure: Results of the MEDIT-AHF Study. *JACC Heart Fail.* **2018**, *6*, 52–62. [CrossRef] [PubMed]
57. Carbone, S.; Billingsley, H.E.; Abbate, A. The Mediterranean diet to treat heart failure: A potentially powerful tool in the hands of providers. *JACC Heart Fail.* **2018**, *6*, 264. [CrossRef] [PubMed]
58. Carbone, S.; Canada, J.M.; Buckley, L.F.; Trankle, C.R.; Billingsley, H.E.; Dixon, D.L.; Mauro, A.G.; Dessie, S.; Kadariya, D.; Mezzaroma, E.; et al. Dietary fat, sugar consumption, and cardiorespiratory fitness in patients with heart failure with preserved ejection fraction. *JACC Basic Transl. Sci.* **2017**, *2*, 513–525. [CrossRef] [PubMed]
59. Dehghan, M.; Mente, A.; Zhang, X.; Swaminathan, S.; Li, W.; Mohan, V.; Iqbal, R.; Kumar, R.; Wentzel-Viljoen, E.; Rosengren, A.; et al. Associations of fats and carbohydrate intake with cardiovascular disease and mortality in 18 countries from five continents (PURE): A prospective cohort study. *Lancet* **2017**, *390*, 2050–2062. [CrossRef]
60. Sacks, F.M.; Lichtenstein, A.H.; Wu, J.H.Y.; Appel, L.J.; Creager, M.A.; Kris-Etherton, P.M.; Miller, M.; Rimm, E.B.; Rudel, L.L.; Robinson, J.G.; et al. Dietary fats and cardiovascular disease: A presidential advisory from the American heart association. *Circulation* **2017**, *136*, e1–e23. [CrossRef] [PubMed]
61. World Health Organization Call for Public Comments on the Draft WHO Guidelines: Saturated Fatty Acid and *Trans*-Fatty Intake for Adults and Children. Available online: http://www.who.int/nutrition/topics/sfa-tfa-public-consultation-4may2018/en/ (assessed on 4 May 2018).
62. Carbone, S.; Billingsley, H.; Abbate, A. Associations of fats and carbohydrates with cardiovascular disease and mortality—PURE and simple? *Lancet* **2018**, *391*, 1679. [CrossRef]
63. Ramsden, C.E.; Domenichiello, A.F. PURE study challenges the definition of a healthy diet: But key questions remain. *Lancet* **2017**, *390*, 2018–2019. [CrossRef]

64. Wang, D.D.; Li, Y.; Chiuve, S.E.; Stampfer, M.J.; Manson, J.E.; Rimm, E.B.; Willett, W.C.; Hu, F.B. Association of specific dietary fats with total and cause-specific mortality. *JAMA Intern. Med.* **2016**, *176*, 1134. [CrossRef] [PubMed]
65. O'Keefe, J.H.; DiNicolantonio, J.J.; Sigurdsson, A.F.; Ros, E. Evidence, not evangelism, for dietary recommendations. *Mayo Clin. Proc.* **2018**, *93*, 138–144. [CrossRef] [PubMed]
66. Kosinski, C.; Jornayvaz, F.R. Effects of ketogenic diets on cardiovascular risk factors: Evidence from animal and human studies. *Nutrients* **2017**, *9*, 517. [CrossRef] [PubMed]
67. Seidelmann, S.B.; Claggett, B.; Cheng, S.; Henglin, M.; Shah, A.; Steffen, L.M.; Folsom, A.R.; Rimm, E.B.; Willett, W.C.; Solomon, S.D. Dietary carbohydrate intake and mortality: A prospective cohort study and meta-analysis. *Lancet Public Health* **2018**, *3*, e419–e428. [CrossRef]
68. Liu, A.G.; Ford, N.A.; Hu, F.B.; Zelman, K.M.; Mozaffarian, D.; Kris-Etherton, P.M. A healthy approach to dietary fats: Understanding the science and taking action to reduce consumer confusion. *Nutr. J.* **2017**, *16*, 53. [CrossRef] [PubMed]
69. KANWU Study Group. Effects of dietary saturated, monounsaturated, and $n-3$ fatty acids on blood pressure in healthy subjects. *Am. J. Clin. Nutr.* **2006**, *83*, 221–226. [CrossRef] [PubMed]
70. Appel, L.J.; Sacks, F.M.; Carey, V.J.; Obarzanek, E.; Swain, J.F.; Miller, E.R., 3rd; Conlin, P.R.; Erlinger, T.P.; Rosner, B.A.; Laranjo, N.M.; et al. Effects of protein, monounsaturated fat, and carbohydrate intake on blood pressure and serum lipids: Results of the OmniHeart randomized trial. *JAMA* **2005**, *294*, 2455–2464. [CrossRef] [PubMed]
71. Gillingham, L.G.; Harris-Janz, S.; Jones, P.J.H. Dietary monounsaturated fatty acids are protective against metabolic syndrome and cardiovascular disease risk factors. *Lipids* **2011**, *46*, 209–228. [CrossRef] [PubMed]
72. Terés, S.; Barceló-Coblijn, G.; Benet, M.; Álvarez, R.; Bressani, R.; Halver, J.E.; Escribá, P. V Oleic acid content is responsible for the reduction in blood pressure induced by olive oil. *Proc. Natl. Acad. Sci. USA* **2008**, *105*, 13811–13816. [CrossRef] [PubMed]
73. Mohammadifard, N.; Salehi-Abargouei, A.; Salas-Salvadó, J.; Guasch-Ferré, M.; Humphries, K.; Sarrafzadegan, N. The effect of tree nut, peanut, and soy nut consumption on blood pressure: A systematic review and meta-analysis of randomized controlled clinical trials. *Am. J. Clin. Nutr.* **2015**, *101*, 966–982. [CrossRef] [PubMed]
74. Sari, I.; Baltaci, Y.; Bagci, C.; Davutoglu, V.; Erel, O.; Celik, H.; Ozer, O.; Aksoy, N.; Aksoy, M. Effect of pistachio diet on lipid parameters, endothelial function, inflammation, and oxidative status: A. prospective study. *Nutrition* **2010**, *26*, 399–404. [CrossRef] [PubMed]
75. Miller, P.E.; Van Elswyk, M.; Alexander, D.D. Long-chain omega-3 fatty acids eicosapentaenoic acid and docosahexaenoic acid and blood pressure: A meta-analysis of randomized controlled trials. *Am. J. Hypertens.* **2014**, *27*, 885–896. [CrossRef] [PubMed]
76. Minihane, A.M.; Armah, C.K.; Miles, E.A.; Madden, J.M.; Clark, A.B.; Caslake, M.J.; Packard, C.J.; Kofler, B.M.; Lietz, G.; Curtis, P.J.; et al. Consumption of fish oil providing amounts of eicosapentaenoic acid and docosahexaenoic acid that can be obtained from the diet reduces blood pressure in adults with systolic hypertension: A retrospective analysis. *J. Nutr.* **2016**, *146*, 516–523. [CrossRef] [PubMed]
77. Jacobson, T.A.; Maki, K.C.; Orringer, C.E.; Jones, P.H.; Kris-Etherton, P.; Sikand, G.; La Forge, R.; Daniels, S.R.; Wilson, D.P.; Morris, P.B.; et al. National lipid association recommendations for patient-centered management of dyslipidemia: Part 2. *J. Clin. Lipidol.* **2015**, *9*. [CrossRef] [PubMed]
78. Covas, M.-I.; de la Torre, R.; Fitó, M. Virgin olive oil: A key food for cardiovascular risk protection. *Br. J. Nutr.* **2015**, *113*, S19–S28. [CrossRef] [PubMed]
79. Bitok, E.; Sabaté, J. Nuts and cardiovascular disease. *Prog. Cardiovasc. Dis.* **2018**, *61*, 33–37. [CrossRef] [PubMed]
80. Sabaté, J.; Oda, K.; Ros, E. Nut consumption and blood lipid levels: A pooled analysis of 25 intervention trials. *Arch. Intern. Med.* **2010**, *170*, 821–827. [CrossRef] [PubMed]
81. Rimm, E.B.; Appel, L.J.; Chiuve, S.E.; Djousse, L.; Engler, M.B.; Kris-Etherton, P.M.; Mozaffarian, D.; Siscovick, D.S.; Lichtenstein, A.H. Seafood long-chain *n*-3 polyunsaturated fatty acids and cardiovascular disease: A science advisory from the american heart association. *Circulation* **2018**, *138*, e35–e47. [CrossRef] [PubMed]
82. Harris, W.S.; Bulchandani, D. Why do omega-3 fatty acids lower serum triglycerides? *Curr. Opin. Lipidol.* **2006**, *17*, 387–393. [CrossRef] [PubMed]

83. Freisling, H.; Noh, H.; Slimani, N.; Chajès, V.; May, A.M.; Peeters, P.H.; Weiderpass, E.; Cross, A.J.; Skeie, G.; Jenab, M.; et al. Nut intake and 5-year changes in body weight and obesity risk in adults: Results from the EPIC-PANACEA study. *Eur. J. Nutr.* **2017**. [CrossRef] [PubMed]
84. Flores-Mateo, G.; Rojas-Rueda, D.; Basora, J.; Ros, E.; Salas-Salvadó, J. Nut intake and adiposity: Meta-analysis of clinical trials. *Am. J. Clin. Nutr.* **2013**, *97*, 1346–1355. [CrossRef] [PubMed]
85. Bes-Rastrollo, M.; Sánchez-Villegas, A.; de la Fuente, C.; de Irala, J.; Martínez, J.A.; Martínez-González, M.A. Olive oil consumption and weight change: The SUN prospective cohort study. *Lipids* **2006**, *41*, 249–256. [CrossRef] [PubMed]
86. Galvão Cândido, F.; Xavier Valente, F.; da Silva, L.E.; Gonçalves Leão Coelho, O.; Gouveia Peluzio, M.D.C.; Gonçalves Alfenas, R.C. Consumption of extra virgin olive oil improves body composition and blood pressure in women with excess body fat: A randomized, double-blinded, placebo-controlled clinical trial. *Eur. J. Nutr.* **2017**. [CrossRef] [PubMed]
87. Rasmussen, L.G.; Larsen, T.M.; Mortensen, P.K.; Due, A.; Astrup, A. Effect on 24-h energy expenditure of a moderate-fat diet high in monounsaturated fatty acids compared with that of a low-fat, carbohydrate-rich diet: A 6-mo controlled dietary intervention trial. *Am. J. Clin. Nutr.* **2007**, *85*, 1014–1022. [CrossRef] [PubMed]
88. Kien, C.L.; Bunn, J.Y.; Tompkins, C.L.; Dumas, J.A.; Crain, K.I.; Ebenstein, D.B.; Koves, T.R.; Muoio, D.M. Substituting dietary monounsaturated fat for saturated fat is associated with increased daily physical activity and resting energy expenditure and with changes in mood. *Am. J. Clin. Nutr.* **2013**, *97*, 689–697. [CrossRef] [PubMed]
89. Worldwide trends in diabetes since 1980: A pooled analysis of 751 population-based studies with 44 million participants. *Lancet* **2016**, *387*, 1513–1530. [CrossRef]
90. Estruch, R.; Martínez-González, M.; Corella, D. Effects of a Mediterranean-style diet on cardiovascular risk factors: A randomized trial. *Ann. Intern. Med.* **2006**, *145*, 1–11. [CrossRef] [PubMed]
91. Billingsley, H.E.; Carbone, S. The antioxidant potential of the Mediterranean diet in patients at high cardiovascular risk: An in-depth review of the PREDIMED. *Nutr. Diabetes* **2018**, *8*. [CrossRef] [PubMed]
92. Paniagua, J.A.; de la Sacristana, A.G.; Sánchez, E.; Romero, I.; Vidal-Puig, A.; Berral, F.J.; Escribano, A.; Moyano, M.J.; Peréz-Martinez, P.; et al. A MUFA-rich diet improves posprandial glucose, lipid and GLP-1 responses in insulin-resistant subjects. *J. Am. Coll. Nutr.* **2007**, *26*, 434–444. [CrossRef] [PubMed]
93. Ericson, U.; Hellstrand, S.; Brunkwall, L.; Schulz, C.-A.; Sonestedt, E.; Wallström, P.; Gullberg, B.; Wirfält, E.; Orho-Melander, M. Food sources of fat may clarify the inconsistent role of dietary fat intake for incidence of type 2 diabetes. *Am. J. Clin. Nutr.* **2015**, *101*, 1065–1080. [CrossRef] [PubMed]
94. Evert, A.B.; Boucher, J.L.; Cypress, M.; Dunbar, S.A.; Franz, M.J.; Mayer-Davis, E.J.; Neumiller, J.J.; Nwankwo, R.; Verdi, C.L.; Urbanski, P.; et al. Nutrition therapy recommendations for the management of adults with diabetes. *Diabetes Care* **2014**, *37*, S120–S143. [CrossRef] [PubMed]
95. Imamura, F.; Micha, R.; Wu, J.H.Y.; de Oliveira Otto, M.C.; Otite, F.O.; Abioye, A.I.; Mozaffarian, D. Effects of saturated fat, polyunsaturated fat, monounsaturated fat, and carbohydrate on glucose-insulin homeostasis: A systematic review and meta-analysis of randomised controlled feeding trials. *PLoS Med.* **2016**, *13*, e1002087. [CrossRef] [PubMed]
96. Turco, J.V.; Inal-Veith, A.; Fuster, V. Cardiovascular Health Promotion. *J. Am. Coll. Cardiol.* **2018**, *72*, 908–913. [CrossRef] [PubMed]
97. Salas-Salvado, J.; Becerra-Tomas, N.; Garcia-Gavilan, J.F.; Bullo, M.; Barrubes, L. Mediterranean Diet and Cardiovascular Disease Prevention: What Do We Know? *Prog. Cardiovasc. Dis.* **2018**, *61*, 62–67. [CrossRef] [PubMed]
98. Jacobs, D.R.J.; Petersen, K.S.; Svendsen, K.; Ros, E.; Sloan, C.B.; Steffen, L.M.; Tapsell, L.C.; Kris-Etherton, P.M. Considerations to facilitate a US study that replicates PREDIMED. *Metabolism* **2018**, *85*, 361–367. [CrossRef] [PubMed]
99. Appel, L.J.; Van Horn, L. Did the PREDIMED trial test a Mediterranean diet? *N. Engl. J. Med.* **2013**, *368*, 1353–1354. [CrossRef] [PubMed]

12

Uncommon Fatty Acids and Cardiometabolic Health

Kelei Li [1], Andrew J. Sinclair [2,3], Feng Zhao [1] and Duo Li [1,3,*]

[1] Institute of Nutrition and Health, Qingdao University, Qingdao 266021, China; likelei@qdu.edu.cn (K.L.); fzhao@qdu.edu.cn (F.Z.)

[2] Faculty of Health, Deakin University, Locked Bag 20000, Geelong, VIC 3220, Australia; andrew.sinclair@deakin.edu.au

[3] Department of Nutrition, Dietetics and Food, Monash University, Notting Hill, VIC 3168, Australia

* Correspondence: duoli@qdu.edu.cn

Abstract: Cardiovascular disease (CVD) is a major cause of mortality. The effects of several unsaturated fatty acids on cardiometabolic health, such as eicosapentaenoic acid (EPA) docosahexaenoic acid (DHA), α linolenic acid (ALA), linoleic acid (LA), and oleic acid (OA) have received much attention in past years. In addition, results from recent studies revealed that several other uncommon fatty acids (fatty acids present at a low content or else not contained in usual foods), such as furan fatty acids, *n*-3 docosapentaenoic acid (DPA), and conjugated fatty acids, also have favorable effects on cardiometabolic health. In the present report, we searched the literature in PubMed, Embase, and the Cochrane Library to review the research progress on anti-CVD effect of these uncommon fatty acids. DPA has a favorable effect on cardiometabolic health in a different way to other long-chain *n*-3 polyunsaturated fatty acids (LC *n*-3 PUFAs), such as EPA and DHA. Furan fatty acids and conjugated linolenic acid (CLNA) may be potential bioactive fatty acids beneficial for cardiometabolic health, but evidence from intervention studies in humans is still limited, and well-designed clinical trials are required. The favorable effects of conjugated linoleic acid (CLA) on cardiometabolic health observed in animal or in vitro cannot be replicated in humans. However, most intervention studies in humans concerning CLA have only evaluated its effect on cardiometabolic risk factors but not its direct effect on risk of CVD, and randomized controlled trials (RCTs) will be required to clarify this point. However, several difficulties and limitations exist for conducting RCTs to evaluate the effect of these fatty acids on cardiometabolic health, especially the high costs for purifying the fatty acids from natural sources. This review provides a basis for better nutritional prevention and therapy of CVD.

Keywords: furan fatty acids; docosapentaenoic acid; conjugated fatty acids; cardiovascular disease; metabolic disease; blood lipids; inflammation; antioxidant

---

1. Introduction

Cardiovascular disease (CVD) is a major cause of mortality [1]. In addition to genetic factors, dyslipidemia [2], poor glycemic control [3], oxidative stress [4], inflammation [5], obesity [6], hyperhomocysteinemia [7], smoking [8], lack of exercise [8], and dietary factors [8] are all related to the development of CVD.

Fatty acids are important structural components of biological membranes and an energy source for living organism. In addition, they also play an important role in regulating many physiological processes, such as inflammation, glycemic control, lipid metabolism and oxidative stress. All these physiological processes are closely related to the development of CVD and metabolic disorders. The beneficial effect of several unsaturated fatty acids, such as eicosapentaenoic acid (EPA) docosahexaenoic acid (DHA), α linolenic acid (ALA), linoleic acid (LA), and oleic acid (OA), on cardiometabolic health has been given much attention [9–19]. However, the effect of several other uncommon fatty acids (fatty acids present at a low content or else not contained in usual foods) on cardiometabolic health, such as furan fatty acids, *n*-3 docosapentaenoic acid (DPA), and conjugated fatty acids, is also worthy of attention. In the present review, we searched PubMed, Embase, and the Cochrane Library for the terms (docosapentaenoic acid OR *n*-3 polyunsaturated fatty acids OR DPA OR furan fatty acids OR CMPF OR conjugated linolenic acid OR conjugated linoleic acid OR conjugated fatty acid OR CLNA OR CLA) in combination with (cardiometabolic health OR cardiovascular disease OR CVD OR blood lipids OR diabetes mellitus OR glucose metabolism OR oxidative stress OR inflammation) up to July 2018, to review the research progress on the effect of these uncommon fatty acids on cardiometabolic health. Studies in humans, animals or in vitro evaluating the relationship between uncommon fatty acids (furan fatty acids, conjugated fatty acids or DPA) and cardiometabolic health were included in the present review. The review should provide a basis for better nutritional prevention and therapy of CVD and metabolic disorders.

2. Furan Fatty Acids and Cardiometabolic Health

2.1. Origin of Furan Fatty Acids

Naturally occurring furan fatty acids are a family of fatty acids consisting of a furan ring with a fatty acid chain on the α1-position, a short straight alkyl group on the α2-position, a methyl group on the β1-position, and either a methyl group or a hydrogen atom on the β2-position [20]. Structures of the most abundant furan fatty acids are shown in Figure 1. Furan fatty acids have been found in different biological species, in low concentrations, including marine and freshwater fish [21], plants [22], algae [23,24], crustaceans [25,26], mammals [27], human tissues [28], fungi [29], ascidian [30], bacteria [31], bivalves [32], and echinoidea [33]. Furan fatty acids are mainly enriched in cholesterol ester and fraction of triacylglycerol (TAG) in liver of mammals, but occur mainly in phosphatidylcholine (PC) and phosphatidylethanolamine (PE) in plasma [34].

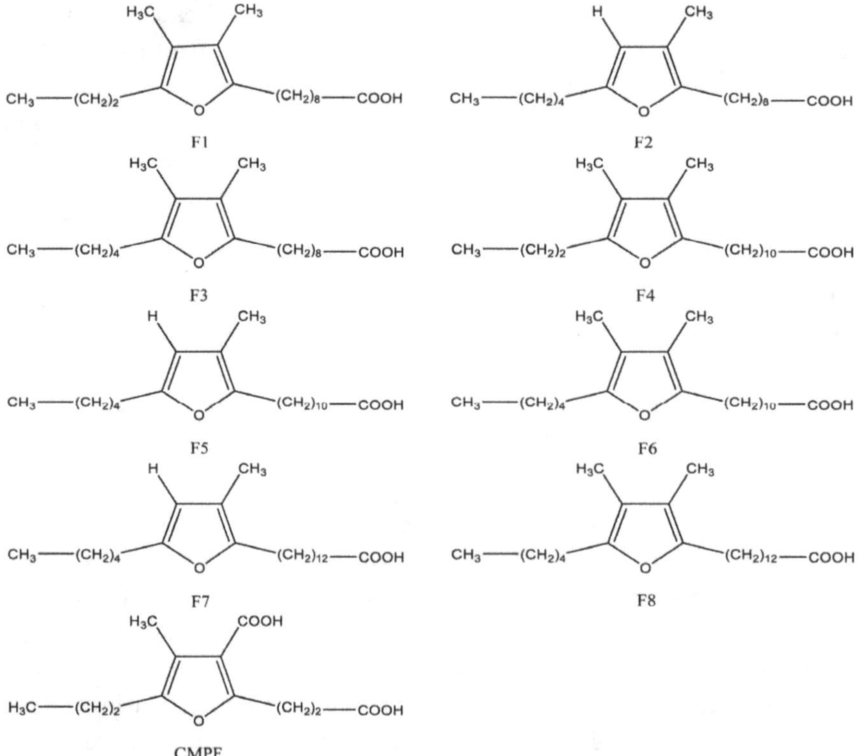

Figure 1. Structure of most abundant furan fatty acids (F1–F8) [35] and their bioactive metabolite 3-carboxy-4-methyl-5-propyl-2-furanpropionic acid (CMPF).

2.2. Evidence from Human Studies

In addition to EPA and DHA, furan fatty acids may be another bioactive constituent of marine food and its oil product beneficial for cardiometabolic health despite its low concentration (around 1% in some species of fish [21,28]). Fish oil consumption significantly increased 3-carboxy-4-methyl-5-propyl-2-furanpropionic acid (CMPF), a metabolite of common furan fatty acids, by 3-fold and 5 to 6-fold in serum and urine of humans, respectively [36]. Our recent randomized controlled trial (RCT) in subjects with type 2 diabetes mellitus (T2DM) indicated that fish oil consumption significantly increased the serum CMPF level, and most importantly, the change of CMPF during intervention was negatively correlated with the change of plasma TAG levels [37]. In another randomized crossover study, a multifunctional diet (MFD) formulated according to the Nordic Nutrition Recommendations improved serum total cholesterol (TC), low density lipoprotein cholesterol (LDLC), triacylglycerol (TAG), ratios of LDL to high density lipoprotein (HDL) and apolipoprotein B (ApoB) to ApoA1, glycated hemoglobin (HbA1c), C-reactive protein (CRP) and systolic blood pressure [38]. Metabolomics analysis indicated that this MFD significantly increased plasma level of four furan fatty acids, including CMPF, 3,4-dimethyl-5-pentyl-2-furanpropanoic acid (a furan fatty acids have been identified in crayfish), and furan fatty acids with molecular weights of 226.084 and 252.172 (accurate structure was not confirmed). Furthermore, a strong inverse correlation of CMPF and 3,4-dimethyl-5-pentyl-2-furanpropanoic acid with TC, LDLC, and the LDLC to HDLC ratio was observed [38]. Furan fatty acids may also have an anti-inflammatory effect: The New Zealand green lipped mussel contains a certain amount of furan fatty acids [32], and our previous RCT indicated a lipid extract from mussels effectively improved clinical conditions of patients with rheumatoid arthritis, significantly decreased levels of tumor necrosis factor α (TNF-α), interleukin 1β (IL-1β) and prostaglandin E2 (PGE2), and significantly increased levels of IL-10 [39].

However, until now, no clinical trials have been conducted to evaluate the effect of furan fatty acids with relatively high purity on cardiometabolic health because they are usually difficult to separate in quantity and high purity from other fatty acids. One previous study indicated that starvation could dramatically increase the weight percentage of furan fatty acids in total lipids of cod liver by more than 34% [21]. A method for isolation of furan fatty acids from fish lipids has been reported, and the process included: lipid extraction by chloroform and methanol (2:1), methylation of fatty acids, hydrogenation of common straight-chain unsaturated fatty acid methyl esters, and removal of saturated fatty acid methyl esters by crystallization as urea complexes [35]. In addition to isolation of furan fatty acids from lipids of food, artificial synthesis is another option to obtain furan fatty acids with relatively high degree of purity [40].

2.3. Evidence from Animal and In Vitro Studies

One recently published animal study indicated that purified CMPF supplementation improved insulin sensitivity, increased beta-oxidation, reduced lipogenic gene expression, and ameliorated steatosis [41]. This suggested that CMPF has a favorable metabolic effect. However, a contradictory result concerning the effect of CMPF on glucose metabolism was observed by another animal study, including glucose intolerance, impaired glucose-stimulated insulin secretion, and decreased glucose utilization [42]. Sand et al. extracted furan fatty acids from northern pike (*Esox lucius*) testes, and supplementation of furan fatty acids to rats led to the appearance of CMPF in urine, indicating that CMPF was a metabolite of common furan fatty acids [43]. Wakimoto et al. extracted furan fatty acids (predominantly F4 and F6) from mussels and compared their anti-inflammatory effect with EPA, commercially available F6, and the anti-inflammatory drug Naproxen in a rat model of adjuvant-induced arthritis, and found that furan fatty acids extracted from mussels had comparable anti-inflammatory effect with Naproxen and commercially available F6; the anti-inflammatory effect of furan fatty acids was more potent than that of EPA [32]. The anti-inflammatory effect of a lipid extract from mussel was also observed in our previous animal study which found that a lipid extract from mussel had an equivalent protective effect to fish oil on intestinal integrity after lipopolysaccharide

(LPS) challenge in mice, by increasing the expression of anti-inflammatory cytokine IL-10, decreasing the expression of pro-inflammatory cytokines TNF-α and IL-1β and downregulating toll-like receptor 4 (TLR-4) signal pathway [39]. These results indicated that furan fatty acids, long neglected, might be one bioactive component responsible for the anti-inflammatory effect of lipid products of marine food. Okada et al. synthesized four kinds of furan fatty acids, F2, F3, F6, and 9,12-epoxyoctadeca-9,11-dienoic acid (NMF), and found that tetra-alkyl substituted furan fatty acids (F3 and F6) had the best antioxidant activity in vitro by decomposing hydroperoxides and scavenging peroxyl radicals; the antioxidant activity of tri-alkyl substituted compound (F2) was about 50% as effective as the tetra-alkyl substituted one, while di-alkyl substituted one (NMF) revealed no significant activity [44]. Another in vitro study by Okada et al. compared the hydroxyl radical scavenging activity of artificially synthesized furan fatty acids (F2, F3, and NMF) with other common hydroxyl radical scavengers, and found that the hydroxyl radical scavenging activity of furan fatty acids was better than mannitol and ethanol, and was comparable with that of histidine and dimethyl sulfoxide (DMSO) [45]. Lipid oxidation is an important aspect in the pathogenesis for CVD [46]. Therefore, furan fatty acids, because of their antioxidant activity, may also play a role in protecting against aspects of CVD.

2.4. *Brief Summary*

Evidence from previous studies implied a favorable effect of furan fatty acids on cardiometabolic health. Clinical trials are required to confirm the direct effect of furan fatty acids on cardiometabolic health by using purified furan fatty acids as treatment.

3. DPA and Cardiometabolic Health

3.1. *Origin of DPA*

DPA is a long chain *n*-3 polyunsaturated fatty acid (LC *n*-3 PUFA) widely existing in marine foods and fish oils, together with EPA and DHA. The structures of DPA, EPA, and DHA are shown in Figure 2. The content of DPA in most fish is typically much less than that of EPA and DHA, and in salmon flesh, fish oil, and seal oil the levels are about 0.3%, 2–5%, and 4–5%, respectively [47]. One previous study dramatically increased DPA content in a marine fish, nibe croaker, from 1.8% to 4.1% by addition of an elongase gene to the fish [48].

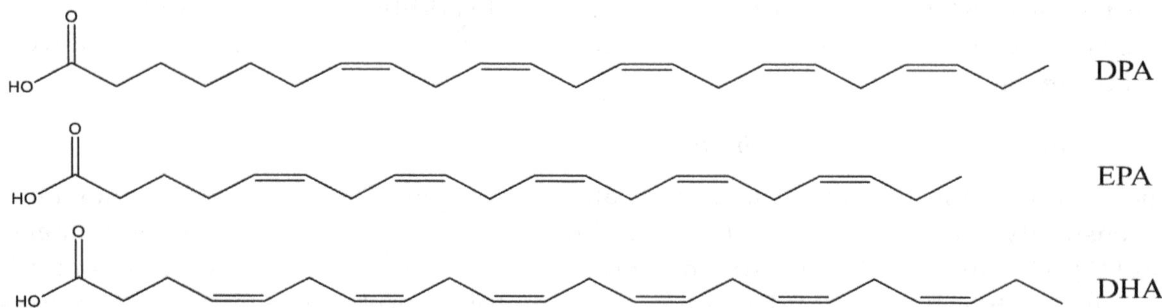

Figure 2. Structure of *n*-3 docosapentaenoic acid (DPA), eicosapentaenoic acid (EPA), and docosahexaenoic acid (DHA).

3.2. *Evidence from Human Studies*

Most previous studies evaluating the effect of LC *n*-3 PUFA on cardiometabolic health did not discriminate between the effect of EPA, DHA, and DPA. Results from recent studies indicated that DPA could also influence cardiometabolic health. Our previous meta-analysis based on 10 prospective cohort studies in 20,460 individuals indicated that the risk of stroke was negatively associated with circulating level of DPA (relative risk (RR) 0.74, 95% confidence interval (CI) 0.60 to 0.92) and DHA (RR 0.78, 95% CI 0.65 to 0.94), but not EPA (RR 0.95, 95% CI 0.82 to 1.12) [49]. Dose–response analysis indicated that 1% increment of DPA and DHA proportions in circulating blood was associated with

25% (RR 0.75, 95% CI 0.64 to 0.87) and 11% (RR 0.89, 95% CI 0.83 to 0.95) reduced risk of stroke, respectively [49]. One meta-analysis based on prospective cohort studies indicated that coronary risk was negatively associated with circulating levels of DPA (RR 0.64, 95% CI 0.47 to 0.87, 7155 subjects in four studies) [50]. Evidence from observational studies indicated that the circulating DPA level was also negatively associated with the risk of cardiovascular mortality (hazard ratio (HR) 0.68, 95% CI 0.52 to 0.89) [51], sudden cardiac death (odds ratio (OR) 0.70, 95% CI 0.51 to 0.97) [52], heart failure (OR 0.81, 95% CI 0.68–0.95) and peripheral arterial disease (OR 0.61, 95% CI 0.45 to 0.82) [53] as well as carotid intimal–medial thickness ($\beta = -0.0002 \pm 0.0007$ (standard error), $p = 0.037$) [54].

Our previous double blind crossover study found that pure DPA supplementation could significantly reduce postprandial plasma chylomicronemia compared with pure EPA or olive oil supplementation in healthy subjects [55]. Another crossover study found that compared with EPA alone, EPA + DPA supplementation could significantly lower TAG, TC, non-high-density lipoprotein cholesterol, very low-density lipoprotein cholesterol (VLDLC), ApoC3, and proprotein convertase subtilisin kexin type 9 (PCSK9) in subjects with severe hypertriglyceridemia [56]. This trial also reported that EPA + DPA supplementation rather than EPA alone could significantly reduce nile red staining of lipids in monocytes, and that both EPA + DPA and EPA alone significantly reduce monocytes surface markers CD11c, CD36, and CCR5, indicating that DPA might protect against atherosclerosis by inhibiting foamy monocyte formation and modulating monocyte phenotype [57]. In addition, DPA can modulate lipid mediator profile in a different way compared with EPA: in a crossover study, DPA supplementation increased 19,20-dihydroxy-DPA (19,20-DiHDoPE), 7,17-DiHDoPE, and 15-keto-prostaglandin E2, while EPA increased monohydroxy-eicosapentaenoic acids (HEPEs), and there was no overlap in PUFA metabolites formed after DPA and EPA supplementation [58]. One RCT found that EPA + DPA supplementation dose-dependently increased erythrocyte membrane DPA content, and DPA level was inversely associated with serum CRP level. A cohort study in 2547 children with elevated risk of type 1 diabetes indicated that erythrocyte membrane DPA content but not EPA or DHA was negatively associated with the risk of islet autoimmunity [59]. Our cross-sectional study in healthy subjects indicated that after adjusting for potential confounding factors, platelet phospholipid DPA content but not EPA was inversely correlated with mean platelet volume, an independent risk factor for acute myocardial infarction [60].

3.3. Evidence from Animal and In Vitro Studies

In a rat model of rheumatoid arthritis, DPA showed a comparable reducing effect with EPA on the progression and severity of arthritic disease as well as pro-inflammatory cytokines, such as IL-17A, IL-1β, IL-6, and TNFα [61]. In addition, DPA and EPA both significantly down-regulated the activation of mitogen-activated protein kinases (p38 MAPK) and nuclear factor-kappa B (NF-κB) pathways and decreased the expression of cyclooxygenase-2 (COX-2), matrix metalloproteinase-2 (MMP-2) and MMP-9 [61]. This can help explain the mechanism for their anti-inflammatory effect. Moreover, pro-resolving mediators derived from DPA can also contribute to its anti-inflammatory effect, but the types of pro-resolving mediators derived from DPA were different from those derived from other LC *n*-3 PUFA, such as EPA and DHA [62]. In mice fed a high-fat diet, purified DPA, EPA, or DHA supplementation improved serum TC, glucose, and liver cholesterol content; only DPA improved insulin resistance rather than EPA or DHA. DPA and DHA but not EPA prevented decreased serum adiponectin and increased serum alanine aminotransferase (ALT) [63]. Either high-fat diet or high-fructose diet significantly decreased plasma DPA and DHA level in rats, and both LC *n*-3 PUFAs were positively associated with insulin sensitivity [64]. Our previous study in rat liver cells indicated that DPA could down-regulate a series of genes involved in fat synthesis, including sterol-regulatory element-binding protein-1c (*SREBP-1c*), 3-hydroxy-3-methyl-glutaryl-coenzyme A reductase (*HMG-CoA reductase*), acetyl coenzyme A carboxylase (*ACC-1*), and fatty acid synthase (*FASn*) [65]. This result can help explain the mechanism for the protecting effect of DPA against hypertriglyceridemia. Reduced platelet aggregation by DPA was also observed in our previous in vitro study [66].

3.4. Brief Summary

DPA has a favorable effect on cardiometabolic health in a different way to the other LC *n*-3 PUFAs, such as EPA and DHA. However, few intervention studies in humans have been conducted to evaluate the direct effect of DPA on risk of CVD. Well-designed RCTs should be conducted by using purified DPA as treatment to clarify this point.

4. Conjugated Fatty Acids and Cardiometabolic Health

4.1. Origin of Conjugated Fatty Acids

Conjugated fatty acids is the general term for positional and geometric isomers of polyunsaturated fatty acids with conjugated double bonds [67]. The most common conjugated fatty acids are conjugated linoleic acids (CLAs), such as *cis*-9,*trans*-11 CLA and *trans*-10,*cis*-12 CLA, and conjugated linolenic acids (CLNAs), such as α-eleostearic acid, punicic acid, and jacaric acid. *cis*-9,*trans*-11 CLA is the main naturally occurring isomer of CLA, and it was first found as an intermediate for the conversion from PUFA to saturated stearic acid by rumen bacteria [68]. This explained its presence in food from ruminant-animal origin, such as beef, sheep and goat meat and dairy products [67]. In addition, CLA has also been found in low proportions in some plant oils and seafood [69]. CLNA naturally occurs in plant seeds, such as tung seed, bitter gourd seed, snake gourd seed, pomegranate seed, trichosanthes seed, pot marigold seed, jacaranda seed, and catalpa seed [70–72]. Several studies in humans and animals indicated that CLNA could be metabolized into CLA in vivo [73,74]. The structures of the most common conjugated fatty acids are shown in Figure 3.

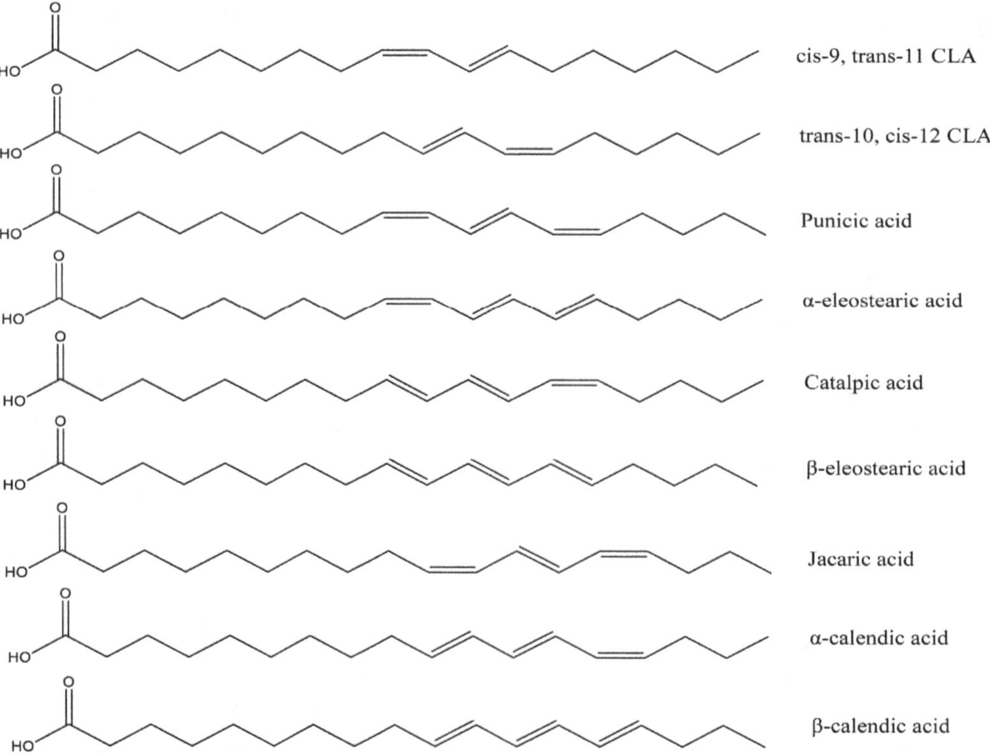

Figure 3. Structure of most abundant conjugated linoleic acids (CLAs) and conjugated linolenic acids (CLNA).

4.2. CLA and Cardiometabolic Health

4.2.1. Evidence from Human Studies

Few significant effects of CLA on CVD and its risk factors have been observed in human studies. Only one case-control study reported a significant negative association between *cis*-9,*trans*-11 CLA in adipose tissue and risk of myocardial infarction [75]. One RCT indicated that 6-month supplementation of *cis*-9,*trans*-11 CLA had no significant influence on blood lipids, glucose, CRP, blood pressure, insulin resistance, body composition and 10-year absolute risk of fatal CVD calculated by the European Systematic Coronary Risk Evaluation (SCORE) formula in overweight and obese subjects [76]. Consistent results concerning CVD risk factors were also observed in another two RCTs in healthy subjects and patients with atherosclerosis [77,78]. In addition, results from RCTs even indicated that *cis*-9,*trans*-11 CLA consumption could increase lipid peroxidation [77,79]. One RCT found that supplementation of another isomer of CLA, *trans*-10,*cis*-12 CLA, significantly increased CRP as well as lipid peroxidation [80]. Only one RCT reported a significant lowering effect of CLA (mixture of *cis*-9,*trans*-11 CLA and *trans*-10,*cis*-12 CLA, 50:50) on CRP in patients with atherosclerosis [81].

4.2.2. Evidence from Animal and in Vitro Studies

Lee et al. first reported that CLA (the isomer of CLA used was not reported) could significantly decrease TC, LDLC, TAG, the ratios of LDLC to HDLC and TC to HDLC and led to less atherosclerosis in rabbits [82]. The protective effect of CLA (*cis*-9,*trans*-11 CLA, *trans*-10,*cis*-12 CLA or their mixture) against atherosclerosis was also observed in other animal studies [83–85]. A more recent study in mice indicated that CLA could inhibit platelet deposition, decrease macrophage accumulation and expression of the macrophage scavenger receptor CD36 in the aorta, and increase apoptosis in atherosclerotic lesions, and thus exert a pre-resolving effect on atherosclerosis [86]. Increased expression of peroxisome proliferators-activated receptor α (PPARα) and PPARγ by CLA may be one possible mechanism for its protective effects against atherosclerosis [86]. CLA could also suppress monocyte adhesion in vitro by targetting β2 integrin expression [87]. This may be another mechanism for the anti-atherosclerotic effect of CLA. CLA (mixture of *cis*-9,*trans*-11 CLA and *trans*-10,*cis*-12 CLA) decreased pro-inflammatory cytokines (including IL-1β, IL-6, and TNFα) expression in mammary epithelial cells treated with LPS by inhibiting reactive oxygen species (ROS) production and up-regulating PPARγ expression [88]. A PPARγ-dependent anti-inflammatory effect of CLA was also observed in mice with inflammatory bowel disease [89]. Moreover, reducing pro-inflammatory eicosanoids release by inhibiting COX expression is also involved in the regulatory effect of CLA on inflammatory responses [90,91]. In addition, CLA could inhibit high glucose-induced hypertrophy and contractile dysfunction in adult rat cardiomyocytes by modulating PPARγ activation [92]. However, an unfavorable effect on cardiometabolic health was also observed: high dose of CLA supplementation increased insulin resistance in rats fed either a low fat or a high fat diet [93].

4.2.3. Brief Summary

Although favorable effects of CLA on cardiometabolic health have been observed in animal studies and an observational study in humans, there is little evidence from RCTs, which supports this opinion, and several RCTs even reported unfavorable results concerning lipid peroxidation and inflammation. However, few intervention studies in humans have been conducted to evaluate the direct effect of CLA on risk of CVD. Well-designed RCTs should be conducted to clarify this point.

4.3. CLNA and Cardiometabolic Health

4.3.1. Evidence from Human Studies

Favorable effects of CLNA on lipid metabolism were observed in one RCT: pomegranate seed oil supplementation (rich in punicic acid (*cis*-9,*trans*-11,*cis*-13 CLNA)) significantly lowered serum

TAG, the ratios of TAG to HDLC and TC to HDLC, and increased serum HDLC in hyperlipidemic subjects [94]. No studies in humans have evaluated the association between CLNA and CVD or other risk factors.

4.3.2. Evidence from Animal and in Vitro Studies

α-eleostearic acid (*cis*-9,*trans*-11,*trans*-13 CLNA) supplementation significantly lowered blood TAG level in diabetic rats [95]. Pomegranate seed oil supplementation, which is rich in punicic acid (*cis*-9,*trans*-11,*cis*-13 CLNA), significantly lowered TC in broilers [96]. Punicic acid (*cis*-9,*trans*-11,*cis*-13 CLNA) also significantly decreased ApoB100 secretion by human HepG2 cell in vitro [97]. ApoB100 is the essential component of very-low density lipoproteins and positively correlated with the incidence of coronary heart disease and atherosclerosis [97]. Bitter gourd oil supplementation, which is rich in α-eleostearic acid (*cis*-9,*trans*-11,*trans*-13 CLNA), decreased blood level of free cholesterol and increased HDLC in rats [98]. Several animal and in vitro studies reported the antioxidative effect of CLNA. Results from an animal study indicated that α-eleostearic acid (*cis*-9,*trans*-11,*trans*-13 CLNA) supplementation could significantly lower LDL-lipid peroxidation and erythrocyte membrane lipid peroxidation in diabetic rats [95]. One in vitro study also demonstrated that both punicic acid (*cis*-9,*trans*-11,*cis*-13 CLNA) and α-eleostearic acid (*cis*-9,*trans*-11,*trans*-13 CLNA) could more effectively scavenge hydroxyl radical and inhibit lipid peroxidation at lower concentrations than at higher concentrations [99]. Another animal study compared the antioxidant effect of punicic acid (*cis*-9,*trans*-11,*cis*-13 CLNA) and α-eleostearic acid (*cis*-9,*trans*-11,*trans*-13 CLNA) in rats, and found that both could effectively decrease oxidative stress and lipid peroxidation induced by sodium arsenite; the antioxidant effect of α-eleostearic acid was more potent than that of punicic acid [100]. However, contradictory results concerning the antioxidative effect of CLNA was observed in another animal study: supplementation of bitter gourd oil (rich in α-eleostearic acid (*cis*-9,*trans*-11,*trans*-13 CLNA)) significantly increased plasma hydroperoxides level [98]. One animal study evaluated the antioxidative effect of punicic acid at different dose, and found punicic acid could act as both pro-oxidant (dose as 1.2% in total fatty acids) and antioxidant (dose as 0.6% in total fatty acids) [101]. Therefore, differences in dose may help explain the inconsistent results concerning antioxidative effects of CLNA observed in previous studies. In addition, CLNA also has an anti-inflammatory effect. Intake of pomegranate seed oil (rich in punicic acid (*cis*-9,*trans*-11,*cis*-13 CLNA)) effectively inhibited neutrophil-activation and protected against trinitrobenzene sulfonic acid (TNBS)-induced colon inflammation in rats; the mechanism involved inhibiting TNF-α induced priming of NADPH oxidase and myeloperoxidase release [102]. One study reported that α-eleostearic acid (*cis*-9,*trans*-11,*trans*-13 CLNA) ameliorated inflammatory bowel disease in mice by activating PPARγ [103]. Down-regulating pro-inflammatory cytokines expression, COX expression and NF-κB signal pathway are potential mechanisms for the anti-inflammatory effects of CLNA [104,105].

4.3.3. Brief Summary

CLNA may have a favorable effect on cardiometabolic health, but evidence from human studies is still very limited, and well-designed RCTs should be conducted to evaluate the effect of CLNA supplementation on CVD and its risk factors.

5. Conclusions and Perspectives

DPA has a favorable effect on cardiometabolic health in a different way to the other LC *n*-3 PUFAs, such as EPA and DHA. Furan fatty acids and CLNA may be potential bioactive components beneficial for cardiometabolic health, but evidence from intervention studies in humans is still limited, and well-designed clinical trials will be required. The favorable effects of CLA on cardiometabolic health observed in animals or in vitro have not been replicated in most studies of humans. However, most intervention studies in humans concerning CLA have only evaluated its effect on cardiometabolic risk factors but not its direct effect on risk of CVD, and RCTs with large sample size are still required to clarify this point. Several difficulties and limitations exist for conducting RCTs to evaluate the effect of these fatty acids on cardiometabolic health, especially the high cost of purifying these fatty acids from natural sources because they occur at low levels in natural oils or foods.

Author Contributions: Conceptualization, K.L., A.J.S., and D.L.; methodology, K.L. and F.Z.; writing—original draft preparation, K.L.; writing—review and editing, A.J.S. and D.L.; supervision, A.J.S. and D.L.; project administration, K.L. and F.Z.; funding acquisition, D.L. and K.L.

References

1. Lloyd-Jones, D.; Adams, R.; Carnethon, M.; De Simone, G.; Ferguson, T.B.; Flegal, K.; Ford, E.; Furie, K.; Go, A.; Greenlund, K.; et al. Heart disease and stroke statistics—2009 update: A report from the American heart association statistics committee and stroke statistics subcommittee. *Circulation* **2009**, *119*, 480–486. [PubMed]
2. Nelson, R.H. Hyperlipidemia as a risk factor for cardiovascular disease. *Prim. Care* **2013**, *40*, 195–211. [CrossRef] [PubMed]
3. Laakso, M.; Kuusisto, J. Insulin resistance and hyperglycaemia in cardiovascular disease development. *Nat. Rev. Endocrinol.* **2014**, *10*, 293–302. [CrossRef] [PubMed]
4. Cai, H.; Harrison, D.G. Endothelial dysfunction in cardiovascular diseases: The role of oxidant stress. *Circ. Res.* **2000**, *87*, 840–844. [CrossRef] [PubMed]
5. Golia, E.; Limongelli, G.; Natale, F.; Fimiani, F.; Maddaloni, V.; Pariggiano, I.; Bianchi, R.; Crisci, M.; D'Acierno, L.; Giordano, R.; et al. Inflammation and cardiovascular disease: From pathogenesis to therapeutic target. *Curr. Atheroscler. Rep.* **2014**, *16*, 435. [CrossRef] [PubMed]
6. Zalesin, K.C.; Franklin, B.A.; Miller, W.M.; Peterson, E.D.; McCullough, P.A. Impact of obesity on cardiovascular disease. *Endocrinol. Metab. Clin. N. Am.* **2008**, *37*, 663–684. [CrossRef] [PubMed]
7. Wald, D.S.; Law, M.; Morris, J.K. Homocysteine and cardiovascular disease: Evidence on causality from a meta-analysis. *BMJ* **2002**, *325*, 1202. [CrossRef] [PubMed]
8. Potvin, L.; Richard, L.; Edwards, A.C. Knowledge of cardiovascular disease risk factors among the Canadian population: Relationships with indicators of socioeconomic status. *CMAJ* **2000**, *162*, S5–S11. [PubMed]
9. Abdelhamid, A.S.; Brown, T.J.; Brainard, J.S.; Biswas, P.; Thorpe, G.C.; Moore, H.J.; Deane, K.H.; AlAbdulghafoor, F.K.; Summerbell, C.D.; Worthington, H.V.; et al. Omega-3 fatty acids for the primary and secondary prevention of cardiovascular disease. *Cochrane Database Syst. Rev.* **2018**, *7*, Cd003177. [CrossRef] [PubMed]
10. Alhassan, A.; Young, J.; Lean, M.E.J.; Lara, J. Consumption of fish and vascular risk factors: A systematic review and meta-analysis of intervention studies. *Atherosclerosis* **2017**, *266*, 87–94. [CrossRef] [PubMed]
11. Chowdhury, R.; Stevens, S.; Gorman, D.; Pan, A.; Warnakula, S.; Chowdhury, S.; Ward, H.; Johnson, L.; Crowe, F.; Hu, F.B.; et al. Association between fish consumption, long chain omega 3 fatty acids, and risk of cerebrovascular disease: Systematic review and meta-analysis. *BMJ* **2012**, *345*, e6698. [CrossRef] [PubMed]
12. Clarke, R.; Daly, L.; Robinson, K.; Naughten, E.; Cahalane, S.; Fowler, B.; Graham, I. Hyperhomocysteinemia: An independent risk factor for vascular disease. *N. Engl. J. Med.* **1991**, *324*, 1149–1155. [CrossRef] [PubMed]
13. Huang, T.; Zheng, J.; Chen, Y.; Yang, B.; Wahlqvist, M.L.; Li, D. High consumption of omega-3 polyunsaturated fatty acids decrease plasma homocysteine: A meta-analysis of randomized, placebo-controlled trials. *Nutrition* **2011**, *27*, 863–867. [CrossRef] [PubMed]
14. Li, K.; Huang, T.; Zheng, J.; Wu, K.; Li, D. Effect of marine-derived n-3 polyunsaturated fatty acids on c-reactive protein, interleukin 6 and tumor necrosis factor alpha: A meta-analysis. *PLoS ONE* **2014**, *9*, e88103.
15. Maki, K.C.; Palacios, O.M.; Bell, M.; Toth, P.P. Use of supplemental long-chain omega-3 fatty acids and risk for cardiac death: An updated meta-analysis and review of research gaps. *J. Clin. Lipidol.* **2017**, *11*, 1152–1160. [CrossRef] [PubMed]

16. Fleming, J.A.; Kris-Etherton, P.M. The evidence for alpha-linolenic acid and cardiovascular disease benefits: Comparisons with eicosapentaenoic acid and docosahexaenoic acid. *Adv. Nutr.* **2014**, *5*, 863s–876s. [CrossRef] [PubMed]
17. Pan, A.; Chen, M.; Chowdhury, R.; Wu, J.H.; Sun, Q.; Campos, H.; Mozaffarian, D.; Hu, F.B. Alpha-linolenic acid and risk of cardiovascular disease: A systematic review and meta-analysis. *Am. J. Clin. Nutr.* **2012**, *96*, 1262–1273. [CrossRef] [PubMed]
18. Farvid, M.S.; Ding, M.; Pan, A.; Sun, Q.; Chiuve, S.E.; Steffen, L.M.; Willett, W.C.; Hu, F.B. Dietary linoleic acid and risk of coronary heart disease: A systematic review and meta-analysis of prospective cohort studies. *Circulation* **2014**, *130*, 1568–1578. [CrossRef] [PubMed]
19. Huth, P.J.; Fulgoni, V.L.; Larson, B.T. A systematic review of high-oleic vegetable oil substitutions for other fats and oils on cardiovascular disease risk factors: Implications for novel high-oleic soybean oils. *Adv. Nutr.* **2015**, *6*, 674–693. [CrossRef] [PubMed]
20. Xu, L.; Sinclair, A.J.; Faiza, M.; Li, D.; Han, X.; Yin, H.; Wang, Y. Furan fatty acids—Beneficial or harmful to health? *Prog. Lipid. Res.* **2017**, *68*, 119–137. [CrossRef] [PubMed]
21. Gunstone, F.D.; Chakra Wijesundera, R.; Scrimgeour, C.M. The component acids of lipids from marine and freshwater species with special reference to furan-containing acids. *J. Sci. Food Agric.* **1978**, *29*, 539–550. [CrossRef]
22. Hannemann, K.; Puchta, V.; Simon, E.; Ziegler, H.; Ziegler, G.; Spiteller, G. The common occurrence of furan fatty acids in plants. *Lipids* **1989**, *24*, 296–298. [CrossRef] [PubMed]
23. Batna, A.; Scheinkönig, J.; Spiteller, G. The occurrence of furan fatty acids in isochrysis sp. and phaeodactylum tricornutum. *Biochim. Biophys. Acta* **1993**, *1166*, 171–176. [CrossRef]
24. Kazlauskas, R.; Murphy, P.; Wells, R.; Gregson, R. Two new furans from the brown alga acrocarpia paniculata: The use of 4-phenyl-4h-1,2,4-triazoline-3,5-dione to determine the substitution pattern of a furan. *Aust. J. Chem.* **1982**, *35*, 165–170. [CrossRef]
25. Ishii, K.; Okajima, H.; Koyamatsu, T.; Okada, Y.; Watanabe, H. The composition of furan fatty acids in the crayfish. *Lipids* **1988**, *23*, 694–700. [CrossRef] [PubMed]
26. Dembitsky, V.M.; Rezanka, T. Furan fatty acids of some brackish invertebrates from the caspian sea. *Comp. Biochem. Physiol. B: Biochem. Mol. Biol.* **1996**, *114*, 317–320. [CrossRef]
27. Schödel, R.; Spiteller, G. Über das vorkommen von F-säuren in Rinderleber und deren enzymatischen Abbau bei Gewebeverletzung. *Liebigs Annalen der Chemie* **1987**, *1987*, 459–462. [CrossRef]
28. Wahl, H.G.N.; Chrzanowski, A.; Mu¨ller, C.; Liebich, H.M.; Hoffmann, A. Identification of furan fatty acids in human blood cells and plasma by multi-dimensional gas chromatography-mass spectrometry. *J. Chromatogr. A* **1995**, *697*, 453–459. [CrossRef]
29. Vetter, W.; Laure, S.; Wendlinger, C.; Mattes, A.; Smith, A.W.T.; Knight, D.W. Determination of furan fatty acids in food samples. *J. Am. Oil Chem. Soc.* **2012**, *89*, 1501–1508. [CrossRef]
30. Vysotskii, M.V.; Ota, T.; Takagi, T. N-3 polyunsaturated fatty acids in lipids of ascidian halocynthia roretzi. *Nippon Suisan Gakkaishi* **1992**, *58*, 953–958. [CrossRef]
31. Norifumi, S.; Kiyohiko, N.; Sakayu, S. Occurrence of a furan fatty acid in marine bacteria. *Biochim. Biophys. Acta* **1995**, *1258*, 225–227. [CrossRef]
32. Wakimoto, T.; Kondo, H.; Nii, H.; Kimura, K.; Egami, Y.; Oka, Y.; Yoshida, M.; Kida, E.; Ye, Y.; Akahoshi, S.; et al. Furan fatty acid as an anti-inflammatory component from the green-lipped mussel perna canaliculus. *Proc. Natl. Acad. Sci. USA* **2011**, *108*, 17533–17537. [CrossRef] [PubMed]
33. Angioni, A.; Addis, P. Characterization of the lipid fraction of wild sea urchin from the Sardinian sea (Western Mediterranean). *J. Food Sci.* **2014**, *79*, C155–C162. [CrossRef] [PubMed]
34. Spiteller, G. Furan fatty acids: Occurrence, synthesis, and reactions. Are furan fatty acids responsible for the cardioprotective effects of a fish diet? *Lipids* **2005**, *40*, 755–771. [CrossRef] [PubMed]
35. Glass, R.L.; Krick, T.P.; Sand, D.M.; Rahn, C.H.; Schlenk, H. Furanoid fatty acids from fish lipids. *Lipids* **1975**, *10*, 695–702. [CrossRef] [PubMed]
36. Wahl, H.G.; Tetschner, B.; Liebich, H.M. The effect of dietary fish oil supplementation on the concentration of 3-carboxy-4-methyl-5-propyl-2-furanpropionic acid in human blood and urine. *J. High. Resolut. Chromatogr.* **1992**, *15*, 815–818. [CrossRef]

37. Zheng, J.S.; Lin, M.; Imamura, F.; Cai, W.; Wang, L.; Feng, J.P.; Ruan, Y.; Tang, J.; Wang, F.; Yang, H.; et al. Serum metabolomics profiles in response to n-3 fatty acids in Chinese patients with type 2 diabetes: A double-blind randomised controlled trial. *Sci. Rep.* **2016**, *6*, 29522. [CrossRef] [PubMed]
38. Tovar, J.; De Mello, V.D.; Nilsson, A.; Johansson, M.; Paananen, J.; Lehtonen, M.; Hanhineva, K.; Bjorck, I. Reduction in cardiometabolic risk factors by a multifunctional diet is mediated via several branches of metabolism as evidenced by nontargeted metabolite profiling approach. *Mol. Nutr. Food Res.* **2017**, *61*. [CrossRef] [PubMed]
39. Fu, Y.; Li, G.; Zhang, X.; Xing, G.; Hu, X.; Yang, L.; Li, D. Lipid extract from hard-shelled mussel (Mytilus coruscus) improves clinical conditions of patients with rheumatoid arthritis: A randomized controlled trial. *Nutrients* **2015**, *7*, 625–645. [CrossRef] [PubMed]
40. Rahn, C.H.; Sand, D.M.; Wedmid, Y.; Schlenk, H.; Krick, T.P.; Glass, R.L. Synthesis of naturally occurring furan fatty acids. *J. Org. Chem.* **1979**, *44*, 3420–3424. [CrossRef]
41. Prentice, K.J.; Wendell, S.G.; Liu, Y.; Eversley, J.A.; Salvatore, S.R.; Mohan, H.; Brandt, S.L.; Adams, A.C.; Serena Wang, X.; Wei, D.; et al. CMPF, a metabolite formed upon prescription omega-3-acid ethyl ester supplementation, prevents and reverses steatosis. *EBioMedicine* **2018**, *27*, 200–213. [CrossRef] [PubMed]
42. Prentice, K.J.; Luu, L.; Allister, E.M.; Liu, Y.; Jun, L.S.; Sloop, K.W.; Hardy, A.B.; Wei, L.; Jia, W.; Fantus, I.G.; et al. The furan fatty acid metabolite CMPF is elevated in diabetes and induces beta cell dysfunction. *Cell Metab.* **2014**, *19*, 653–666. [CrossRef] [PubMed]
43. Sand, D.M.; Schlenk, H.; Thoma, H.; Spiteller, G. Catabolism of fish furan fatty acids to urofuran acids in the rat. *Biochim. Biophys. Acta* **1983**, *751*, 455–461. [CrossRef]
44. Okada, Y.; Okajima, H.; Konishi, H.; Terauchi, M.; Ishii, K.; Liu, I.-M.; Watanabe, H. Antioxidant effect of naturally occurring furan fatty acids on oxidation of linoleic acid in aqueous dispersion. *J. Am. Oil Chem. Soc.* **1990**, *67*, 858–862. [CrossRef]
45. Okada, Y.; Kaneko, M.; Okajima, H. Hydroxyl radical scavenging activity of naturally occurring furan fatty acids. *Biol. Pharm. Bull.* **1996**, *19*, 1607–1610. [CrossRef] [PubMed]
46. McIntyre, T.M.; Hazen, S.L. Lipid oxidation and cardiovascular disease: Introduction to a review series. *Circ. Res.* **2010**, *107*, 1167–1169. [CrossRef] [PubMed]
47. Kaur, G.; Guo, X.F.; Sinclair, A.J. Short update on docosapentaenoic acid: A bioactive long-chain n-3 fatty acid. *Curr. Opin. Clin. Nutr. Metab. Care* **2016**, *19*, 88–91. [CrossRef] [PubMed]
48. Kabeya, N.; Takeuchi, Y.; Yamamoto, Y.; Yazawa, R.; Haga, Y.; Satoh, S.; Yoshizaki, G. Modification of the n-3 HUFA biosynthetic pathway by transgenesis in a marine teleost, nibe croaker. *J. Biotechnol.* **2014**, *172*, 46–54. [CrossRef] [PubMed]
49. Yang, B.; Ren, X.L.; Huang, H.; Guo, X.J.; Ma, A.G.; Li, D. Circulating long-chain n-3 polyunsaturated fatty acid and incidence of stroke: A meta-analysis of prospective cohort studies. *Oncotarget* **2017**, *8*, 83781–83791. [CrossRef] [PubMed]
50. Chowdhury, R.; Warnakula, S.; Kunutsor, S.; Crowe, F.; Ward, H.A.; Johnson, L.; Franco, O.H.; Butterworth, A.S.; Forouhi, N.G.; Thompson, S.G.; et al. Association of dietary, circulating, and supplement fatty acids with coronary risk: A systematic review and meta-analysis. *Ann. Intern. Med.* **2014**, *160*, 398–406. [CrossRef] [PubMed]
51. Mozaffarian, D.; Lemaitre, R.N.; King, I.B.; Song, X.; Huang, H.; Sacks, F.M.; Rimm, E.B.; Wang, M.; Siscovick, D.S. Plasma phospholipid long-chain omega-3 fatty acids and total and cause-specific mortality in older adults: A cohort study. *Ann. Intern. Med.* **2013**, *158*, 515–525. [CrossRef] [PubMed]
52. Friedman, A.N.; Yu, Z.; Denski, C.; Tamez, H.; Wenger, J.; Thadhani, R.; Li, Y.; Watkins, B. Fatty acids and other risk factors for sudden cardiac death in patients starting hemodialysis. *Am. J. Nephrol.* **2013**, *38*, 12–18. [CrossRef] [PubMed]
53. Leng, G.C.; Horrobin, D.F.; Fowkes, F.G.; Smith, F.B.; Lowe, G.D.; Donnan, P.T.; Ells, K. Plasma essential fatty acids, cigarette smoking, and dietary antioxidants in peripheral arterial disease. A population-based case-control study. *Arterioscler. Thromb.* **1994**, *14*, 471–478. [CrossRef] [PubMed]
54. Hino, A.; Adachi, H.; Toyomasu, K.; Yoshida, N.; Enomoto, M.; Hiratsuka, A.; Hirai, Y.; Satoh, A.; Imaizumi, T. Very long chain n-3 fatty acids intake and carotid atherosclerosis: An epidemiological study evaluated by ultrasonography. *Atherosclerosis* **2004**, *176*, 145–149. [CrossRef] [PubMed]

55. Linderborg, K.M.; Kaur, G.; Miller, E.; Meikle, P.J.; Larsen, A.E.; Weir, J.M.; Nuora, A.; Barlow, C.K.; Kallio, H.P.; Cameron-Smith, D.; et al. Postprandial metabolism of docosapentaenoic acid (DPA, 22:5n-3) and eicosapentaenoic acid (EPA, 20:5n-3) in humans. *Prostaglandins Leukot. Essent. Fatty Acids* **2013**, *88*, 313–319. [CrossRef] [PubMed]
56. Maki, K.C.; Bobotas, G.; Dicklin, M.R.; Huebner, M.; Keane, W.F. Effects of mat9001 containing eicosapentaenoic acid and docosapentaenoic acid, compared to eicosapentaenoic acid ethyl esters, on triglycerides, lipoprotein cholesterol, and related variables. *J. Clin. Lipidol.* **2017**, *11*, 102–109. [CrossRef] [PubMed]
57. Dai Perrard, X.Y.; Lian, Z.; Bobotas, G.; Dicklin, M.R.; Maki, K.C.; Wu, H. Effects of n-3 fatty acid treatment on monocyte phenotypes in humans with hypertriglyceridemia. *J. Clin. Lipidol.* **2017**, *11*, 1361–1371. [CrossRef] [PubMed]
58. Markworth, J.F.; Kaur, G.; Miller, E.G.; Larsen, A.E.; Sinclair, A.J.; Maddipati, K.R.; Cameron-Smith, D. Divergent shifts in lipid mediator profile following supplementation with n-3 docosapentaenoic acid and eicosapentaenoic acid. *FASEB J.* **2016**, *30*, 3714–3725. [CrossRef] [PubMed]
59. Norris, J.M.; Kroehl, M.; Fingerlin, T.E.; Frederiksen, B.N.; Seifert, J.; Wong, R.; Clare-Salzler, M.; Rewers, M. Erythrocyte membrane docosapentaenoic acid levels are associated with islet autoimmunity: The diabetes autoimmunity study in the young. *Diabetologia* **2014**, *57*, 295–304. [CrossRef] [PubMed]
60. Li, D.; Turner, A.; Sinclair, A.J. Relationship between platelet phospholipid FA and mean platelet volume in healthy men. *Lipids* **2002**, *37*, 901–906. [CrossRef] [PubMed]
61. Morin, C.; Blier, P.U.; Fortin, S. Eicosapentaenoic acid and docosapentaenoic acid monoglycerides are more potent than docosahexaenoic acid monoglyceride to resolve inflammation in a rheumatoid arthritis model. *Arthritis Res. Ther.* **2015**, *17*, 142. [CrossRef] [PubMed]
62. Vik, A.; Dalli, J.; Hansen, T.V. Recent advances in the chemistry and biology of anti-inflammatory and specialized pro-resolving mediators biosynthesized from n-3 docosapentaenoic acid. *Bioorg. Med. Chem. Lett.* **2017**, *27*, 2259–2266. [CrossRef] [PubMed]
63. Guo, X.F.; Sinclair, A.J.; Kaur, G.; Li, D. Differential effects of EPA, DPA and DHA on cardio-metabolic risk factors in high-fat diet fed mice. *Prostaglandins Leukot. Essent. Fatty Acids* **2017**. [CrossRef] [PubMed]
64. Huang, J.P.; Cheng, M.L.; Hung, C.Y.; Wang, C.H.; Hsieh, P.S.; Shiao, M.S.; Chen, J.K.; Li, D.E.; Hung, L.M. Docosapentaenoic acid and docosahexaenoic acid are positively associated with insulin sensitivity in rats fed high-fat and high-fructose diets. *J. Diabetes* **2017**, *9*, 936–946. [CrossRef] [PubMed]
65. Kaur, G.; Sinclair, A.J.; Cameron-Smith, D.; Barr, D.P.; Molero-Navajas, J.C.; Konstantopoulos, N. Docosapentaenoic acid (22:5n-3) down-regulates the expression of genes involved in fat synthesis in liver cells. *Prostaglandins Leukot. Essent. Fatty Acids* **2011**, *85*, 155–161. [CrossRef] [PubMed]
66. Phang, M.; Garg, M.L.; Sinclair, A.J. Inhibition of platelet aggregation by omega-3 polyunsaturated fatty acids is gender specific-redefining platelet response to fish oils. *Prostaglandins Leukot. Essent. Fatty Acids* **2009**, *81*, 35–40. [CrossRef] [PubMed]
67. Yuan, G.; Chen, X.; Li, D. Modulation of peroxisome proliferator-activated receptor gamma (PPAR gamma) by conjugated fatty acid in obesity and inflammatory bowel disease. *J. Agric. Food Chem.* **2015**, *63*, 1883–1895. [CrossRef] [PubMed]
68. Kepler, C.R.; Hirons, K.P.; McNeill, J.J.; Tove, S.B. Intermediates and products of the biohydrogenation of linoleic acid by butyrinvibrio fibrisolvens. *J. Biol. Chem.* **1966**, *241*, 1350–1354. [PubMed]
69. Chin, S.F.; Liu, W.; Storkson, J.M.; Ha, Y.L.; Pariza, M.W. Dietary sources of conjugated dienoic isomers of linoleic acid, a newly recognized class of anticarcinogens. *J. Food Compost. Anal.* **1992**, *5*, 185–197. [CrossRef]
70. Özgül-Yücel, S. Determination of conjugated linolenic acid content of selected oil seeds grown in Turkey. *J. Am. Oil Chem. Soc.* **2005**, *82*, 893–897. [CrossRef]
71. Takagi, T.; Itabashi, Y. Occurrence of mixtures of geometrical isomers of conjugated octadecatrienoic acids in some seed oils: Analysis by open-tubular gas liquid chromatography and high performance liquid chromatography. *Lipids* **1981**, *16*, 546–551. [CrossRef]
72. Chisholm, M.J.; Hopkins, C.Y. Isolation and structure of a new conjugated triene fatty acid 1. *J. Org. Chem.* **1962**, *27*, 3137–3139. [CrossRef]
73. Kijima, R.; Honma, T.; Ito, J.; Yamasaki, M.; Ikezaki, A.; Motonaga, C.; Nishiyama, K.; Tsuduki, T. Jacaric acid is rapidly metabolized to conjugated linoleic acid in rats. *J. Oleo Sci.* **2013**, *62*, 305–312. [CrossRef] [PubMed]

74. Yuan, G.; Sinclair, A.J.; Xu, C.; Li, D. Incorporation and metabolism of punicic acid in healthy young humans. *Mol. Nutr. Food Res.* **2009**, *53*, 1336–1342. [CrossRef] [PubMed]
75. Smit, L.A.; Baylin, A.; Campos, H. Conjugated linoleic acid in adipose tissue and risk of myocardial infarction. *Am. J. Clin. Nutr.* **2010**, *92*, 34–40. [CrossRef] [PubMed]
76. Sluijs, I.; Plantinga, Y.; De Roos, B.; Mennen, L.I.; Bots, M.L. Dietary supplementation with *cis*-9,*trans*-11 conjugated linoleic acid and aortic stiffness in overweight and obese adults. *Am. J. Clin. Nutr.* **2010**, *91*, 175–183. [CrossRef] [PubMed]
77. Raff, M.; Tholstrup, T.; Basu, S.; Nonboe, P.; Sorensen, M.T.; Straarup, E.M. A diet rich in conjugated linoleic acid and butter increases lipid peroxidation but does not affect atherosclerotic, inflammatory, or diabetic risk markers in healthy young men. *J. Nutr.* **2008**, *138*, 509–514. [CrossRef] [PubMed]
78. Eftekhari, M.; Aliasghari, F.; Beigi, M.A.; Hasanzadeh, J. The effect of conjugated linoleic acids and omega-3 fatty acids supplementation on lipid profile in atherosclerosis. *Adv. Biomed. Res.* **2014**, *3*, 15. [PubMed]
79. Riserus, U.; Vessby, B.; Arnlov, J.; Basu, S. Effects of *cis*-9,*trans*-11 conjugated linoleic acid supplementation on insulin sensitivity, lipid peroxidation, and proinflammatory markers in obese men. *Am. J. Clin. Nutr.* **2004**, *80*, 279–283. [CrossRef] [PubMed]
80. Riserus, U.; Basu, S.; Jovinge, S.; Fredrikson, G.N.; Arnlov, J.; Vessby, B. Supplementation with conjugated linoleic acid causes isomer-dependent oxidative stress and elevated c-reactive protein: A potential link to fatty acid-induced insulin resistance. *Circulation* **2002**, *106*, 1925–1929. [CrossRef] [PubMed]
81. Hassan Eftekhari, M.; Aliasghari, F.; Babaei-Beigi, M.A.; Hasanzadeh, J. Effect of conjugated linoleic acid and omega-3 fatty acid supplementation on inflammatory and oxidative stress markers in atherosclerotic patients. *ARYA Atheroscler.* **2013**, *9*, 311–318. [PubMed]
82. Lee, K.N.; Kritchevsky, D.; Pariza, M.W. Conjugated linoleic acid and atherosclerosis in rabbits. *Atherosclerosis* **1994**, *108*, 19–25. [CrossRef]
83. Kritchevsky, D.; Tepper, S.A.; Wright, S.; Czarnecki, S.K.; Wilson, T.A.; Nicolosi, R.J. Conjugated linoleic acid isomer effects in atherosclerosis: Growth and regression of lesions. *Lipids* **2004**, *39*, 611–616. [CrossRef] [PubMed]
84. Kritchevsky, D.; Tepper, S.A.; Wright, S.; Tso, P.; Czarnecki, S.K. Influence of conjugated linoleic acid (CLA) on establishment and progression of atherosclerosis in rabbits. *J. Am. Coll. Nutr.* **2000**, *19*, 472S–477S. [CrossRef] [PubMed]
85. Kritchevsky, D.; Tepper, S.A.; Wright, S.; Czarnecki, S.K. Influence of graded levels of conjugated linoleic acid (CLA) on experimental atherosclerosis in rabbits. *Nutr. Res.* **2002**, *22*, 1275–1279. [CrossRef]
86. Toomey, S.; Harhen, B.; Roche, H.M.; Fitzgerald, D.; Belton, O. Profound resolution of early atherosclerosis with conjugated linoleic acid. *Atherosclerosis* **2006**, *187*, 40–49. [CrossRef] [PubMed]
87. De Gaetano, M.; Dempsey, E.; Marcone, S.; James, W.G.; Belton, O. Conjugated linoleic acid targets beta2 integrin expression to suppress monocyte adhesion. *J. Immunol.* **2013**, *191*, 4326–4336. [CrossRef] [PubMed]
88. Dipasquale, D.; Basirico, L.; Morera, P.; Primi, R.; Troscher, A.; Bernabucci, U. Anti-inflammatory effects of conjugated linoleic acid isomers and essential fatty acids in bovine mammary epithelial cells. *Animal* **2018**, *12*, 2108–2114. [CrossRef] [PubMed]
89. Bassaganya-Riera, J.; Reynolds, K.; Martino-Catt, S.; Cui, Y.; Hennighausen, L.; Gonzalez, F.; Rohrer, J.; Benninghoff, A.U.; Hontecillas, R. Activation of PPAR gamma and delta by conjugated linoleic acid mediates protection from experimental inflammatory bowel disease. *Gastroenterology* **2004**, *127*, 777–791. [CrossRef] [PubMed]
90. Whigham, L.D.; Cook, E.B.; Stahl, J.L.; Saban, R.; Bjorling, D.E.; Pariza, M.W.; Cook, M.E. CLA reduces antigen-induced histamine and PGE2 release from sensitized guinea pig tracheae. *Am. J. Physiol. Regul. Integr. Comp. Physiol.* **2001**, *280*, R908–R912. [CrossRef] [PubMed]
91. Whigham, L.D.; Higbee, A.; Bjorling, D.E.; Park, Y.; Pariza, M.W.; Cook, M.E. Decreased antigen-induced eicosanoid release in conjugated linoleic acid-fed guinea pigs. *Am. J. Physiol. Regul. Integr. Comp. Physiol.* **2002**, *282*, R1104–R1112. [CrossRef] [PubMed]
92. Aloud, B.M.; Raj, P.; O'Hara, K.; Shao, Z.; Yu, L.; Anderson, H.D.; Netticadan, T. Conjugated linoleic acid prevents high glucose-induced hypertrophy and contractile dysfunction in adult rat cardiomyocytes. *Nutr. Res.* **2016**, *36*, 134–142. [CrossRef] [PubMed]

93. Bezan, P.N.; Holland, H.; De Castro, G.S.; Cardoso, J.F.R.; Ovidio, P.P.; Calder, P.C.; Jordao, A.A. High dose of a conjugated linoleic acid mixture increases insulin resistance in rats fed either a low fat or a high fat diet. *Exp. Clin. Endocrinol. Diabetes* **2018**, *126*, 379–386. [CrossRef] [PubMed]
94. Mirmiran, P.; Fazeli, M.R.; Asghari, G.; Shafiee, A.; Azizi, F. Effect of pomegranate seed oil on hyperlipidaemic subjects: A double-blind placebo-controlled clinical trial. *Br. J. Nutr.* **2010**, *104*, 402–406. [CrossRef] [PubMed]
95. Dhar, P.; Bhattacharyya, D.; Bhattacharyya, D.K.; Ghosh, S. Dietary comparison of conjugated linolenic acid (9 *cis*, 11 *trans*, 13 *trans*) and alpha-tocopherol effects on blood lipids and lipid peroxidation in alloxan-induced diabetes mellitus in rats. *Lipids* **2006**, *41*, 49–54. [CrossRef] [PubMed]
96. Manterys, A.; Franczyk-Zarow, M.; Czyzynska-Cichon, I.; Drahun, A.; Kus, E.; Szymczyk, B.; Kostogrys, R.B. Haematological parameters, serum lipid profile, liver function and fatty acid profile of broiler chickens fed on diets supplemented with pomegranate seed oil and linseed oil. *Br. Poult. Sci.* **2016**, *57*, 771–779. [CrossRef] [PubMed]
97. Arao, K.; Yotsumoto, H.; Han, S.Y.; Nagao, K.; Yanagita, T. The 9 *cis*, 11 *trans*, 13 *cis* isomer of conjugated linolenic acid reduces apolipoprotein b100 secretion and triacylglycerol synthesis in hepg2 cells. *Biosci. Biotechnol. Biochem.* **2004**, *68*, 2643–2645. [CrossRef] [PubMed]
98. Noguchi, R.; Yasui, Y.; Suzuki, R.; Hosokawa, M.; Fukunaga, K.; Miyashita, K. Dietary effects of bitter gourd oil on blood and liver lipids of rats. *Arch. Biochem. Biophys.* **2001**, *396*, 207–212. [CrossRef] [PubMed]
99. Saha, S.S.; Patra, M.; Ghosh, M. In vitro antioxidant study of vegetable oils containing conjugated linolenic acid isomers. *LWT-Food Sci. Technol.* **2012**, *46*, 10–15. [CrossRef]
100. Saha, S.S.; Ghosh, M. Comparative study of antioxidant activity of α-eleostearic acid and punicic acid against oxidative stress generated by sodium arsenite. *Food Chem. Toxicol.* **2009**, *47*, 2551–2556. [CrossRef] [PubMed]
101. Mukherjee, C.; Bhattacharyya, S.; Ghosh, S.; Bhattacharyya, D.K. Dietary effects of punicic acid on the composition and peroxidation of rat plasma lipid. *J. Oleo Sci.* **2002**, *51*, 513–522. [CrossRef]
102. Boussetta, T.; Raad, H.; Letteron, P.; Gougerot-Pocidalo, M.A.; Marie, J.C.; Driss, F.; El-Benna, J. Punicic acid a conjugated linolenic acid inhibits tnfalpha-induced neutrophil hyperactivation and protects from experimental colon inflammation in rats. *PLoS ONE* **2009**, *4*, e6458. [CrossRef] [PubMed]
103. Lewis, S.N.; Brannan, L.; Guri, A.J.; Lu, P.; Hontecillas, R.; Bassaganya-Riera, J.; Bevan, D.R. Dietary alpha-eleostearic acid ameliorates experimental inflammatory bowel disease in mice by activating peroxisome proliferator-activated receptor-gamma. *PLoS ONE* **2011**, *6*, e24031. [CrossRef] [PubMed]
104. Saha, S.S.; Ghosh, M. Antioxidant and anti-inflammatory effect of conjugated linolenic acid isomers against streptozotocin-induced diabetes. *Br. J. Nutr.* **2012**, *108*, 974–983. [CrossRef] [PubMed]
105. Mashhadi, Z.; Boeglin, W.E.; Brash, A.R. Robust inhibitory effects of conjugated linolenic acids on a cyclooxygenase-related linoleate 10s-dioxygenase: Comparison with cox-1 and cox-2. *Biochim. Biophys. Acta* **2015**, *1851*, 1346–1352. [CrossRef] [PubMed]

13

The Role of *n*-3 Long Chain Polyunsaturated Fatty Acids in Cardiovascular Disease Prevention and Interactions with Statins

Julia K. Bird [1,*], Philip C. Calder [2,3] and Manfred Eggersdorfer [1]

1 DSM Nutritional Products, 4303 Kaiseraugst, Switzerland; manfred.eggersdorfer@dsm.com
2 Human Development and Health Academic Unit, Faculty of Medicine, University of Southampton, Southampton SO16 6YD, UK; pcc@soton.ac.uk
3 NIHR Southampton Biomedical Research Centre, University Hospital Southampton NHS Foundation Trust and University of Southampton, Southampton SO16 6YD, UK
* Correspondence: julia.bird@dsm.com

Abstract: Decreases in global cardiovascular disease (CVD) mortality and morbidity in recent decades can be partly attributed to cholesterol reduction through statin use. *n*-3 long chain polyunsaturated fatty acids are recommended by some authorities for primary and secondary CVD prevention, and for triglyceride reduction. The residual risk of CVD that remains after statin therapy may potentially be reduced by *n*-3 long chain polyunsaturated fatty acids. However, the effects of concomitant use of statins and *n*-3 long chain polyunsaturated fatty acids are not well understood. Pleiotropic effects of statins and *n*-3 long chain polyunsaturated fatty acids overlap. For example, cytochrome P450 enzymes that metabolize statins may affect *n*-3 long chain polyunsaturated fatty acid metabolism and vice versa. Clinical and mechanistic study results show both synergistic and antagonistic effects of statins and *n*-3 long chain polyunsaturated fatty acids when used in combination.

Keywords: omega-3; cardiovascular disease; statins

---

1. Introduction

Cardiovascular diseases (CVDs) are the leading cause of global mortality, accounting for 32% of the 56 million deaths in 2015 [1]. Despite declines in age-adjusted mortality rates of 22% over the last few decades, mostly in high income countries [2], mortality rates are expected to rise again due to shifts from infectious to chronic disease over the next decades [3]. CVDs contribute not only to mortality, but cause a considerable disease burden in healthy life years lost [4]. Reductions in cardiovascular risk factors such as smoking have contributed to half the drop in mortality, whereas the other half can be attributed to medical therapies that include the use of medications such as statins, niacin and fibrates in both primary and secondary prevention [5].

Statins are 3-hydroxy-3-methylglutaryl coenzyme A (HMG-CoA) reductase inhibitors and are currently considered standard of care in both primary and secondary prevention of CVD. Their main mode of action is to lower circulating cholesterol, mainly low-density lipoprotein (LDL) cholesterol, concentrations, thereby slowing or even reversing the development of atherosclerotic plaques [6]. A recent meta-analysis found that statins used as primary prevention reduced all-cause mortality by 14%, CVD by 25% and stroke events by 22% [7]. While lipid-lowering monotherapy has reduced overall cardiovascular mortality risk, even patients with a successful, aggressive reduction in LDL-cholesterol levels have a residual risk of myocardial infarction [8]. Risk factors other than elevated LDL-cholesterol have a marked influence on CVD incidence and mortality.

n-3 polyunsaturated fatty acids (PUFAs) have cardioprotective effects, particularly the two *n*-3 long chain (LC) PUFAs eicosapentaenoic acid (EPA) and docosahexaenoic acid (DHA) [9]. A landmark study comparing the diets and CVD rates of Greenland Inuit to the Danish population triggered the initial interest in the role of marine-derived *n*-3 PUFAs in CVD [10], and this was supported by epidemiological research associating fish consumption with a reduction in CVD mortality in other populations [11,12]. Various mechanisms have been proposed to explain the modest reductions in cardiovascular risk by *n*-3 LC PUFAs: these include preventing cardiac arrhythmias, lowering plasma triglycerides, reducing blood pressure, decreasing platelet aggregation, and reducing inflammation. Early randomized, controlled trials showed a reduction in risk of cardiovascular mortality after increasing consumption of fatty fish or *n*-3 LC PUFA dietary supplements [13–15]. However, some more recent intervention studies did not show significant effects of EPA and/or DHA supplementation [16].

One reason postulated for the lack of effect of *n*-3 LC PUFA supplements in the more recent secondary prevention studies conducted is the frequent use of statin therapy in study patients [17]. The mechanisms of action of *n*-3 LC PUFAs overlap with the pleiotropic effects of statins, such as improving endothelial function, and anti-thrombotic and antioxidant effects [18]. In addition, statins may affect PUFA concentrations and the production of eicosanoids through interactions with cytochrome P450 (CYP) enzymes. The use of statins may therefore interfere with the effects of *n*-3 LC PUFAs. The aim of this review is to explore the interrelationship between statins and *n*-3 LC PUFAs in the context of CVD.

2. Statins: Mode of Action

Statins decrease LDL-cholesterol levels and are classed as anti-dyslipidemic drugs. The mode of action common to all statins is the competitive inhibition of the activity of HMG-CoA reductase (HMGCR), the rate-limiting step in the endogenous production of cholesterol. The structure of statins mimics that of the cholesterol precursor HMG-CoA. Statins compete for binding sites on the HMGCR enzyme, slowing the rate of mevalonate production from HMG-CoA in the liver, which leads to a reduction in overall cholesterol production and also of other products downstream of mevalonate [19]. Statins consist of a HMG-like moiety with chemical side groups that affect their pharmacokinetics, lipophilicity, affinity to HMGCR, rate of entry into the liver and non-target cells, and associated side effects.

Pleiotropic effects of statins include improving endothelial function, inhibiting vascular inflammation, and the stabilization of atherosclerotic plaques [20]. Plaque stabilization and regression through statins may be caused by activation of peroxisome proliferator-activated receptors (PPARs). These effects may be related to the inhibition of isoprenoid synthesis by statins, which ultimately inhibits various intracellular signaling molecules.

Seven statins are approved for use in the United States and Europe for primary prevention of CVD in patients with hypercholesteremia or an elevated risk of CVD, and in secondary prevention in pre-existing CVD. Table 1 provides an overview of these statins and their classification. Of the marketed statins, fluvastatin, atorvastatin, rosuvastatin, and pitavastatin are synthetic molecules, while lovastatin, pravastatin and simvastatin are derived from compounds found in nature. Statin types have differing effects on LDL-cholesterol reduction and may be further classified as "weak" statins (pravastatin, simvastatin) and "strong" statins (rosuvastatin, pitavastatin, atorvastatin), loosely based on their ability to lower the concentration of LDL-cholesterol. Weak statins lower cholesterol by up to 25%, with strong statins achieving a greater reduction [21]. The degree of hydrophilicity is a further point of differentiation between statins as it affects their absorption, tissue selectivity, and metabolism by CYP enzymes in the liver [22]. The choice of statin is generally guided by the desired reduction in LDL-cholesterol concentration.

Table 1. Statin classifications.

Statin Name	Origin [23]	Structure [23]	Lipophilicity [23]	Generation [23]	CYP Metabolism [22,24,25]
Fluvastatin	Synthetic	Fluorophenyl group	Lipophilic	I	CYP2C9
Atorvastatin	Synthetic	Fluorophenyl group	Lipophilic	II	CYP3A4
Rosuvastatin	Synthetic	Fluorophenyl group	Lipophobic	III	CYP2C9
Pitavastatin	Synthetic	Fluorophenyl group	Lipophilic	II	Marginal [26]
Lovastatin	Fungal	Butyryl group	Lipophilic	I	CYP3A4
Pravastatin	Fungal	Butyryl group	Lipophobic	I	CYP2C9
Simvastatin	Fungal	Butyryl group	Lipophilic	II	CYP3A4

Cytochrome P450 (CYP).

The effectiveness of statins for both cholesterol-lowering and prevention of cardiovascular mortality was recently confirmed once again with a systematic review and meta-analysis [27]. There was a dose-dependent reduction in CVD with LDL-cholesterol lowering. Across 27 trials, all-cause mortality was reduced by 10% per 1.0 mmol/L (approximately 40 mg/dL) LDL-cholesterol lowering, with LDL-cholesterol lowering largely reflecting a significant decrease in deaths due to coronary heart disease [27].

Even so, a residual CVD risk remains after statins are used, particularly in high-risk patients such as type II diabetics. Cardiovascular events occur even in patients that are adherent to intensive statin therapy and who achieve a large reduction in LDL-cholesterol to below 100 mg/dL [28]. CVD is multifactorial, and various risk factors that work through numerous mechanisms in the cardiovascular system affect the severity of disease risk. Statins mainly affect circulating concentrations of LDL-cholesterol, but other parameters of the lipid profile or markers of inflammation independently affect CVD progression and outcomes, such as HDL-cholesterol, LDL-cholesterol particle distribution, and elevated C-reactive protein and triglyceride concentrations [28,29]. The remaining risk of CVD outcomes in statin-treated patients is related to the independent effects of these risk factors and residual atherosclerosis. Combination therapy offers a means to treat other atherogenic components of the lipid profile, and also other risk factors. Common combinations include treatment with a fibrate to simultaneously lower triglyceride concentrations or with niacin to increase HDL-cholesterol [28].

3. Epidemiology of Statin Use

Since the introduction of lovastatin into clinical practice in 1987, statins have become one of the most widely prescribed classes of drugs in the world. The extensive use of statins has lowered LDL-cholesterol levels in the general population in high-income countries, and statins are considered to be one of the direct causes of the global reduction in cardiovascular events and mortality that has taken place in recent decades [30].

The largest markets for statins globally are the United States and Europe; however, the loss of patent exclusivity of the major brands since 2001 has opened the market for developing countries. In the United States, 93% of users of cholesterol-lowering prescription medication used a statin. 25% of adults aged 45 years and over used a statin in the period 2005–2008, equivalent to around 30 million adults [31], but usage varied widely depending on age and existence of CVD or diabetes [32]. Statin use varies greatly within Europe, with usage in countries such as Sweden, Ireland and the Netherlands four times greater than that in Austria or Italy [33]. The pattern of statin types prescribed also shows considerable variation among countries in the European Union [33]. In the United Kingdom, statins accounted for 94% of all prescriptions in the anti-dyslipidemic class in 2010: this corresponds to 55.1 million statin prescriptions dispensed in primary care. 72% of these prescriptions were for generic simvastatin [31]. Even so, treatment rates are still considered sub-optimal, and there is a considerable opportunity to reduce CVD through greater use in populations [30,32].

4. *n*-3 LC PUFAs: Mode of Action in CVD Prevention

The PUFAs linoleic acid (LA, *n*-6) and alpha-linolenic acid (ALA, *n*-3) are essential fatty acids: they are unable to be synthesized *de novo* by humans and must therefore be provided by the diet [34]. Intakes of LA and ALA less than 0.5% of energy are associated with deficiency symptoms, which include impaired barrier function and wound healing, failure to thrive, and can lead to poor neurological and visual development in infants [34]. Most vegetable oils are a good source of LA, and ALA may be obtained from selected vegetable oils including flaxseed, canola and soybean [34]. Dietary LA can function as a precursor for arachidonic acid (ARA). Likewise, ALA is a precursor for EPA and DHA, although conversion is rather poor in humans. Pre-formed EPA and DHA from fatty fish remains a more important dietary source of *n*-3 LC-PUFAs [35,36]. The *n*-3 LC PUFA DHA is regarded as conditionally essential for neonates for normal visual and cognitive development [34]. For adults, intakes of 250–2000 mg per day of EPA + DHA contribute to coronary heart disease prevention, and possibly to prevention of other chronic, degenerative diseases [34].

n-3 LC PUFAs are incorporated into triglycerides, phospholipids, and cholesteryl esters in plasma after absorption. There is a high correlation between EPA + DHA in erythrocytes, whole blood and plasma [37]. DHA is the most abundant *n*-3 fatty acid in cell membranes, being present in all organs, particularly in the cerebral cortex, the retina and in sperm [38]. EPA is also present in cells and tissues, albeit at considerably lower concentrations than DHA [36]. Both human plasma and tissues respond dose-dependently to supplementation with ALA, EPA and DHA [36]. Steady-state concentrations are reached after 1 month in plasma, and after 4–6 months in red blood cells; higher doses also lead to a faster response [36]. Interconversion from ALA to EPA and DHA is achieved in the liver via the sequential addition of 2-carbon units to the fatty acid backbone using elongation and desaturation enzymes until the chain length reaches 24 carbon units (Figure 1). The final step of conversion to DHA requires peroxisomal beta-oxidation. This last step is highly inefficient, particularly for men, with less than 1% of ALA intake ultimately converted to DHA [36]. Increasing doses of ALA will increase ALA and EPA concentrations in plasma but result in no discernable change in DHA concentrations [36]. The same enzyme system is also used for the elongation of *n*-6 PUFAs, therefore high background *n*-6 PUFA intakes reduce interconversion of *n*-3 PUFAs through competition (see Figure 1). Retroconversion of DHA to shorter chain *n*-3 PUFAs also occurs, albeit at a low rate of approximately 1.4% of a single dose [39]. Higher rates of retroconversion above 10% are suggested in individuals with high chronic intakes of DHA [40,41].

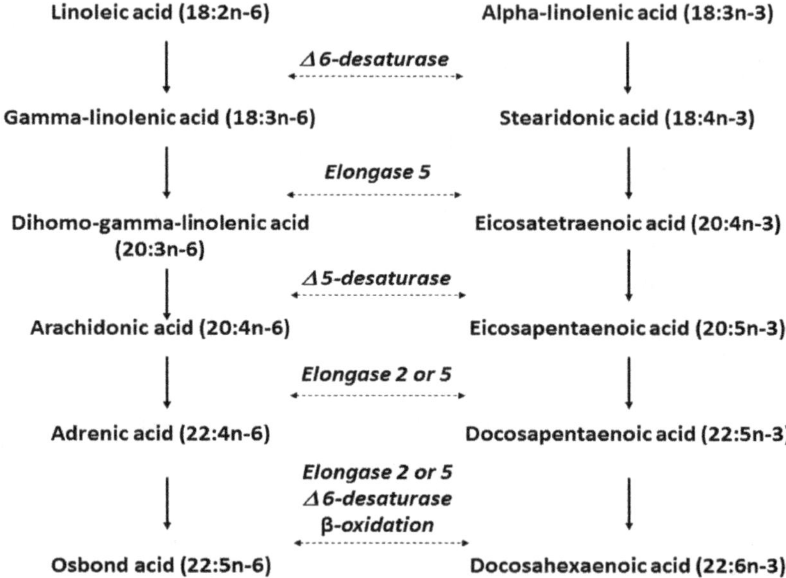

Figure 1. Pathway of metabolic interconversion of omega-6 and omega-3 polyunsaturated fatty acids. Abbreviation used: Δ, delta.

The ratio of EPA + DHA to total fatty acids is considered to be important as supplementation with EPA + DHA displaces ARA from plasma and tissues [36]. The saturation of the fatty acids and their chain length in the phospholipid bilayer of cell membranes affect its permeability, and physical state which in turn influences receptor function and the efficiency of signaling pathways [37]. The chain length of incorporated PUFAs affects membrane order; transmembrane protein activity is conferred by longer molecules with a greater number of double bonds. Of importance to CVD prevention, *n*-3 LC PUFAs reduce blood triglycerides, modulate the excitability of myocytes to reduce arrhythmias after damage to the heart, slow the progression of atherosclerosis, are mildly hypotensive, anti-inflammatory and promote endothelial relaxation, are anti-thrombotic, and are associated with a modest reduction in risk of cardiac death [17,34,42,43].

The effect of both EPA and DHA on lowering blood triglyceride concentrations is well established and is the basis for the use of ethyl esters of both molecules as a prescription medication for patients with hypertriglyceridemia [44]. The mechanisms of action are not completely understood; however, it is thought that a combination of reduced triglyceride synthesis and increased oxidation of triglycerides induced by *n*-3 LC PUFAs act to lower circulating triglyceride concentrations. *n*-3 LC PUFAs inhibit the hepatic synthesis and secretion of VLDL-triglycerides, mediated by decreases in transcription factors controlling the expression of enzymes involved in the assembly of triglycerides. Some studies link the down-regulation of sterol regulatory element-binding proteins (SREBPs), transcription factors required for the biosynthesis of both cholesterol and fatty acids, with reduced triglyceride synthesis in animal models seen following fish oil feeding. An increase in acyl-coenzyme A oxidase gene expression induced by PPAR-α may increase rates of peroxisomal β-oxidation of fatty acids. While both EPA and DHA lower triglycerides, head-to-head studies find that supplementation with DHA alone can raise LDL-cholesterol to a small extent but EPA does not [45]. The atherogenic potential of this increase in LDL-cholesterol may be mitigated by a shift in LDL particle size towards larger, more buoyant LDL particles after DHA supplementation [46,47]. On the other hand, DHA supplementation was associated with a modest increase in HDL-cholesterol, while increases due to EPA were comparatively minor [45].

The reduction in mortality found in some supplementation studies with *n*-3 LC PUFAs is attributed primarily to reductions in sudden cardiac deaths from decreased arrhythmogenesis [9,17,42]. Specifically, *n*-3 LC PUFAs are incorporated into the phospholipids of myocyte plasma membranes, where they have the ability to modulate cellular ion currents. EPA reduced myocyte excitability by increasing the time taken to return sodium channels in the membrane to their active state; however, this only occurs in cells that have become hyper-excitable due to damage such as ischemia [43]. Small to medium-sized intervention studies with *n*-3 LC PUFAs in secondary prevention support this mechanism by showing a reduction in both atrial fibrillation and ventricular arrhythmias in patients with frequent premature ventricular complexes or after coronary artery bypass surgery [42]. This may explain why a reduced risk of coronary heart disease with EPA + DHA from food or supplements was found in a recent meta-analysis, particularly in people with a higher risk of CVD [48]. *n*-3 LC PUFAs may therefore be most effective in reducing sudden cardiac death when cardiac tissue has already been injured.

A reduction in the risk of stroke is a clinically relevant outcome of the anti-thrombogenic and hypotensive effects of *n*-3 LC PUFAs [49,50], although results from some intervention studies have been indeterminate or only applicable to certain sub-groups [51–53]. Anti-thrombotic effects are thought to be primarily caused by the exchange of ARA with EPA in membrane phospholipids of blood platelets, causing favorable reductions in thrombogenicity due to enhanced production of non-aggregatory eicosanoids from EPA. The promotion of endothelial relaxation through stimulating nitric oxide synthesis in the endothelium has been demonstrated [54], but other effects on vascular reactivity independent of the endothelium are considered to be important contributors to the reduction in blood pressure found in intervention trials with *n*-3 LC PUFAs [55]. The slowing of atherosclerosis progression is related to the modulation of the expression and transcription of genes involved in the inflammatory response. Both EPA and DHA affect the nuclear factor-κB signal transduction pathway to reduce inflammation: EPA decreases the expression of tumor necrosis factor-α by impeding phosphorylation of nuclear factor-κB, while DHA reduces the ability of nuclear factor-κB to bind to

DNA in an ischemia–reperfusion model [54]. It is likely that synergy between anti-inflammatory mechanisms, triglyceride lowering, improving membrane order, anti-thrombotic and anti-arrhythmic effects contributes to the overall reduction in CVD risk from *n*-3 LC PUFAs.

5. Use of *n*-3 LC PUFAs as Dietary Supplements in the General Population

Dietary supplements containing *n*-3 LC PUFAs are used widely in North America, Europe, and the Asia-Pacific region. The main sources of these products include fatty fish, krill, and fermentation-derived microalgal oils. Demand for *n*-3 LC PUFAs for human nutrition is projected to grow 4.1% annually on a volume basis over the coming decade [56]. An international survey of *n*-3 LC PUFA supplement users in ten countries (U.S., U.K., Germany, Italy, China, South Korea, Russia, Australia, Brazil, Mexico) found that usage varied from 14% of the adult population in Germany to 38% in Australia [57]. A high proportion of *n*-3 LC PUFA supplement use has also been found by other researchers [58]. In most countries, users started taking supplements due to advice from a physician. The main reasons given for taking supplements are for overall or cardiovascular health [57]. *n*-3 LC PUFA supplements are taken by 10% of the U.S. adult population aged 20 years or more, most commonly for heart health [59].

6. Interactions between LC PUFAs and Statins, and Effects on Dyslipidemia, CVD and Mortality

In addition to distinct effects on dyslipidemia, the pleiotropic effects of statins overlap with those of *n*-3 LC PUFAs. Similar mechanisms include enhancing endothelial nitric oxide synthesis, inhibiting the production of pro-inflammatory cytokines, and the lowering of LDL-cholesterol via repression in activity and mRNA expression of the HMG-CoA reductase enzyme [60,61]. Given these commonalities in actions, statins and *n*-3 LC PUFAs may interact, either competing with or complementing each other. Statins may also augment the metabolism of LC PUFAs and their metabolites [60]. These interactions are summarized in Figure 2.

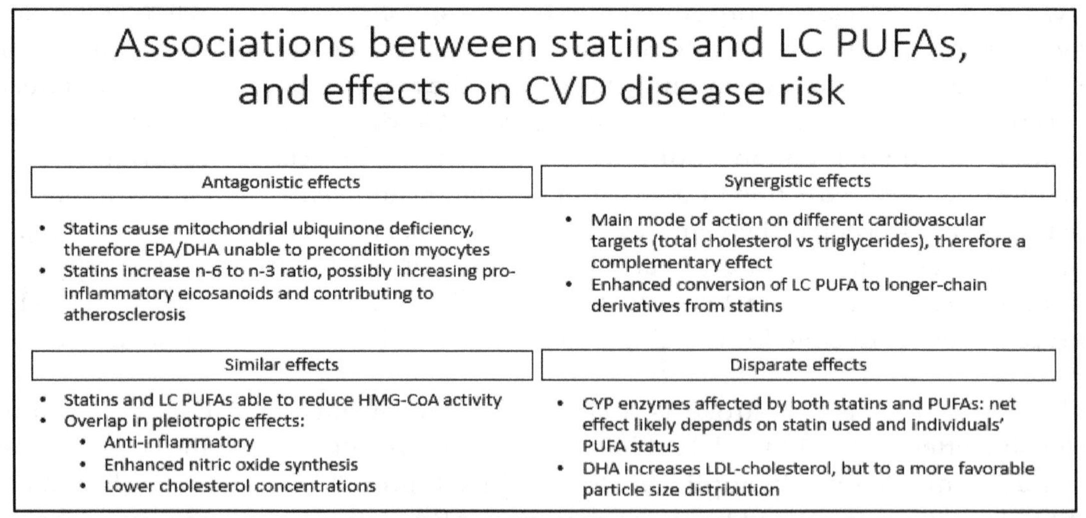

Figure 2. Overview of the interaction between statins and *n*-3 LC PUFAs on cardiovascular risk factor.

6.1. Effects of Dietary Fatty Acids and Statin Co-Administration on Dyslipidemia

There is a well-established link between dietary fat type and the blood lipid profile. Dietary manipulation of fatty acid unsaturation affects both total circulating cholesterol concentration and various cholesterol fractions. For example, replacement of saturated fats in the diet with polyunsaturated and monounsaturated fats lowers total cholesterol and LDL-cholesterol concentrations [25,34]. The LDL-cholesterol lowering effect is thought to be due to the increased expression of LDL-cholesterol receptors in response to a higher concentration of unsaturated fatty acids. In contrast, saturated fatty acids maintain a lower expression of LDL-cholesterol receptors and thus LDL-cholesterol concentrations remain high [25], with the notable exception of LDL-cholesterol-lowering stearic acid [62].

Cholesterol levels may also be affected by EFA status through the modulation of HMG CoA reductase activity. In animal models, EFA deficiency increased the activity of HMG CoA reductase, possibly to help maintain barrier function and integrity when the supply of EFA is low [63]. Reversing deficiency normalized HMG CoA reductase activity [63]. Likewise, feeding studies in rodents show reduced HMG CoA reductase activity or expression after *n*-3 LC PUFA administration [64–67].

Dietary fatty acids can influence statin pharmacokinetics. When combined with simvastatin treatment, patients consuming a diet using olive oil as the primary culinary fat had a more favorable change in calculated risk of CVD, based on serum lipid and lipoprotein concentrations, than patients using sunflower oil. The higher concentrations of linoleic acid in sunflower oil compared to olive oil was postulated to cause a comparatively greater activation of cytochrome P450 enzymes, leading to a reduction in statin half-life, affecting its ability to lower cholesterol [25].

In clinical studies investigating the effect of various statins with *n*-3 LC PUFAs on cardiovascular risk factors, predominantly performed in patients with elevated cholesterol and triglycerides, combined treatment resulted in decreases in triglycerides, total cholesterol, and thrombotic potential compared to statin-only [25]. In general, concomitant therapy with statin medication and *n*-3 LC PUFAs is considered to be complementary, and alongside a reduction in both elevated triglycerides and LDL-cholesterol, there is a trend to lower LDL-cholesterol particle size and a more favorable lipoprotein distribution [68].

6.2. Effects of Statins on n-3 LC PUFA Concentrations

Statins and EFAs interact to modulate fatty acid synthesis and metabolism. In particular, statins have the ability to alter *n*-3 LC PUFA concentrations [69]. Statins have differential effects on the activities of the Δ6- and Δ5-desaturase enzymes, and studies indicate increases in activity (simvastatin, rosuvastatin and pitavastatin [70,71]) or decreases (atorvastatin [72]), and PPARs can be activated [20]. This can lead to changes in the relative proportions of longer chain PUFAs.

In vitro studies show that statins increase concentrations of ARA and other LC PUFAs, possibly because elongation activity is enhanced [73,74]. A dietary intervention study conducted in 120 hypercholesterolemic men found marked changes in the fatty acid profile after treatment with simvastatin, notably ARA, which suggested that there were changes in the activity of enzymes involved in the elongation and desaturation of fatty acids [71]. Another clinical trial in 57 men with coronary heart disease found that simvastatin treatment increased circulating concentrations of ARA, with no effect on *n*-3 LC PUFAs or saturated fatty acids [75].

A rat model was used to determine the effect of atorvastatin on *n*-3 PUFAs in plasma, blood, and erythrocyte membranes [72]. While *n*-3 LC PUFA concentrations remained the same or increased in plasma and erythrocyte membranes, there were significant reductions in liver *n*-3 LC PUFA concentrations as a result of atorvastatin treatment. These changes in *n*-3 LC PUFAs in the liver coincided with decreases in the mRNA expression of fatty acid desaturase (*FADS*) 1 and 2 genes, which encode Δ5-desaturase and Δ6-desaturase, respectively, and of *ELOVL5* gene, which encodes a key fatty acid elongation enzyme [76].

A study of 1723 Japanese cardiology patients showed that use of any statin increased circulating ARA and reduced circulating concentrations of DHA relative to ARA, without affecting EPA [77]. Differential effects were seen with simvastatin compared to rosuvastatin or pitavastatin. In 106 hypercholesterolemic adults and in in vitro experiments, simvastatin appeared to enhance the conversion of linoleic acid and EPA to ARA and DHA, respectively [69,78]. On the other hand, rosuvastatin or pitavastatin decreased serum DHA levels without affecting ARA or EPA, and thereby increased the ARA/DHA ratio in 46 dyslipidemic patients [70]. A further study in 46 coronary artery disease (CAD) patients found that atorvastatin, rosuvastatin or pitavastatin reduced EPA and DHA concentrations in serum, in proportion to reductions in LDL-cholesterol, while concentrations of ARA were unchanged [79]. There was a correlation between reduction in serum EPA + DHA and LDL-lowering, producing counteractive effects on risk factors for atherosclerosis. This has led some researchers to conclude that "weak" statins (simvastatin, pravastatin) increase the ARA/EPA ratio, while "strong" statins (atorvastatin, rosuvastatin or pitavastatin) increase the ARA/DHA ratio. Hydrophilic statins may require a higher dose to affect linoleic acid conversion than lipophilic statins [74]. In any case, statin use in general appears to favor *n*-6 over *n*-3 LC PUFA content [77], which may result in a net increase in inflammation and thrombogenesis [80].

6.3. Interactions between Statins and n-3 LC PUFAs on Mitochondrial Function

There may be a counteracting effect of statins and *n*-3 LC PUFAs on mitochondrial function [80]. Myocardial mitochondria provide energy for ischemic pre-conditioning in cardiomyocytes prior to myocardial infarction, which may reduce the size of the infarction, reduce post-ischemic arrhythmias and result in better patient survival. Dietary *n*-3 LC PUFAs are able to induce a chronic state of cardiac preconditioning, associated with increases in *n*-3 LC PUFA accumulation in plasma as well as cardiac mitochondria [80]. On the other hand, a known side-effect of statin usage is muscle pain and weakness, linked to disrupted mitochondria in muscles [22]. Endogenous production of ubiquinone, used primarily to generate energy in mitochondria, is decreased by statin administration, as its biosynthesis requires the HMG-CoA reductase enzyme [81]. Therefore, in the presence of statins, *n*-3 LC PUFAs may not be able to precondition cardiomyocytes due to a reduction in mitochondrial function arising from intrinsic ubiquinone deficiency.

6.4. Inhibition of CYP Enzymes by Statins and Effects on Eicosanoid Production

An important biological function of LC PUFAs is the production of eicosanoids, lipid mediators with cardioprotective, vasodilatory, inflammatory and allergic properties [82]. ARA is considered the traditional precursor of eicosanoids; however the CYP enzymes responsible for metabolizing ARA have broad substrate specificities and accept most *n*-3 and *n*-6 LC PUFAs [82]. Increasing the availability of EPA and DHA to the CYP enzymes shifts eicosanoid production to EPA- and DHA-derived metabolites, possibly having a favorable effect on CVD risk [83]. However, statins can inhibit or induce the activity of particular CYP enzymes [22,24,84], and thus the production of CYP-derived eicosanoids. For example, fluvastatin is both a substrate for, and potent inhibitor of, CYP2C9 [84]. CYP2C9 is found in human cardiovascular tissue [85], where it catalyzes the conversion of ARA, EPA and DHA to epoxyeicosatrienoic acids (EETs), epoxyeicosatetraenoic acids (EpETE) and epoxydocosapentaenoic acids (EpDPE), respectively [86]. EpETE and EpDPE show in vitro anti-inflammatory and cardioprotective properties [82]. Use of fluvastatin may reduce the overall production of PUFA-derived eicosanoids, with differential effects on CVD risk depending on the ultimate shift in PUFA-derived eicosanoids that occurs. When underlying *n*-3 LC PUFA concentrations are high, statins may lower the effectiveness of EPA or DHA in reducing CVD risk by inhibiting the production of EpETEs and EpDPE. On the other hand, when *n*-6 LC PUFA concentrations are high, a reduction in the production of ARA-derived inflammatory metabolites through CYP2C9 inhibition by certain statins may be beneficial. As a complicating factor, different statins affect different CYP enzymes, and some have no effect. In populations using a range of different statins, disparate effects on eicosanoid production may increase variability in the effect of PUFA on cardiovascular risk. Clearly, further work is needed in this area.

6.5. Effects of Statins and n-3 LC PUFAs on Clinical and Mechanistic Endpoints

The effect of *n*-3 LC PUFAs and statins on various clinically relevant endpoints has been addressed in several observational and interventional studies. Clinical study results are summarized in Table 2. Three large studies contrasted the effects of *n*-3 LC PUFAs in statin users compared to non-users. The Southern Cohort Community study is a prospective cohort investigation into risk factors for chronic disease in the Southwestern USA [87]. Among 69,559 participants, there was a statistically significant reduction in all-cause mortality across quintiles of increasing *n*-3 fatty acid intakes in non-statin users only; there was no effect in statin users. The Alpha Omega clinical trial in the Netherlands tested the effect of margarines that provided 4153 participants with a randomly-selected dose of 400 mg EPA + DHA, 2 g ALA, a combination, or placebo on major cardiovascular events [88]. There was no effect of the fatty acid type on risk of composite cardiovascular endpoints in statin users. In non-users, there were non-significant decreases in cardiovascular events in all treatment groups compared to placebo, and the reduction bordered on significance in the adjusted model for the combined EPA + DHA + ALA group ($p = 0.051$). On the other hand, in a retrospective cohort study conducted in 11,269 survivors of acute myocardial infarction from five Italian Local Health Units, a significant reduction in recurrent myocardial infarction was only seen in users of concurrent *n*-3 LC PUFA supplements and statins [89]. Statin use did not affect all-cause mortality in this study, however; there was a significant reduction in both statin users (HR 0.52 [0.40–0.68]) and statin non-users (HR 0.39 [0.20–0.75]) who were taking the *n*-3 LC PUFA supplements.

Table 2. Clinical studies with a combination of *n*-3 LC PUFAs and statins.

Study Name (*n*)	Study Type/Treatments	Main Results	Reference
Southern cohort community study ($n = 69{,}559$)	Prospective cohort study	Modest inverse associations between *n*-3 PUFA and *n*-6 PUFA intake with mortality among non-statin users but not among statin users.	[87]
($n = 14{,}704$)	Retrospective cohort study	As compared with statins alone, combined treatment with statins and *n*-3 LC PUFAs was associated with an adjusted higher survival rate, survival free of atrial fibrillation and survival free of new heart failure development, but not with re-infarction.	[90]
JELIS ($n = 18{,}645$)	RCT Treatment: 1800 mg EPA + statin Control: statin alone	The incidence of MCE was significantly lower in the EPA group. Compared to patients with normal serum TG and HDL-C levels, those with abnormal had significantly higher CAD hazard ratio. In this higher risk group, EPA treatment suppressed the risk of CAD by 53%.	[91,92]
Alpha Omega ($n = 4153$)	Post hoc analysis of RCT Treatments: 400 mg EPA + DHA 2 g ALA Both Control: Placebo margarine	In statin users, *n*-3 fatty acids did not reduce cardiovascular events. In statin non-users, only 9% of those who received EPA-DHA plus ALA experienced an event compared with 18% in the placebo group.	[88]
CHERRY ($n = 193$)	RCT Treatment: 1,800 mg EPA + 4 mg pitavastatin Control: Pitavastatin (Pitavastatin) 4 mg	The prevalence rate of plaque regression was significantly higher in Pitavastatin/EPA group than in Pitavastatin group (50% vs. 24%, $p < 0.001$).	[93]
Kagawa hospital study ($n = 241$)	Prospective, open-label, randomized trial Treatment: 1,800 mg EPA + 2 mg Pitavastatin Control: 2 mg Pitavastatin	Significant reduction in composite endpoint of cardiovascular death, MI, stroke, or coronary revascularization at 1 year: 9.2% in the EPA group and 20.2% in the control group (absolute risk reduction, 11.0%; HR, 0.42; 95% CI, 0.21–087; $p = 0.02$), in acute coronary syndrome patients.	[94]
($n = 11{,}269$)	Retrospective cohort study	*n*-3 LC PUFA supplement users had a reduced risk of all-cause mortality (HR 0.76 [0.59 to 0.97]). Statin use did not affect all-cause mortality reduction, however a reduction in recurrent myocardial infarction was only seen in statin users.	[89]
($n = 77{,}776$)	Meta-regression	Lower control group statin use and higher DHA/EPA ratio was associated with higher reduction in total mortality.	[18]
HEARTS ($n = 285$)	RCT in patients with stable statin therapy Treatment: 1860 mg EPA + 1500 mg DHA Control: Placebo	EPA + DHA in addition to low-dose statin treatment prevented progression of atherosclerotic plaques, compared to low-dose statin treatment alone.	[95]

Abbreviations: coronary artery disease (CAD), alpha-linolenic acid (ALA, *n*-3), randomized clinical trial (RCT), major coronary event (MCE), triglycerides (TG), coronary artery disease (CAD), myocardial infarction (MI), eicosapentaenoic acid (EPA), hazard ratio (HR), docosahexaenoic acid (DHA).

Further clinical studies have investigated the effect of combined treatment with *n*-3 LC PUFAs and statins compared to treatment with statins alone on cardiovascular events. In a large retrospective cohort study conducted across Italy, combined treatment with a statin and *n*-3 LC PUFAs (non-specified) after acute myocardial infarction was associated with improved survival in both crude and adjusted estimates for major outcomes compared to treatment with only a statin [90]. The large randomized controlled study JELIS, conducted in Japanese patients with hypercholesterolemia, tested the effect of adding 1800 mg EPA daily to existing statin treatment (10 mg pravastatin or 5 mg simvastatin) [91]. Compared to statin treatment alone, patients randomized to additional EPA had a lower incidence of major coronary events. In a recent open-label, randomized, controlled trial, acute coronary syndrome patients who were randomized to EPA + statin (1800 mg EPA ethyl ester and 2 mg pitavastatin daily) had approximately half the rate of a composite endpoint consisting of cardiovascular death, MI, stroke, or coronary revascularization at 1 year, compared to patients randomized to the statin treatment alone [94].

Several studies conducted in patients taking statins show that *n*-3 LC PUFA use in addition to statins affects CVD mechanisms. In 20 adults with familial hypercholesterolemia on stable statin therapy, an 8-week intervention with 4 g per day *n*-3 LC PUFAs (46% EPA and 38% DHA) resulted in improved arterial elasticity, and reduced blood pressure, apolipoprotein B and triglycerides, compared to statin therapy alone. In this risk group for premature CVD, *n*-3 LC PUFAs improved several independent predictors of CVD in addition to the normalization of cholesterol from statins [96]. In a small study that explored the mechanisms of cardiovascular risk factors in 200 patients treated with pitavastatin both alone and combined with 1800 mg EPA, there was a significantly higher rate of plaque regression in the combination group compared to pitavastatin alone [93]. In a similar recent RCT of patients with stable coronary artery disease on statin therapy, adherent patients randomized to 3.4 g EPA + DHA per day had less progression of fibrous coronary plaques, compared to statin therapy alone [95]. Both these studies show that atherosclerotic plaques regressed when a combination of *n*-3 LC PUFAs and statins were used.

Combination therapy of *n*-3 LC PUFAs and statins has shown some potential for patients who show poor tolerability or a lack of response to statin treatment. For example, in patients with moderate hypertriglyceridemia despite statin treatment, a combination of low dose rosuvastatin (10 mg) and *n*-3 LC PUFAs (2 g EPA + DHA) reduced total cholesterol and triglycerides compared to baseline [97]. While this reduction was not as great as for high dose rosuvastatin (40 mg), it showed clinical benefit and may be an option for patients with poor tolerability for high dose rosuvastatin. Another small clinical trial investigating the use of *n*-3 LC PUFAs and phytochemicals as complementary therapy to reduce statin dose used a personalized approach. In the first phase of the study, patients responding to treatment with 1.7 g *n*-3 LC PUFAs were identified and assigned to receive a halved statin dose in the second phase of the study. Despite a marked reduction in dose, there were no significant changes in the lipid profile in responders taking the combination therapy [98].

The research involving clinical and mechanistic endpoints is equivocal: some studies show that the combination of *n*-3 LC PUFAs and statins is beneficial, while others show no difference in outcomes, and yet others find that *n*-3 LC PUFAs only affect outcomes in statin non-users. Yet, in the period in which statin use has transitioned to becoming a first-line medication for reducing mortality derived from hypercholesterolemia, the results of supplementation studies with *n*-3 LC PUFAs have changed from showing a significant reduction in all-cause mortality increasingly to a null-effect [52], although a modest reduction in cardiac death or coronary heart disease risk has been found in two recent meta-analyses [17,48]. The disparate results of meta-analyses arise at least partly from variations in inclusion criteria, with Maki et al. reporting that their inclusion of smaller trials contributed to the robustness of the meta-analysis results [17]. Differences in *n*-3 LC PUFA doses used and the formulation or dosage form may be important: lower doses are less effective in raising circulating fatty acid concentrations, and the bioavailability from a food matrix may be subject to greater variability than from a dietary supplement. In addition, the distinct effects of DHA compared to EPA cannot be elucidated due to a paucity of comparative studies [55]. Furthermore, the effect size of *n*-3 LC PUFAs on mortality may have become smaller against a background of increasing statin use in the general population, leading to a higher likelihood of type I error. Overlapping or even counteractive effects of combined treatment with statins and *n*-3 LC PUFAs may be confounding outcomes of clinical trials.

7. Conclusions

Both statins and *n*-3 LC PUFAs are recommended for CVD prevention. While each treatment has a distinct mode of action, pleiotropic effects of the two overlap. In addition, statins and *n*-3 LC PUFAs interact, potentially affecting net cardiovascular risk (Figure 2). Statins may cause a mitochondrial ubiquinone deficiency, which blocks the ability of *n*-3 LC PUFAs to precondition myocytes, reducing their effectiveness in reducing cardiac arrhythmias. Statins appear to increase concentrations of LC PUFAs: when LA intakes are high, this could lead to a rise in concentrations of pro-inflammatory eicosanoids from ARA. The main effect of statins is to block the activity of HMG-CoA reductase; however *n*-3 LC PUFAs are also capable of HMG-CoA reductase inhibition, albeit less effectively, resulting in a smaller effect size for the combination. Both competition for, and activation of, CYP enzymes could be a further confounding factor in the metabolism of statins and the production of eicosanoids from *n*-3 LC PUFAs, but this may depend on the type of statin used. Post hoc analyses of clinical studies have yielded mixed results, with some results indicating that *n*-3 LC PUFA supplementation is only beneficial in statin non-users and others showing combined use of *n*-3 LC PUFA and statins is beneficial. Prospective intervention studies that stratify for statin use are warranted to explore the interaction further.

Author Contributions: Conceptualization, M.E.; Writing-Original Draft Preparation, J.K.B.; Writing-Review and Editing, J.K.B. and P.C.C.

Acknowledgments: We acknowledge the critical reviews of the manuscript by Norman Salem Jr, Karin Yurko-Mauro and Mary van Elswyk.

References

1. GBD Mortality Causes of Death Collaborators. Global, regional, and national life expectancy, all-cause mortality, and cause-specific mortality for 249 causes of death, 1980–2015: A systematic analysis for the Global Burden of Disease Study 2015. *Lancet* **2016**, *388*, 1459–1544. [CrossRef]
2. Bowry, A.D.; Lewey, J.; Dugani, S.B.; Choudhry, N.K. The Burden of Cardiovascular Disease in Low- and Middle-Income Countries: Epidemiology and Management. *Can. J. Cardiol.* **2015**, *31*, 1151–1159. [CrossRef] [PubMed]
3. Institute of Medicine. *Promoting Cardiovascular Health in the Developing World: A Critical Challenge to Achieve Global Health*; National Academies Press (US): Washington, DC, USA, 2010.
4. Vos, T.; Barber, R.M.; Bell, B.; Bertozzi-Villa, A.; Biryukov, S.; Bolliger, I.; Charlson, F.; Davis, A.; Degenhardt, L.; Dicker, D.; et al. Global, regional, and national incidence, prevalence, and years lived with disability for 301 acute and chronic diseases and injuries in 188 countries, 1990–2013: A systematic analysis for the Global Burden of Disease Study 2013. *Lancet* **2015**, *386*, 743–800. [CrossRef]
5. Ford, E.S.; Ajani, U.A.; Croft, J.B.; Critchley, J.A.; Labarthe, D.R.; Kottke, T.E.; Giles, W.H.; Capewell, S. Explaining the decrease in U.S. deaths from coronary disease, 1980–2000. *N. Engl. J. Med.* **2007**, *356*, 2388–2398. [CrossRef] [PubMed]
6. Koskinas, K.C.; Windecker, S.; Raber, L. Regression of coronary atherosclerosis: Current evidence and future perspectives. *Trends Cardiovasc. Med.* **2016**, *26*, 150–161. [CrossRef] [PubMed]
7. Taylor, F.; Huffman, M.D.; Macedo, A.F.; Moore, T.H.; Burke, M.; Davey Smith, G.; Ward, K.; Ebrahim, S. Statins for the primary prevention of cardiovascular disease. *Cochrane Database Syst. Rev.* **2013**, *1*, CD004816. [CrossRef] [PubMed]

8. Superko, H.R.; King, S., 3rd. Lipid management to reduce cardiovascular risk: A new strategy is required. *Circulation* **2008**, *117*, 560–568. [CrossRef] [PubMed]
9. Breslow, J.L. *n*-3 fatty acids and cardiovascular disease. *Am. J. Clin. Nutr.* **2006**, *83*, 1477S–1482S. [CrossRef] [PubMed]
10. Bang, H.O.; Dyerberg, J.; Sinclair, H.M. The composition of the Eskimo food in north western Greenland. *Am. J. Clin. Nutr.* **1980**, *33*, 2657–2661. [CrossRef] [PubMed]
11. Daviglus, M.L.; Stamler, J.; Orencia, A.J.; Dyer, A.R.; Liu, K.; Greenland, P.; Walsh, M.K.; Morris, D.; Shekelle, R.B. Fish consumption and the 30-year risk of fatal myocardial infarction. *N. Engl. J. Med.* **1997**, *336*, 1046–1053. [CrossRef] [PubMed]
12. Kromhout, D.; Bosschieter, E.B.; de Lezenne Coulander, C. The inverse relation between fish consumption and 20-year mortality from coronary heart disease. *N. Engl. J. Med.* **1985**, *312*, 1205–1209. [CrossRef] [PubMed]
13. Burr, M.L.; Fehily, A.M.; Gilbert, J.F.; Rogers, S.; Holliday, R.M.; Sweetnam, P.M.; Elwood, P.C.; Deadman, N.M. Effects of changes in fat, fish, and fibre intakes on death and myocardial reinfarction: Diet and reinfarction trial (DART). *Lancet* **1989**, *2*, 757–761. [CrossRef]
14. Singh, R.B.; Niaz, M.A.; Sharma, J.P.; Kumar, R.; Rastogi, V.; Moshiri, M. Randomized, double-blind, placebo-controlled trial of fish oil and mustard oil in patients with suspected acute myocardial infarction: the Indian experiment of infarct survival—4. *Cardiovasc. Drugs Ther.* **1997**, *11*, 485–491. [CrossRef] [PubMed]
15. Gruppo Italiano per lo Studio della Sopravvivenza nell'Infarto miocardico. Dietary supplementation with *n*-3 polyunsaturated fatty acids and vitamin E after myocardial infarction: Results of the GISSI-Prevenzione trial. *Lancet* **1999**, *354*, 447–455. [CrossRef]
16. Kromhout, D.; Yasuda, S.; Geleijnse, J.M.; Shimokawa, H. Fish oil and omega-3 fatty acids in cardiovascular disease: do they really work? *Eur. Heart J.* **2012**, *33*, 436–443. [CrossRef] [PubMed]
17. Maki, K.C.; Palacios, O.M.; Bell, M.; Toth, P.P. Use of supplemental long-chain omega-3 fatty acids and risk for cardiac death: An updated meta-analysis and review of research gaps. *J. Clin. Lipidol.* **2017**, *11*, 1152.e2–1160.e2. [CrossRef] [PubMed]
18. Sethi, A.; Bajaj, A.; Khosla, S.; Arora, R.R. Statin Use Mitigate the Benefit of Omega-3 Fatty Acids Supplementation-A Meta-Regression of Randomized Trials. *Am. J. Ther.* **2016**, *23*, e737–e748. [CrossRef] [PubMed]
19. Istvan, E. Statin inhibition of HMG-CoA reductase: A 3-dimensional view. *Atheroscler. Suppl.* **2003**, *4*, 3–8. [CrossRef]
20. Zhou, Q.; Liao, J.K. Pleiotropic effects of statins—Basic research and clinical perspectives. *Circ. J.* **2010**, *74*, 818–826. [CrossRef] [PubMed]
21. Grundy, S.M. Primary prevention of cardiovascular disease with statins: Assessing the evidence base behind clinical guidance. *Clin. Pharm.* **2016**, *8*, 57.
22. Neuvonen, P.J. Drug interactions with HMG-CoA reductase inhibitors (statins): the importance of CYP enzymes, transporters and pharmacogenetics. *Curr. Opin. Investig. Drugs* **2010**, *11*, 323–332. [PubMed]
23. Maji, D.; Shaikh, S.; Solanki, D.; Gaurav, K. Safety of statins. *Indian J. Endocrinol. Metab.* **2013**, *17*, 636–646. [CrossRef] [PubMed]
24. Shitara, Y.; Sugiyama, Y. Pharmacokinetic and pharmacodynamic alterations of 3-hydroxy-3-methylglutaryl coenzyme A (HMG-CoA) reductase inhibitors: drug-drug interactions and interindividual differences in transporter and metabolic enzyme functions. *Pharmacol. Ther.* **2006**, *112*, 71–105. [CrossRef] [PubMed]
25. Vaquero, M.P.; Sanchez Muniz, F.J.; Jimenez Redondo, S.; Prats Olivan, P.; Higueras, F.J.; Bastida, S. Major diet-drug interactions affecting the kinetic characteristics and hypolipidaemic properties of statins. *Nutr. Hosp.* **2010**, *25*, 193–206. [PubMed]
26. Corsini, A.; Ceska, R. Drug-drug interactions with statins: Will pitavastatin overcome the statins' Achilles' heel? *Curr. Med. Res. Opin.* **2011**, *27*, 1551–1562. [CrossRef] [PubMed]
27. Fulcher, J.; O'Connell, R.; Voysey, M.; Emberson, J.; Blackwell, L.; Mihaylova, B.; Simes, J.; Collins, R.; Kirby, A.; Colhoun, H.; et al. Efficacy and safety of LDL-lowering therapy among men and women: meta-analysis of individual data from 174,000 participants in 27 randomised trials. *Lancet* **2015**, *385*, 1397–1405. [CrossRef] [PubMed]
28. Cziraky, M.J.; Watson, K.E.; Talbert, R.L. Targeting low HDL-cholesterol to decrease residual cardiovascular risk in the managed care setting. *J. Manag. Care Pharm.* **2008**, *14*, S3–S28; quiz S30–S21. [CrossRef] [PubMed]

29. Nishikido, T.; Oyama, J.; Keida, T.; Ohira, H.; Node, K. High-dose statin therapy with rosuvastatin reduces small dense LDL and MDA-LDL: The Standard versus high-dose therApy with Rosuvastatin for lipiD lowering (SARD) trial. *J. Cardiol.* **2016**, *67*, 340–346. [CrossRef] [PubMed]
30. Mann, D.; Reynolds, K.; Smith, D.; Muntner, P. Trends in statin use and low-density lipoprotein cholesterol levels among US adults: impact of the 2001 National Cholesterol Education Program guidelines. *Ann. Pharmacother.* **2008**, *42*, 1208–1215. [CrossRef] [PubMed]
31. Falkingbridge, S. *The Cardiovascular Market Outlook to 2017: Competitive Landscape, Global Market Analysis, Key Trends, and Pipeline Analysis*; Informa: London, UK, 2012; pp. 58–61.
32. Robinson, J.G.; Booth, B. Statin use and lipid levels in older adults: National Health and Nutrition Examination Survey, 2001 to 2006. *J. Clin. Lipidol.* **2010**, *4*, 483–490. [CrossRef] [PubMed]
33. Walley, T.; Folino-Gallo, P.; Stephens, P.; Van Ganse, E. Trends in prescribing and utilization of statins and other lipid lowering drugs across Europe 1997-2003. *Br. J. Clin. Pharmacol.* **2005**, *60*, 543–551. [CrossRef] [PubMed]
34. Food and Agriculture Organization of the United Nations. *Fats and Fatty Acids in Human Nutrition: Report of an Expert Consultation*; Food and Agriculture Organization of the United Nations: Rome, Italy, 2010; Available online: http://www.fao.org/3/a-i1953e.pdf (accessed on 5 April 2016).
35. Stark, K.D.; Van Elswyk, M.E.; Higgins, M.R.; Weatherford, C.A.; Salem, N., Jr. Global survey of the omega-3 fatty acids, docosahexaenoic acid and eicosapentaenoic acid in the blood stream of healthy adults. *Prog. Lipid Res.* **2016**, *63*, 132–152. [CrossRef] [PubMed]
36. Arterburn, L.M.; Hall, E.B.; Oken, H. Distribution, interconversion, and dose response of *n*-3 fatty acids in humans. *Am. J. Clin. Nutr.* **2006**, *83*, 1467S–1476S. [CrossRef] [PubMed]
37. Stark, K.D.; Aristizabal Henao, J.J.; Metherel, A.H.; Pilote, L. Translating plasma and whole blood fatty acid compositional data into the sum of eicosapentaenoic and docosahexaenoic acid in erythrocytes. *Prostaglandins Leukot. Essent. Fatty Acids* **2016**, *104*, 1–10. [CrossRef] [PubMed]
38. Brenna, J.T.; Salem, N., Jr.; Sinclair, A.J.; Cunnane, S.C.; for the International Society for the Study of Fatty Acids and Lipids; ISSFAL. alpha-Linolenic acid supplementation and conversion to *n*-3 long-chain polyunsaturated fatty acids in humans. *Prostaglandins Leukot. Essent. Fatty Acids* **2009**, *80*, 85–91. [CrossRef] [PubMed]
39. Brossard, N.; Croset, M.; Pachiaudi, C.; Riou, J.P.; Tayot, J.L.; Lagarde, M. Retroconversion and metabolism of (13C)22:6*n*-3 in humans and rats after intake of a single dose of (13C)22:6*n*-3-triacylglycerols. *Am. J. Clin. Nutr.* **1996**, *64*, 577–586. [CrossRef] [PubMed]
40. Conquer, J.A.; Holub, B.J. Supplementation with an algae source of docosahexaenoic acid increases (*n*-3) fatty acid status and alters selected risk factors for heart disease in vegetarian subjects. *J. Nutr.* **1996**, *126*, 3032–3039. [CrossRef] [PubMed]
41. Conquer, J.A.; Holub, B.J. Dietary docosahexaenoic acid as a source of eicosapentaenoic acid in vegetarians and omnivores. *Lipids* **1997**, *32*, 341–345. [CrossRef] [PubMed]
42. Calo, L.; Martino, A.; Tota, C. The anti-arrhythmic effects of *n*-3 PUFAs. *Int. J. Cardiol.* **2013**, *170*, S21–S27. [CrossRef] [PubMed]
43. Leaf, A.; Kang, J.X.; Xiao, Y.F.; Billman, G.E. Clinical prevention of sudden cardiac death by *n*-3 polyunsaturated fatty acids and mechanism of prevention of arrhythmias by *n*-3 fish oils. *Circulation* **2003**, *107*, 2646–2652. [CrossRef] [PubMed]
44. Weintraub, H. Update on marine omega-3 fatty acids: management of dyslipidemia and current omega-3 treatment options. *Atherosclerosis* **2013**, *230*, 381–389. [CrossRef] [PubMed]
45. Jacobson, T.A.; Glickstein, S.B.; Rowe, J.D.; Soni, P.N. Effects of eicosapentaenoic acid and docosahexaenoic acid on low-density lipoprotein cholesterol and other lipids: A review. *J. Clin. Lipidol.* **2012**, *6*, 5–18. [CrossRef] [PubMed]
46. Davidson, M.H. Omega-3 fatty acids: New insights into the pharmacology and biology of docosahexaenoic acid, docosapentaenoic acid, and eicosapentaenoic acid. *Curr. Opin. Lipidol.* **2013**, *24*, 467–474. [CrossRef] [PubMed]
47. Ryan, A.S.; Keske, M.A.; Hoffman, J.P.; Nelson, E.B. Clinical overview of algal-docosahexaenoic acid: effects on triglyceride levels and other cardiovascular risk factors. *Am. J. Ther.* **2009**, *16*, 183–192. [CrossRef] [PubMed]

48. Alexander, D.D.; Miller, P.E.; Van Elswyk, M.E.; Kuratko, C.N.; Bylsma, L.C. A Meta-Analysis of Randomized Controlled Trials and Prospective Cohort Studies of Eicosapentaenoic and Docosahexaenoic Long-Chain Omega-3 Fatty Acids and Coronary Heart Disease Risk. *Mayo Clin. Proc.* **2017**, *92*, 15–29. [CrossRef] [PubMed]
49. Saber, H.; Yakoob, M.Y.; Shi, P.; Longstreth, W.T., Jr.; Lemaitre, R.N.; Siscovick, D.; Rexrode, K.M.; Willett, W.C.; Mozaffarian, D. Omega-3 Fatty Acids and Incident Ischemic Stroke and Its Atherothrombotic and Cardioembolic Subtypes in 3 US Cohorts. *Stroke* **2017**, *48*, 2678–2685. [CrossRef] [PubMed]
50. Woodman, R.J.; Mori, T.A.; Burke, V.; Puddey, I.B.; Barden, A.; Watts, G.F.; Beilin, L.J. Effects of purified eicosapentaenoic acid and docosahexaenoic acid on platelet, fibrinolytic and vascular function in hypertensive type 2 diabetic patients. *Atherosclerosis* **2003**, *166*, 85–93. [CrossRef]
51. Casula, M.; Soranna, D.; Catapano, A.L.; Corrao, G. Long-term effect of high dose omega-3 fatty acid supplementation for secondary prevention of cardiovascular outcomes: A meta-analysis of randomized, placebo controlled trials (corrected). *Atheroscler. Suppl.* **2013**, *14*, 243–251. [CrossRef]
52. Rizos, E.C.; Ntzani, E.E.; Bika, E.; Kostapanos, M.S.; Elisaf, M.S. Association between omega-3 fatty acid supplementation and risk of major cardiovascular disease events: A systematic review and meta-analysis. *JAMA* **2012**, *308*, 1024–1033. [CrossRef] [PubMed]
53. Cheng, P.; Huang, W.; Bai, S.; Wu, Y.; Yu, J.; Zhu, X.; Qi, Z.; Shao, W.; Xie, P. BMI Affects the Relationship between Long Chain *n*-3 Polyunsaturated Fatty Acid Intake and Stroke Risk: A Meta-Analysis. *Sci. Rep.* **2015**, *5*, 14161. [CrossRef] [PubMed]
54. Mollace, V.; Gliozzi, M.; Carresi, C.; Musolino, V.; Oppedisano, F. Re-assessing the mechanism of action of *n*-3 PUFAs. *Int. J. Cardiol.* **2013**, *170*, S8–S11. [CrossRef] [PubMed]
55. Innes, J.K.; Calder, P.C. The Differential Effects of Eicosapentaenoic Acid and Docosahexaenoic Acid on Cardiometabolic Risk Factors: A Systematic Review. *Int. J. Mol. Sci.* **2018**, *19*. [CrossRef] [PubMed]
56. Frost and Sullivan. *The State of the Global Omega-3 Ingredients Market in 2015. A Market at a Crossroad*; Frost and Sullivan: New York, NY, USA, 2015; pp. 4–33.
57. DSM Nutritional Products; TNS Canada Market Research. *2014 Omega-3 Usage & Attitude Study*; DSM Nutritional Products: Heerlen, The Netherland, 2015; pp. 5–35.
58. Burnett, A.J.; Livingstone, K.M.; Woods, J.L.; McNaughton, S.A. Dietary Supplement Use among Australian Adults: Findings from the 2011–2012 National Nutrition and Physical Activity Survey. *Nutrients* **2017**, *9*, 1248. [CrossRef] [PubMed]
59. Bailey, R.L.; Gahche, J.J.; Miller, P.E.; Thomas, P.R.; Dwyer, J.T. Why US adults use dietary supplements. *JAMA Intern. Med.* **2013**, *173*, 355–361. [CrossRef] [PubMed]
60. Das, U.N. Essential fatty acids as possible mediators of the actions of statins. *Prostaglandins Leukot. Essent. Fatty Acids* **2001**, *65*, 37–40. [CrossRef] [PubMed]
61. Mori, T.A.; Woodman, R.J. The independent effects of eicosapentaenoic acid and docosahexaenoic acid on cardiovascular risk factors in humans. *Curr. Opin. Clin. Nutr. Metab. Care* **2006**, *9*, 95–104. [CrossRef] [PubMed]
62. Hunter, J.E.; Zhang, J.; Kris-Etherton, P.M. Cardiovascular disease risk of dietary stearic acid compared with trans, other saturated, and unsaturated fatty acids: a systematic review. *Am. J. Clin. Nutr.* **2010**, *91*, 46–63. [CrossRef] [PubMed]
63. Proksch, E.; Feingold, K.R.; Elias, P.M. Epidermal HMG CoA reductase activity in essential fatty acid deficiency: barrier requirements rather than eicosanoid generation regulate cholesterol synthesis. *J. Investig. Dermatol.* **1992**, *99*, 216–220. [CrossRef] [PubMed]
64. Notarnicola, M.; Messa, C.; Refolo, M.G.; Tutino, V.; Miccolis, A.; Caruso, M.G. Polyunsaturated fatty acids reduce fatty acid synthase and hydroxy-methyl-glutaryl CoA-reductase gene expression and promote apoptosis in HepG2 cell line. *Lipids Health Dis.* **2011**, *10*, 10. [CrossRef] [PubMed]
65. Oh, H.T.; Chung, M.J.; Kim, S.H.; Choi, H.J.; Ham, S.S. Masou salmon (*Oncorhynchus masou*) ethanol extract decreases 3-hydroxy-3-methylglutaryl coenzyme A reductase expression in diet-induced obese mice. *Nutr. Res.* **2009**, *29*, 123–129. [CrossRef] [PubMed]
66. Shirai, N.; Suzuki, H. Effect of docosahexaenoic acid on brain 3-hydroxy-3-methylglutaryl -coenzyme A reductase activity in male ICR mice. *J. Nutr. Biochem.* **2007**, *18*, 488–494. [CrossRef] [PubMed]

67. Ihara-Watanabe, M.; Umekawa, H.; Takahashi, T.; Furuichi, Y. Effects of dietary alpha- or gamma-linolenic acid on levels and fatty acid compositions of serum and hepatic lipids, and activity and mRNA abundance of 3-hydroxy-3-methylglutaryl CoA reductase in rats. *Comp. Biochem. Physiol. Part A Mol. Integr. Physiol.* **1999**, *122*, 213–220. [CrossRef]
68. Wang, H.; Blumberg, J.B.; Chen, C.Y.; Choi, S.W.; Corcoran, M.P.; Harris, S.S.; Jacques, P.F.; Kristo, A.S.; Lai, C.Q.; Lamon-Fava, S.; et al. Dietary modulators of statin efficacy in cardiovascular disease and cognition. *Mol. Aspects Med.* **2014**, *38*, 1–53. [CrossRef] [PubMed]
69. Harris, J.I.; Hibbeln, J.R.; Mackey, R.H.; Muldoon, M.F. Statin treatment alters serum *n*-3 and *n*-6 fatty acids in hypercholesterolemic patients. *Prostaglandins Leukot. Essent. Fatty Acids* **2004**, *71*, 263–269. [CrossRef] [PubMed]
70. Nozue, T.; Michishita, I. Statin treatment alters serum *n*-3 to *n*-6 polyunsaturated fatty acids ratio in patients with dyslipidemia. *Lipids Health Dis.* **2015**, *14*, 67. [CrossRef] [PubMed]
71. Jula, A.; Marniemi, J.; Ronnemaa, T.; Virtanen, A.; Huupponen, R. Effects of diet and simvastatin on fatty acid composition in hypercholesterolemic men: a randomized controlled trial. *Arterioscler. Thromb. Vasc. Biol.* **2005**, *25*, 1952–1959. [CrossRef] [PubMed]
72. Al Mamun, A.; Hashimoto, M.; Katakura, M.; Tanabe, Y.; Tsuchikura, S.; Hossain, S.; Shido, O. Effect of dietary *n*-3 fatty acids supplementation on fatty acid metabolism in atorvastatin-administered SHR.Cg-Leprcp/NDmcr rats, a metabolic syndrome model. *Biomed. Pharmacother.* **2017**, *85*, 372–379. [CrossRef] [PubMed]
73. Risé, P.; Pazzucconi, F.; Sirtori, C.R.; Galli, C. Statins enhance arachidonic acid synthesis in hypercholesterolemic patients. *Nutr. Metab. Cardiovasc. Dis.* **2001**, *11*, 88–94. [PubMed]
74. Risé, P.; Ghezzi, S.; Galli, C. Relative potencies of statins in reducing cholesterol synthesis and enhancing linoleic acid metabolism. *Eur. J. Pharmacol.* **2003**, *467*, 73–75. [CrossRef]
75. De Lorgeril, M.; Salen, P.; Guiraud, A.; Zeghichi, S.; Boucher, F.; de Leiris, J. Lipid-lowering drugs and essential omega-6 and omega-3 fatty acids in patients with coronary heart disease. *Nutr. Metab. Cardiovasc. Dis.* **2005**, *15*, 36–41. [CrossRef] [PubMed]
76. Green, C.D.; Ozguden-Akkoc, C.G.; Wang, Y.; Jump, D.B.; Olson, L.K. Role of fatty acid elongases in determination of de novo synthesized monounsaturated fatty acid species. *J. Lipid Res.* **2010**, *51*, 1871–1877. [CrossRef] [PubMed]
77. Takahashi, M.; Ando, J.; Shimada, K.; Nishizaki, Y.; Tani, S.; Ogawa, T.; Yamamoto, M.; Nagao, K.; Hirayama, A.; Yoshimura, M.; et al. The ratio of serum *n*-3 to *n*-6 polyunsaturated fatty acids is associated with diabetes mellitus in patients with prior myocardial infarction: A multicenter cross-sectional study. *BMC Cardiovasc. Disord.* **2017**, *17*, 41. [CrossRef] [PubMed]
78. Risé, P.; Colombo, C.; Galli, C. Effects of simvastatin on the metabolism of polyunsaturated fatty acids and on glycerolipid, cholesterol, and de novo lipid synthesis in THP-1 cells. *J. Lipid Res.* **1997**, *38*, 1299–1307. [PubMed]
79. Kurisu, S.; Ishibashi, K.; Kato, Y.; Mitsuba, N.; Dohi, Y.; Nishioka, K.; Kihara, Y. Effects of lipid-lowering therapy with strong statin on serum polyunsaturated fatty acid levels in patients with coronary artery disease. *Heart Vessels* **2013**, *28*, 34–38. [CrossRef] [PubMed]
80. De Lorgeril, M.; Salen, P.; Defaye, P.; Rabaeus, M. Recent findings on the health effects of omega-3 fatty acids and statins, and their interactions: Do statins inhibit omega-3? *BMC Med.* **2013**, *11*, 5. [CrossRef] [PubMed]
81. Banach, M.; Serban, C.; Ursoniu, S.; Rysz, J.; Muntner, P.; Toth, P.P.; Jones, S.R.; Rizzo, M.; Glasser, S.P.; Watts, G.F.; et al. Statin therapy and plasma coenzyme Q10 concentrations—A systematic review and meta-analysis of placebo-controlled trials. *Pharmacol. Res.* **2015**, *99*, 329–336. [CrossRef] [PubMed]
82. Schunck, W.H.; Konkel, A.; Fischer, R.; Weylandt, K.H. Therapeutic potential of omega-3 fatty acid-derived epoxyeicosanoids in cardiovascular and inflammatory diseases. *Pharmacol. Ther.* **2018**, *183*, 177–204. [CrossRef] [PubMed]
83. Fleming, I. The pharmacology of the cytochrome P450 epoxygenase/soluble epoxide hydrolase axis in the vasculature and cardiovascular disease. *Pharmacol. Rev.* **2014**, *66*, 1106–1140. [CrossRef] [PubMed]
84. Cohen, L.H.; van Leeuwen, R.E.; van Thiel, G.C.; van Pelt, J.F.; Yap, S.H. Equally potent inhibitors of cholesterol synthesis in human hepatocytes have distinguishable effects on different cytochrome P450 enzymes. *Biopharm. Drug Dispos.* **2000**, *21*, 353–364. [CrossRef] [PubMed]

85. Jamieson, K.L.; Endo, T.; Darwesh, A.M.; Samokhvalov, V.; Seubert, J.M. Cytochrome P450-derived eicosanoids and heart function. *Pharmacol. Ther.* **2017**, *179*, 47–83. [CrossRef] [PubMed]
86. Spector, A.A.; Kim, H.Y. Cytochrome P450 epoxygenase pathway of polyunsaturated fatty acid metabolism. *Biochim. Biophys. Acta* **2015**, *1851*, 356–365. [CrossRef] [PubMed]
87. Kiage, J.N.; Sampson, U.K.; Lipworth, L.; Fazio, S.; Mensah, G.A.; Yu, Q.; Munro, H.; Akwo, E.A.; Dai, Q.; Blot, W.J.; et al. Intake of polyunsaturated fat in relation to mortality among statin users and non-users in the Southern Community Cohort Study. *Nutr. Metab. Cardiovasc. Dis.* **2015**, *25*, 1016–1024. [CrossRef] [PubMed]
88. Eussen, S.R.; Geleijnse, J.M.; Giltay, E.J.; Rompelberg, C.J.; Klungel, O.H.; Kromhout, D. Effects of *n*-3 fatty acids on major cardiovascular events in statin users and non-users with a history of myocardial infarction. *Eur. Heart J.* **2012**, *33*, 1582–1588. [CrossRef] [PubMed]
89. Greene, S.J.; Temporelli, P.L.; Campia, U.; Vaduganathan, M.; Degli Esposti, L.; Buda, S.; Veronesi, C.; Butler, J.; Nodari, S. Effects of Polyunsaturated Fatty Acid Treatment on Postdischarge Outcomes After Acute Myocardial Infarction. *Am. J. Cardiol.* **2016**, *117*, 340–346. [CrossRef] [PubMed]
90. Macchia, A.; Romero, M.; D'Ettorre, A.; Tognoni, G.; Mariani, J. Exploratory analysis on the use of statins with or without *n*-3 PUFA and major events in patients discharged for acute myocardial infarction: an observational retrospective study. *PLoS ONE* **2013**, *8*, e62772. [CrossRef] [PubMed]
91. Matsuzaki, M.; Yokoyama, M.; Saito, Y.; Origasa, H.; Ishikawa, Y.; Oikawa, S.; Sasaki, J.; Hishida, H.; Itakura, H.; Kita, T.; et al. Incremental effects of eicosapentaenoic acid on cardiovascular events in statin-treated patients with coronary artery disease. *Circ. J.* **2009**, *73*, 1283–1290. [CrossRef] [PubMed]
92. Saito, Y.; Yokoyama, M.; Origasa, H.; Matsuzaki, M.; Matsuzawa, Y.; Ishikawa, Y.; Oikawa, S.; Sasaki, J.; Hishida, H.; Itakura, H.; et al. Effects of EPA on coronary artery disease in hypercholesterolemic patients with multiple risk factors: Sub-analysis of primary prevention cases from the Japan EPA Lipid Intervention Study (JELIS). *Atherosclerosis* **2008**, *200*, 135–140. [CrossRef] [PubMed]
93. Watanabe, T.; Ando, K.; Daidoji, H.; Otaki, Y.; Sugawara, S.; Matsui, M.; Ikeno, E.; Hirono, O.; Miyawaki, H.; Yashiro, Y.; et al. A randomized controlled trial of eicosapentaenoic acid in patients with coronary heart disease on statins. *J. Cardiol.* **2017**, *70*, 537–544. [CrossRef] [PubMed]
94. Nosaka, K.; Miyoshi, T.; Iwamoto, M.; Kajiya, M.; Okawa, K.; Tsukuda, S.; Yokohama, F.; Sogo, M.; Nishibe, T.; Matsuo, N.; et al. Early initiation of eicosapentaenoic acid and statin treatment is associated with better clinical outcomes than statin alone in patients with acute coronary syndromes: 1-year outcomes of a randomized controlled study. *Int. J. Cardiol.* **2017**, *228*, 173–179. [CrossRef] [PubMed]
95. Alfaddagh, A.; Elajami, T.K.; Ashfaque, H.; Saleh, M.; Bistrian, B.R.; Welty, F.K. Effect of Eicosapentaenoic and Docosahexaenoic Acids Added to Statin Therapy on Coronary Artery Plaque in Patients With Coronary Artery Disease: A Randomized Clinical Trial. *J. Am. Heart Assoc.* **2017**, *6*. [CrossRef] [PubMed]
96. Chan, D.C.; Pang, J.; Barrett, P.H.; Sullivan, D.R.; Mori, T.A.; Burnett, J.R.; van Bockxmeer, F.M.; Watts, G.F. Effect of omega-3 fatty acid supplementation on arterial elasticity in patients with familial hypercholesterolaemia on statin therapy. *Nutr. Metab. Cardiovasc. Dis.* **2016**, *26*, 1140–1145. [CrossRef] [PubMed]
97. Ballantyne, C.M.; Braeckman, R.A.; Bays, H.E.; Kastelein, J.J.; Otvos, J.D.; Stirtan, W.G.; Doyle, R.T., Jr.; Soni, P.N.; Juliano, R.A. Effects of icosapent ethyl on lipoprotein particle concentration and size in statin-treated patients with persistent high triglycerides (the ANCHOR Study). *J. Clin. Lipidol.* **2015**, *9*, 377–383. [CrossRef] [PubMed]
98. Scolaro, B.; Nogueira, M.S.; Paiva, A.; Bertolami, A.; Barroso, L.P.; Vaisar, T.; Heffron, S.P.; Fisher, E.A.; Castro, I.A. Statin dose reduction with complementary diet therapy: A pilot study of personalized medicine. *Mol. Metab.* **2018**, *11*, 137–144. [CrossRef] [PubMed]

14

Quality of Dietary Fat Intake and Body Weight and Obesity in a Mediterranean Population: Secondary Analyses within the PREDIMED Trial

Yvette Beulen [1], Miguel A. Martínez-González [2,3], Ondine van de Rest [1], Jordi Salas-Salvadó [3,4], José V. Sorlí [3,5], Enrique Gómez-Gracia [6], Miquel Fiol [3,7], Ramón Estruch [3,8], José M. Santos-Lozano [3,9], Helmut Schröder [10,11], Angel Alonso-Gómez [3,12], Luis Serra-Majem [3,13], Xavier Pintó [3,14], Emilio Ros [3,15], Nerea Becerra-Tomas [3,4], José I. González [3,5], Montserrat Fitó [3,10], J. Alfredo Martínez [3,16] and Alfredo Gea [2,*]

1. Division of Human Nutrition, Wageningen University, 6708 Wageningen, The Netherlands; yvette.beulen@wur.nl (Y.B.); ondine.vanderest@wur.nl (O.v.d.R.)
2. Department of Preventive Medicine & Public Health, University of Navarra, 31008 Pamplona, Spain; mamartinez@unav.es
3. CIBER Fisiopatología de la Obesidad y Nutrición (CIBEROBN), Instituto de Salud Carlos III (ISCIII), Spanish Government, 28029 Madrid, Spain; jordi.salas@urv.cat (J.S.-S.); sorli@uv.es (J.V.S.); mfiol@hsd.es (M.F.); restruch@clinic.cat (R.E.); josemanuel.santos@ono.com (J.M.S.-L.); angelmago13@gmail.com (A.A.-G.); lluis.serra@ulpgc.es (L.S.-M.); xpinto@bellvitgehospital.cat (X.P.); eros@clinic.cat (E.R.); nerea.becerra@urv.cat (N.B.-T.); arraez@uv.es (J.I.G.); mfito@imim.es (M.F.); jalfmtz@unav.es (J.A.M.)
4. Human Nutrition Unit, Faculty of Medicine and Health Sciences, Pere Virgili Health Research Institute, Rovira i Virgili University, 43002 Reus, Spain
5. Department of Preventive Medicine, University of Valencia, 46010 Valencia, Spain
6. Department of Preventive Medicine, University of Málaga, 29016 Málaga, Spain; egomezgracia@uma.es
7. Institute of Health Sciences IUNICS, University of Balearic Islands and Hospital Son Espases, 07010 Palma de Mallorca, Spain
8. Department of Internal Medicine, Department of Endocrinology and Nutrition Biomedical Research Institute August Pi Sunyer (IDI- BAPS), Hospital Clinic, University of Barcelona, 08036 Barcelona, Spain
9. Department of Family Medicine, Research Unit, Distrito Sanitario Atención Primaria Sevilla, Centro de Salud Universitario San Pablo, 41013 Sevilla, Spain
10. Cardiovascular and Nutrition Research Group (Regicor Study Group), Hospital del Mar Research Institute (IMIM), 08003 Barcelona, Spain; hschoeder@imim.es
11. CIBER Epidemiología y Salud Pública (CIBERESP), Instituto de Salud Carlos III (ISCIII), Spanish Government, 28029 Madrid, Spain
12. Department of Cardiology, University Hospital of Alava, 48940 Vitoria, Spain
13. Research Institute of Biomedical and Health Sciences (IUIBS), University of Las Palmas de Gran Canaria and Service of Preventive Medicine, Complejo Hospitalario Universitario Insular Materno Infantil (CHUIMI), Canary Health Service, 35016 Las Palmas de Gran Canaria, Spain
14. Lipids and Vascular Risk Unit, Internal Medicine, Hospital Universitario de Bellvitge, Hospitalet de Llobregat, 08907 Barcelona, Spain
15. Lipid Clinic, Department of Endocrinology and Nutrition Biomedical Research Institute August Pi Sunyer (IDIBAPS), Hospital Clinic, University of Barcelona, 08036 Barcelona, Spain
16. Department of Nutrition and Food Sciences and Physiology, University of Navarra, 31008 Pamplona, Spain

* Correspondence: ageas@unav.es

Abstract: A moderately high-fat Mediterranean diet does not promote weight gain. This study aimed to investigate the association between dietary intake of specific types of fat and obesity and body weight. A prospective cohort study was performed using data of 6942 participants in the PREDIMED trial, with yearly repeated validated food-frequency questionnaires, and anthropometric outcomes (median follow-up: 4.8 years). The effects of replacing dietary fat subtypes for one another, proteins or carbohydrates were estimated using generalized estimating equations substitution models. Replacement of 5% energy from saturated fatty acids (SFA) with monounsaturated fatty acids (MUFA) or polyunsaturated fatty acids (PUFA) resulted in weight changes of −0.38 kg (95% Confidece Iinterval (CI): −0.69, −0.07), and −0.51 kg (95% CI: −0.81, −0.20), respectively. Replacing proteins with MUFA or PUFA decreased the odds of becoming obese. Estimates for the daily substitution of one portion of red meat with white meat, oily fish or white fish showed weight changes up to −0.87 kg. Increasing the intake of unsaturated fatty acids at the expense of SFA, proteins, and carbohydrates showed beneficial effects on body weight and obesity. It may therefore be desirable to encourage high-quality fat diets like the Mediterranean diet instead of restricting total fat intake.

Keywords: fat; obesity; body weight; cohort study; substitution models

---

1. Introduction

Obesity is one of the most important risk factors of noncommunicable diseases. The epidemic has been described extensively in scientific literature, providing cogent evidence for its role in the development of cardiovascular diseases, diabetes, musculoskeletal disorders, and certain types of cancer [1]. Dietary fat intake has long been believed to be an important predictor of obesity as it is the most energy-dense macronutrient, providing about 9 kcal per gram versus 4 kcal/g from proteins or carbohydrates. Consequently, to control obesity, dietary guidelines have focused on reducing total fat intake for almost four decades [2]. Even after a large body of evidence showed the beneficial health effects of unsaturated fatty acids [3,4], total fat restrictions remained [5], as well as the gradual increase in the global prevalence of overweight and obesity [6].

Currently, some aspects of guidelines are being revised. A report of the third FAO (Food and Agriculture Organization of the United Nations)/WHO (World Health Organization) Expert Consultation on Fats and Fatty Acids in Human Nutrition (Geneva, 2008) showed the focus is clearly shifting from fat quantity to quality [7]. Additionally, the latest US Dietary Guidelines Advisory Committee (DGAC) report concluded that emphasis should be put on optimizing types of dietary fat and not reducing total fat [5]. The quality of fat is generally specified by the relative intake of monounsaturated (MUFA) and polyunsaturated fatty acids (PUFA) versus saturated (SFA) and trans fatty acids. Furthermore, PUFA may be subdivided into plant-derived linoleic (C18:2n-6) and α-linolenic acid (ALA, C18:3n-3) and marine-derived eicosapentaenoic (EPA, 20:5n-3) and docosahexaenoic acid (DHA, C22:6n-3) [8].

The Mediterranean diet (MeDiet) is typically high in fat and there is evidence about its role in the prevention of cardiovascular disease [9,10], in which the proportions of unsaturated and saturated fatty acids have been shown to play an important role [11]. Moreover, multiple systematic reviews and meta-analyses have shown a MeDiet does not promote weight gain [12–15]. In fact, it may even result in greater and more long-lasting weight loss than low-fat diets and be protective against increases in waist circumference [12–15]. This outcome has also been shown for nut intake, a predominant food product in the MeDiet [16–18]. Other food, more specific components of the MeDiet, and their association with obesity-related outcomes have not received as much attention to date.

Although assessing a complete dietary pattern provides insight into the cumulative effects of consuming certain products, determining which nutrients or food items induce the greatest change may lead to better understanding of the associations. The main objective of this study is therefore to investigate the association between dietary fat intake of both specific types of fatty acids and of food items within the MeDiet and body weight and obesity.

2. Materials and Methods

2.1. Study Population

This prospective study was a secondary analysis using data of the large, randomized controlled trial PREDIMED (prevención con dieta Mediterránea, prevention with Mediterranean diet). Participants within the PREDIMED study were Spanish men and women at high risk for cardiovascular disease, recruited from multiple centers across the country between October 2003 and June 2009. After inclusion, participants were assigned to two groups receiving a MeDiet supplemented with either extra virgin olive oil or mixed nuts, and—in the case of the control group—solely receiving advice on following a low-fat diet. The PREDIMED protocol was approved by institutional review boards and all participants provided written informed consent. Further details on the design and protocol of the study have been described elsewhere [19,20].

The trial was stopped in December 2010 and included 7447 participants. After exclusion of participants without food-frequency questionnaire (FFQ) data, without BMI follow-up data, with implausible energy intakes (<800 or >4200 kcal/day in men <500 and >3500 kcal/day in women) [21] or without other data necessary to perform the analyses, the population available for the present analyses included 6942 participants with a median follow-up of 4.8 years (interquartile range: 2.9 to 5.8).

2.2. Dietary Exposure Assessment

At baseline and yearly thereafter, a semiquantitative 137-item food-frequency questionnaire (FFQ) was collected and reviewed by trained, registered dieticians. The used FFQ was repeatedly validated and found to be highly reproducible and have a reasonably good validity with regard to nutrient intake reported [22,23]. Spanish food-composition tables were used to derive energy and nutrient intake [24]. Dietary intakes were considered as the cumulative average of all available data, from baseline to each follow-up measurement, to optimally represent long-term intake and reduce measurement error [25].

2.3. Outcome Assessment

Anthropometric measurements were taken by trained personnel once a year. Weight was measured on a calibrated scale, without shoes and with light clothing. Height was determined using a wall-mounted stadiometer.

Participants with a BMI $\geq$25 and <30 kg/m^2 were classified as overweight and $\geq$30 kg/m^2 as obese. Substantial weight gain or loss was defined as a change $\geq$10% when compared to baseline body weight [26]. Body weight was analyzed as continuous outcomes and dichotomized using this cut-off (a change $\geq$10%), additional to the dichotomous variables for incidence (increasing to a BMI $\geq$30 kg/m^2) and reversion of obesity (decreasing to a BMI <30 kg/m^2).

2.4. Assessment of Other Variables

At each yearly visit, sociodemographic variables and risk factors like educational level and working, marital, and smoking status were assessed using in a general questionnaire. Physical activity was assessed using the Spanish version of Minnesota Leisure-Time Physical Activity, validated in both sexes [27,28]. Based on frequency and duration of 67 activities, a MET (Metabolic equivalents) score was assigned to each participant. The analyses considered updated the measurements of these covariates and in case of missing data, the last observations were carried forward to prevent participants being excluded from the analyses.

2.5. Statistical Analyses

Participant characteristics were reported according to extreme quintiles of fatty acid intakes, as mean (SD) for continuous variables and % for categorical variables.

Generalized estimating equations (GEE) were fit to analyze the association between the cumulative average of yearly measured consumption of dietary fatty acids and body weight. For these continuous outcomes, the distribution was set to Gaussian and link function to identity. Effects of isocaloric substitution of fat types for one another, carbohydrates, and proteins were estimated as the difference between β coefficients of macronutrients exchanged per 5% of energy from these sources. Logistic GEE regression models were used to determine odds ratios for incidence and reversion of obesity and ≥10% changes in body weight. The effects of replacing specific high-fat food products for other, higher-quality options were estimated using non-isocaloric substitution models, by considering the replacement of single portions of meat, fish and seafood (100 g), oils, butter and margarine (10 g), and nuts (30 g). For all GEE models, an exchangeable correlation structure was assumed.

The model included intakes of all energy delivering dietary variables except for one (the last one being omitted as they add up to 100% for any person) and was adjusted for age, sex, intervention group, baseline BMI or body weight, leisure-time physical activity (quintiles of MET-min/week), smoking status (never, former, current smoker), educational level (none/primary, secondary, academic/graduate), working status (employed, unemployed, housewife, retired), marital status (single/widowed, married), and dietary fiber intake (continuous).

Sensitivity analyses were performed using mixed-effects models instead of GEE models and both observed and updated measurements of exposure instead of cumulative averages. Missing values of dietary variables and weight were imputed using multilevel multiple imputation in the GEE model with body weight as the continuous outcome. Data were assumed to be MAR (missing at random) and m = 20 datasets were created using multivariate normal (MVN) as the imputation algorithm [29].

All statistical analyses were performed using STATA/SE V.12.1 (StataCorp, College Station, TX, USA) and p-values < 0.05 were considered statistically significant.

3. Results

3.1. Baseline Characteristics

The population available for the analyses consisted of 6942 participants with a mean age of 67 (SD: 6) years and of which a proportion of 47% was obese at baseline. Table 1 shows the baseline characteristics of participants. Mean total fat intake was 30.5% of total energy intake (EN%) in the lowest quintile versus 50.6 EN% in the highest.

3.2. Substitution of Fat Subtypes

3.2.1. Body Weight Differences

The results of GEE substitution models presented in Table 2 show the predicted effects of replacing 5% of energy from a specific fat subtype for 5 EN% of another fat subtype, proteins or carbohydrates. The results suggested consuming PUFA is associated with a significant weight difference when replacing SFA (mean change −0.51 kg; 95% confidence interval (CI): −0.81, −0.20), proteins (−0.27 kg; 95% CI: −0.49, −0.04) or carbohydrates (−0.20 kg; 95% CI: −0.37, −0.02). Additionally, isocaloric substitution of 5 EN% of SFA with MUFA was inversely associated with body weight (−0.38, 95% CI: −0.69, −0.07). Increasing SFA at the expense of carbohydrates was found to be directly associated with body weight (0.31 kg; 95% CI: 0.06, 0.56).

Table 1. Participant characteristics according to extreme quintiles of total fat (in EN%) at baseline [1].

	Q1	Q5
Participants, n	1391	1387
Age (year)	67 (6)	67 (6)
Women (%)	53.9	62.5
Control group (%)	35.6	32.2
Physical activity (MET-min/week)	249 (259)	216 (226)
Smoking habit: Never smoker (%)	61.0	64.4
Smoking habit: Former smoker (%)	24.4	22.4
Smoking habit: Current smoker (%)	14.6	13.2
Marital status: Married (%)	75.0	76.5
Marital status: Single/widowed (%)	25.0	23.5
Educational level: Lower than high school (%)	80.5	75.3
Educational level: High school (%)	11.9	17.7
Educational level: University (%)	7.6	7.0
Employment status: Employed/housewife	41.6	51.8
Employment status: Unemployed (%)	3.5	3.5
Employment status: Retired (%)	54.9	44.7
Total energy intake (kcal/day)	2262 (573)	2163 (513)
Carbohydrates (EN%)	51.6 (5.8)	35.1 (4.5)
Protein (EN%)	17.4 (3.1)	16.7 (2.8)
Total fat (EN%)	27.7 (3.2)	46.5 (3.7)
MUFAs (EN%)	14.4 (2.4)	26.3 (3.4)
PUFAs (EN%)	5.0 (1.6)	7.9 (2.4)
SFAs (EN%)	8.1 (1.7)	12.1 (2.1)
trans fat (EN%)	0.18 (0.12)	0.28 (0.17)
Alcohol (g/day)	11.2 (18.7)	5.1 (9.2)
Dietary fiber (g/day)	28.9 (10.1)	21.7 (6.6)

[1] Q, quintile; MET, metabolic equivalent task; EN%, energy as a proportion of total energy intake. Data are mean (SD) unless otherwise stated.

Table 2. Estimated mean changes (95% confidence interval) [1] in body weight (kg) after isocaloric substitutions of 5% energy from MUFA, PUFA, and SFA, proteins, and carbohydrates.

Substitution	**↑MUFA**	**↑PUFA**	**↑SFA**
↓PUFA	0.13 (−0.09, 0.34)	-	-
↓SFA	−0.38 (−0.69, −0.07) *	−0.51 (−0.81, −0.20) *	-
↓proteins	−0.14 (−0.30, 0.02)	−0.27 (−0.49, −0.04) *	0.24 (−0.08, 0.56)
↓carbohydrates	−0.07 (−0.17, 0.03)	−0.20 (−0.37, −0.02) *	0.31 (0.06, 0.56) *

[1] Adjusted for age, sex, baseline weight, recruitment center, intervention group, cumulative average of total energy intake, BMI, leisure-time physical activity (metabolic equivalent task in min/day), smoking status (never, former, current smoker), educational level (primary education, high school, university), working status (employed, unemployed, housewife, retired), and marital status (single, married). * $p < 0.05$. ↑ means increases, ↓ means decreases.

3.2.2. Obesity Incidence and Reversion, Substantial Weight Gain and Loss

In a total number of 3700 initially non-obese participants, 657 incident cases of obesity were observed during follow-up. Table 3 shows the results of the logistic GEE investigating the association between nutrient substitution and 2 dichotomous outcomes: Obesity incidence and substantial weight gain (≥10%).

Table 3. Estimated odds ratios (95% confidence interval) [1] for incidence of obesity and substantial weight gain (≥10%) after isocaloric substitution of 5% energy from MUFA, PUFA, and SFA, proteins, and carbohydrates.

Substitution	Obesity Incidence	Weight Gain (≥10%)
↑MUFA, ↓PUFA	1.36 (1.02, 1.81) *	1.16 (0.82, 1.65)
↑MUFA, ↓SFA	1.04 (0.69, 1.56)	1.11 (0.71, 1.65)
↑MUFA, ↓Proteins	0.85 (0.69, 1.03)	0.82 (0.66, 1.02)
↑MUFA, ↓Carbohydrates	1.08 (0.95, 1.23)	1.02 (0.87, 1.18)
↑PUFA, ↓SFA	0.77 (0.51, 1.15)	0.96 (0.62, 1.47)
↑PUFA, ↓Proteins	0.62 (0.47, 0.83) *	0.70 (0.50, 0.99) *
↑PUFA, ↓Carbohydrates	0.80 (0.63, 1.01)	0.87 (0.67, 1.15)
↑SFA, ↓Proteins	0.81 (0.53, 1.24)	0.73 (0.46, 1.17)
↑SFA, ↓Carbohydrates	1.04 (0.75, 1.24)	0.91 (0.63, 1.31)

[1] Adjusted for age, sex, baseline weight, recruitment center, intervention group, cumulative average of total energy intake, BMI, leisure-time physical activity (metabolic equivalent task in min/day), smoking status (never, former, current smoker), educational level (primary education, high school, university), working status (employed, unemployed, housewife, retired), and marital status (single, married). * $p < 0.05$.

Replacing 5 EN% of proteins with 5 EN% of PUFA decreased the odds of obesity incidence (OR: 0.62, 95% CI: 0.47, 0.83) and ≥10% weight gain (OR: 0.70, 95% CI: 0.50, 0.99). The odds ratio (95% CI) for obesity incidence was 1.36 (1.02, 1.81) when 5 EN% of PUFA was replaced by MUFA. Reversion of obesity occurred 819 times within the 3242 participants who were obese at baseline. Note that in Figure 1 an odds ratio (OR) >1 indicates increased odds of reversion of obesity or weight loss (≥10%), so desirable changes.

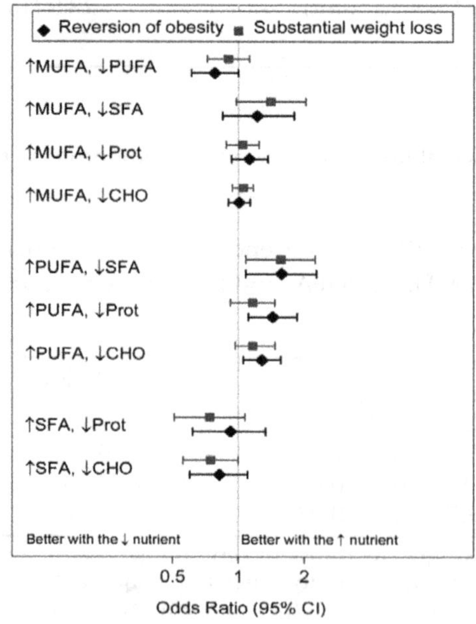

Figure 1. Estimated odds ratios (95% confidence interval) for reversion of obesity (grey squares) and substantial weight loss (≥10%, black diamonds) after isocaloric substitution of 5% energy from MUFA, PUFA, and SFA, proteins (Prot), and carbohydrates (CHO). Adjusted for the same confounders as the analyses in Table 3.

Replacing SFA with PUFA significantly increased the odds of the reversion of obesity (OR: 1.57, 95% CI: 1.09, 2.25) and substantial weight loss (OR: 1.58, 95% CI: 1.09, 2.28). Slightly less strong but significant associations were found for the odds of substantial weight loss when PUFA intake was increased at the expense of proteins (OR: 1.44, 95% CI: 1.12, 1.86) or carbohydrates (OR: 1.29, 95% CI: 1.06, 1.57). Increasing MUFA at the expense of PUFA resulted in an OR of 0.78 (0.61, 1.00) for a

≥10% weight loss. As a summary, all significant results in Table 3 and Figure 1 advocate for a higher PUFA intake.

3.3. Substitution of Food Items

The estimated effects of non-isocaloric food item substitutions on body weight are shown in Table 4. Significant weight difference estimates were observed when daily replacing a 100 g portion of red meat with white meat (−0.64 kg, 95% CI: −0.94, −0.35), oily fish (−0.75 kg, 95% CI: −1.13, −0.38) or white fish (−0.87 kg, 95% CI −1.17, −0.56).

Table 4. Estimated mean changes in body weight (kg) (95% confidence interval) [1] after substitution of one daily portion of high-fat food items in the MeDiet for a priori healthier options.

Substitution	Mean Body Weight (kg) Difference (95% Confidence Interval)
↓Red meat, ↑White meat	−0.64 (−0.94, −0.35) *
↓Red meat, ↑Oily fish	−0.75 (−1.13, −0.38) *
↓Red meat, ↑White fish	−0.87 (−1.17, −0.56) *
↓Butter, ↑Olive oil	−0.25 (−0.56, 0.06)
↓Butter, ↑Other vegetable oils	−0.11 (−0.44, 0.22)
↓Margarine, ↑Olive oil	0.04 (−0.18, 0.25)
↓Margarine, ↑Other vegetable oils	0.26 (0.02, 0.50) *
↓Mixed nuts, ↑Walnuts	−0.15 (−0.61, 0.32)

[1] Substitutions of a portion of 100, 10 and 30 g for meat/fish, butter/margarine/oils, and nuts, respectively. Adjusted for age, sex, baseline weight, recruitment center, intervention group, cumulative average of total energy intake, BMI, leisure-time physical activity (metabolic equivalent task in min/day), smoking status (never, former, current smoker), educational level (primary education, high school, university), working status (employed, unemployed, housewife, retired), and marital status (single, married). * $p < 0.05$. ↑ means increases, ↓ means decreases.

Replacing a 10 g portion of margarine with vegetable oils other than olive oil resulted in a significant estimate, suggesting a weight gain of 0.26 kg (95% CI: 0.02, 0.50). No significant associations were observed for the replacement of butter and margarine with olive oil or replacing 30 g of mixed nuts with an equivalent portion of walnuts.

Estimates of nutrient substitutions for continuous outcomes were consistent when using mixed-effects models with random intercepts for recruitment center and identity level. Mixed-effects models are a little more conservative, however, thus showing wider confidence intervals (data not shown).

4. Discussion

The results of this prospective study suggest that increasing the intake of unsaturated fatty acids (especially PUFA) at the expense of SFA, proteins, and carbohydrates may have beneficial effects on body weight and obesity. Reversing obesity seems to be especially successful when replacing SFA with PUFA, and replacing proteins with PUFA lowers the risk of becoming obese in the first place. Increasing MUFA at the expense of PUFA, on the other hand, shows a significantly increased risk of becoming obese. These findings are in line with previous research [30], although there is still controversy [31]. Most prior research on the association between dietary fat and overweight/obesity merely considered total fat intake or the MeDiet as a whole. Evidence from 53 randomized controlled trials summarized in a systematic review and meta-analysis did not support low-fat diets over other dietary interventions for long-term weight loss, when compared with dietary interventions of similar intensity [15]. A systematic review of 5 RCTs found the MeDiet resulted in greater weight loss than low-fat diet at ≥12 months but produced results similar to other comparator diets, like a low-carbohydrate diet [14]. These results are in line with an earlier meta-analysis [13]. Although the results of the included studies were inconsistent and the meta-analyses reported significant heterogeneity, the evidence ultimately points towards a role of a high-quality, moderately high-fat diet like the MeDiet in the prevention of overweight and obesity. Results of the PREDIMED trial supported that the intervention did not have a differential effect on body weight compared to the control group [32].

One prospective study in a Spanish sample of the EPIC (European Prospective Investigation into Cancer and Nutrition) study further focused on dietary fat subtypes and concluded that the association between consumption of specific types of dietary fat, olive oil, and obesity in Spain was not very important [33]. However, the design of the study was cross-sectional. Ten years later, the results of the EPIC–PANACEA study showed the MeDiet may prevent weight gain and the development of obesity. Unfortunately, this study did not distinguish between types of fat [34].

Previous PREDIMED studies showed a protective effect of MeDiet interventions supplemented by olive oil or nuts and of dairy consumption [35,36]. Moreover, extensive evidence was found that nut consumption does not increase body weight and obesity incidence and may even be inversely associated with these outcomes [17,37,38]. Most nuts are especially high in MUFA, whereas walnuts are rich in PUFA. Adherence to the MeDiet in general has also been shown to be directly associated with fulfilling nutrient recommendations [39,40].

Another important finding of our study, in the context of substitution models, is that reductions in red meat consumption coupled with respective increases in white meat or fish would lead to less weight gain. This is important because it represents a translation of fat substitution models into food item replacement models and it generates a comprehensible and easily understandable message for the population. This is in accordance with the concept of the MeDiet, which fosters the preference for white meat consumption over red meat and includes regular fish consumption. It is also important to focus on specific food groups or items, since different foods rich in a specific fat subtype may have different effects on body weight [41].

The satiating effect of the MeDiet may explain some beneficial effects on body weight, especially in a longer term. Furthermore, evidence shows mono- and polyunsaturated fatty acids are more readily oxidized than saturated fatty acids and have a greater thermogenic effect, which can lead to reduced fat accumulation [42]. The quantity and quality of dietary fat have also been shown to induce differential lipid storage and processing gene expression, influencing adipokines release, but this process and regulation is still only partially understood [43]. Adherence to MeDiet may also be inversely correlated with proinflammatory biomarkers [44], and another potential important mechanism is the influence on adipose tissue metabolism and secretory functions [45].

The major strengths of the present research include its prospective design, large sample size, and repeated measurements of exposure, outcomes, and confounders over a long follow-up period. Due to comprehensive data records, most relevant confounders could be controlled for. Nevertheless, residual confounding is possible. Genetic determinants for instance may influence measures of obesity and were not available in the dataset [46]. Systematic error may be present due to the large proportion of obese individuals, known to have a tendency to underestimate their dietary intakes (in particular total energy intake) and overestimate physical activity; however, this error will probably be nondifferential [47]. Furthermore, well-known measurement errors as a result of methodological issues in the memory-based assessment of dietary factors and physical activity may bias the results. The study of waist circumference as a potential outcome measure was also considered and would shine light on the matter, but the risk of substantial measurement error, especially in overweight and obese participants [48], makes it worthy of special attention and more complex analyses are warranted, so we decided not to include it in this manuscript for the sake of simplicity. Both the FFQ and physical activity questionnaire have been validated, however [22,23,27,28]. Energy-adjusted intraclass correlation coefficients for MUFAs, PUFAs, and SFAs in four 3-day dietary records and the FFQ were 0.61, 0.60, and 0.75, respectively [22]. Analyses of trans fatty acids were considered. Intake of this fat subtype was very low in this study, however (0.47 ± 0.13 EN%); thus, these investigations may be more effective in a different population.

This study cannot fully demonstrate causality of the observed associations. Obesity and body weight may be susceptible to reverse causation in the sense that once their body changes, participants adjust their eating habits [49]. The use of a generalized estimating equation was chosen for all of the analyses. An alternative could have been multilevel mixed-effects models. Both GEE and mixed-effect methods are appropriate for longitudinal data as they account for within-subject correlations occurring as a result of repeated measurements, but GEE models are more flexible. For linear regression models with continuous outcomes, the random effects assumption is equivalent to an exchangeable correlation structure in GEE [50]. The sensitivity analyses confirmed this as estimates were very similar, though the outcomes of the mixed-effects models were more conservative with wider confidence intervals. Models assessing the effect of actual changes in diet on changes in weight may lead to more interpretable results and better conclusions [41].

Although a lot of effort was put into collecting complete data, missing data are unavoidable in longitudinal studies. Throughout the years, this problem has been well documented and a range of solutions have been proposed [29]. In this case, multiple imputation was used only for the GEE model with body weight as a continuous outcome, to verify that the results obtained by complete case analyses with covariate adjustment were indeed unbiased. Multiple imputation is flexible when it comes to assumptions regarding the randomness of the missing data, which makes it suitable for sensitivity analyses in the case of MNAR scenarios. Complete case analysis was used for further analyses as the results were similar and this method is less time-consuming, more transparent, and at least as efficient as multiple imputation [29].

The population of this study consisted of older participants at high risk of cardiovascular disease and (almost all) overweight or obese at baseline, which may affect the generalizability of the findings. The number of subjects was, however, very large, and subjects came from different social levels and geographical areas and biological mechanisms will be similar in other populations. Moreover, mean total fat intake represented 40.5% of the total energy intake in this study population, which is comparable to the intake observed in a pooled analysis of studies across Spain [51]. Mean intakes of fat subtypes were slightly more desirable than intakes measured previously in Spain: MUFA 20.2 in the present study versus 15.9 EN%, PUFA 6.5 versus 5.6 EN% and SFA 10.3 versus 12.0 EN%.

Lastly, body weight was a secondary outcome in the PREDIMED trial. Neither energy restriction nor increased physical activity were advised for any treatment arm, as the intervention was not designed with the intention of causing weight loss. It should also be noted that one diet does not fit all, and weight control strategies should be based on personal goals. The MeDiet could, however, be a useful method to achieve personal goals, due to its high palatability and satiating effects and, therefore, better adherence [46]. Integrating energy restriction and increased physical activity could further enhance weight loss and health benefits [38]. Currently, data are being collected for the PREDIMED-Plus trial, including an intensive lifestyle intervention program with an energy-restricted MeDiet, increased physical activity, and behavioral treatment.

5. Conclusions

In conclusion, this study provides evidence that increasing MUFA and PUFA intakes at the expense of SFA, proteins, and carbohydrate intakes may contribute to losing weight and reverse the state of obesity in an older and overweight/obese Spanish population. It could therefore be recommendable to encourage a high-quality, moderately high-fat eating pattern like the MeDiet, which means increasing the quality of dietary fat instead of restricting total fat intake in the prevention of obesity.

Author Contributions: Conceptualization, Y.B., A.G., and M.A.M.-G.; formal analysis, Y.B., A.G.; investigation, M.A.M.-G., J.S.-S., J.V.S., E.G.-G., M.F. (Miquel Fiol), R.E., J.M.S.-L., H.S., A.A.-G., L.S.-M., X.P., E.R., N.B.-T., J.I.G., M.F. (Montserrat Fitó), J.A.M.; writing—original draft preparation, Y.B., A.G.; writing—review and editing, all authors; visualization, Y.B., A.G.; supervision, A.G., M.A.M.-G., O.v.d.R.; project administration, M.A.M.-G., J.S.-S., R.E., E.R., M.F. (Montserrat Fitó); funding acquisition, M.A.M.-G., J.S.-S., J.V.S., E.G.-G., M.F. (Miquel Fiol), R.E., J.M.S.-L., H.S., A.A.-G., L.S.-M., X.P., E.R., N.B.-T., J.I.G., M.F. (Montserrat Fitó), J.A.M.

Acknowledgments: In this section you can acknowledge any support given which is not covered by the author contribution or funding sections. This may include administrative and technical support, or donations in kind (e.g., materials used for experiments).

References

1. World Health Organization. *Factsheet Obesity and Overweight. Fact sheet N°311*; World Health Organization: Geneva, Switzerland, 2012.
2. Ludwig, D.S. Lowering the bar on the low-fat diet. *JAMA* **2016**, *316*, 2087–2088. [CrossRef]
3. Field, A.E.; Willett, W.C.; Lissner, L.; Colditz, G.A. Dietary fat and weight gain among women in the Nurses' Health Study. *Obesity* **2007**, *15*, 967–976. [CrossRef]
4. Liu, X.; Li, Y.; Tobias, D.K.; Wang, D.D.; Manson, J.E.; Willett, W.C.; Hu, F.B. Changes in types of dietary fats influence long-term weight change in US women and men. *J. Nutr.* **2018**, *148*, 1821–1829. [CrossRef] [PubMed]
5. Mozaffarian, D.; Ludwig, D.S. The 2015 US Dietary Guidelines: Lifting the Ban on Total Dietary Fat. *JAMA* **2015**, *313*, 2421–2422. [CrossRef]
6. Ng, M.; Fleming, T.; Robinson, M.; Thomson, B.; Graetz, N.; Margono, C.; Mullany, E.C.; Biryukov, S.; Abbafati, C.; Abera, S.F.; et al. Global, regional, and national prevalence of overweight and obesity in children and adults during 1980–2013: A systematic analysis for the Global Burden of Disease Study 2013. *Lancet* **2014**, *384*, 766–781. [CrossRef]
7. FAO. *Fats and Fatty Acids in Human Nutrition*; Report of an Expert Consultation; FAO: Rome, Italy, 2010; Volume 91, pp. 1–166, ISBN 978-92-5-106733-8.
8. Schwab, U.; Lauritzen, L.; Tholstrup, T.; Haldorsson, T.I.; Riserus, U.; Uusitupa, M.; Becker, W. Effect of the amount and type of dietary fat on cardiometabolic risk factors and risk of developing type 2 diabetes, cardiovascular diseases, and cancer: A systematic review. *Food Nutr. Res.* **2014**, *58*, 25145. [CrossRef] [PubMed]
9. Ros, E.; Martínez-González, M.A.; Estruch, R.; Salas-Salvadó, J.; Fitó, M.; Martínez, J.A.; Corella, D. Mediterranean diet and cardiovascular health: Teachings of the PREDIMED study. *Adv. Nutr.* **2014**, *5*, 330S–336S. [CrossRef] [PubMed]
10. Sofi, F.; Abbate, R.; Gensini, G.F.; Casini, A. Accruing evidence on benefits of adherence to the Mediterranean diet on health: An updated systematic review and meta-analysis. *Am. J. Clin. Nutr.* **2010**, *92*, 1189–1196. [CrossRef] [PubMed]
11. Guasch-Ferré, M.; Babio, N.; Martínez-González, M.A.; Corella, D.; Ros, E.; Martín-Peláez, S.; Estruch, R.; Arós, F.; Gómez-Gracia, E.; Fiol, M.; et al. Dietary fat intake and risk of cardiovascular disease and all-cause mortality in a population at high risk of cardiovascular disease. *Am. J. Clin. Nutr.* **2015**, *102*, 1563–1573. [CrossRef] [PubMed]
12. Kastorini, C.M.; Milionis, H.J.; Esposito, K.; Giugliano, D.; Goudevenos, J.A.; Panagiotakos, D.B. The effect of Mediterranean diet on metabolic syndrome and its components: A meta-analysis of 50 studies and 534,906 individuals. *J. Am. Coll. Cardiol.* **2011**, *57*, 1299–1313. [CrossRef] [PubMed]
13. Esposito, K.; Kastorini, C.M.; Panagiotakos, D.B.; Giugliano, D. Mediterranean diet and weight loss: Meta-analysis of randomized controlled trials. *Metab. Syndr. Relat. Disord.* **2011**, *9*, 1–12. [CrossRef] [PubMed]
14. Mancini, J.G.; Filion, K.B.; Atallah, R.; Eisenberg, M.J. Systematic Review of the Mediterranean Diet for Long-Term Weight Loss. *Am. J. Med.* **2016**, *129*, 407–415.e4. [CrossRef]
15. Tobias, D.K.; Chen, M.; Manson, J.E.; Ludwig, D.S.; Willett, W.; Hu, F.B. Effect of low-fat diet interventions versus other diet interventions on long-term weight change in adults: A systematic review and meta-analysis. *Lancet Diabetes Endocrinol.* **2015**, *3*, 968–979. [CrossRef]
16. Fernández-Montero, A.; Bes-Rastrollo, M.; Barrio-López, M.T.; de la Fuente-Arrillaga, C.; Salas-Salvadó, J.; Moreno-Galarraga, L.; Martínez-González, M.A. Nut consumption and 5-y all-cause mortality in a Mediterranean cohort: The SUN project. *Nutrition* **2014**, *30*, 1022–1027. [CrossRef] [PubMed]
17. Martínez-González, M.A.; Bes-Rastrollo, M. Nut consumption, weight gain and obesity: Epidemiological evidence. *Nutr. Metab. Cardiovasc. Dis.* **2011**, *21* (Suppl. 1), S40–S45. [CrossRef]
18. Jackson, C.L.; Hu, F.B. Long-term associations of nut consumption with body weight and obesity. *Am. J. Clin. Nutr.* **2014** *100* (Suppl. 1), 408S–411S. [CrossRef]

19. Estruch, R.; Martínez-González, M.A.; Corella, D.; Salas-Salvadó, J.; Ruiz-Gutiérrez, V.; Covas, M.I.; Fiol, M.; Gómez-Gracia, E.; López-Sabater, M.C.; Vinyoles, E.; et al. Effects of a Mediterranean-style diet on cardiovascular risk factors: A randomized trial. *Ann. Intern. Med.* **2006**, *145*, 1–11. [CrossRef]
20. Martínez-González, M.A.; Corella, D.; Salas-Salvadó, J.; Ros, E.; Covas, M.I.; Fiol, M.; Wärnberg, J.; Arós, F.; Ruíz-Gutiérrez, V.; Lamuela-Raventós, R.M.; et al. Cohort profile: Design and methods of the PREDIMED study. *Int. J. Epidemiol.* **2012**, *41*, 377–385. [CrossRef]
21. Willett, W.C. Issues in analysis and presentation of dietary data. In *Nutritional Epidemiology*, 3rd ed.; Willett, W.C., Ed.; Oxford University Press: New York, NY, USA, 2012; pp. 321–346, ISBN 9780199754038.
22. Fernández-Ballart, J.D.; Piñol, J.L.; Zazpe, I.; Corella, D.; Carrasco, P.; Toledo, E.; Perez-Bauer, M.; Martínez-González, M.Á.; Salas-Salvadó, J.; Martín-Moreno, J.M. Relative validity of a semi-quantitative food-frequency questionnaire in an elderly Mediterranean population of Spain. *Br. J. Nutr.* **2010**, *103*, 1808–1816. [CrossRef]
23. Martin-Moreno, J.M.; Boyle, P.; Gorgojo, L.; Maisonneuve, P.; Fernandez-rodriguez, J.C.; Salvini, S.; Willett, W.C. Development and validation of a food frequency questionnaire in Spain. *Int. J. Epidemiol.* **1993**, *22*, 512–519. [CrossRef]
24. Moreiras, O.; Carbajal, A.; Cabrera, L.; Cuadrado, C. *Tablas de Composición de Alimentos*, 9th ed.; Pirámide: Madrid, Spain, 2005; ISBN 978-84-368-3947-0.
25. Hu, F.B.; Stampfer, M.J.; Manson, J.E.; Rimm, E.; Colditz, G.A.; Rosner, B.A.; Hennekens, C.H.; Willett, W.C. Dietary fat intake and the risk of coronary heart disease in women. *N. Engl. J. Med.* **1997**, *337*, 1491–1499. [CrossRef] [PubMed]
26. Wing, R.R.; Hill, J.O. Successful weight loss maintenance. *Annu. Rev. Nutr.* **2001**, *21*, 323–341. [CrossRef] [PubMed]
27. Elosua, R.; Marrugat, J.; Molina, L.; Pons, S.; Pujol, E. Validation of the Minnesota Leisure Time Physical Activity Questionnaire in Spanish men. The MARATHOM Investigators. *Am. J. Epidemiol.* **1994**, *139*, 1197–1209. [CrossRef] [PubMed]
28. Elosua, R.; Garcia, M.; Aguilar, A.; Molina, L.; Covas, M.I.; Marrugat, J. Validation of the Minnesota Leisure Time Physical Activity Questionnaire in Spanish Women. Investigators of the MARATDON Group. *Med. Sci. Sports Exerc.* **2000**, *32*, 1431–1437. [CrossRef] [PubMed]
29. Groenwold, R.H.; Donders, A.R.; Roes, K.C.; Harrell, F.E.; Moons, K.G. Dealing with missing outcome data in randomized trials and observational studies. *Am. J. Epidemiol.* **2012**, *175*, 210–217. [CrossRef]
30. DiNicolantonio, J.J.; O'Keefe, J.H. Good Fats versus Bad Fats: A Comparison of Fatty Acids in the Promotion of Insulin Resistance, Inflammation, and Obesity. *Mo. Med.* **2017**, *114*, 303–307.
31. Hannon, B.A.; Thompson, S.V.; An, R.; Teran-Garcia, M. Clinical Outcomes of Dietary Replacement of Saturated Fatty Acids with Unsaturated Fat Sources in Adults with Overweight and Obesity: A Systematic Review and Meta-Analysis of Randomized Control Trials. *Ann. Nutr. Metab.* **2017**, *71*, 107–117. [CrossRef]
32. González, C.A.; Pera, G.; Quirós, J.R.; Lasheras, C.; Tormo, M.J.; Rodriguez, M.; Navarro, C.; Martinez, C.; Dorronsoro, M.; Chirlaque, M.D.; et al. Types of fat intake and body mass index in a Mediterranean country. *Public Health Nutr.* **2000**, *3*, 329–336. [CrossRef]
33. Romaguera, D.; Norat, T.; Vergnaud, A.C.; Mouw, T.; May, A.M.; Agudo, A.; Buckland, G.; Slimani, N.; Rinaldi, S.; Couto, E.; et al. Mediterranean dietary patterns and prospective weight change in participants of the EPIC-PANACEA project. *Am. J. Clin. Nutr.* **2010**, *92*, 912–921. [CrossRef]
34. Estruch, R.; Martínez-González, M.A.; Corella, D.; Salas-Salvadó, J.; Fitó, M.; Chiva-Blanch, G.; Fiol, M.; Gómez-Gracia, E.; Arós, F.; Lapetra, J.; et al. Effect of a high-fat Mediterranean diet on bodyweight and waist circumference: A prespecified secondary outcome analysis of the PREDIMED randomised controlled trial. *Lancet Diabetes Endocrinol.* **2016**, *4*, 666–676. [CrossRef]
35. Babio, N.; Toledo, E.; Estruch, R.; Ros, E.; Martínez-González, M.A.; Castañer, O.; Bulló, M.; Corella, D.; Arós, F.; Gómez-Gracia, E.; et al. Mediterranean diets and metabolic syndrome status in the PREDIMED randomized trial. *CMAJ* **2014**, *186*, E649–E657. [CrossRef] [PubMed]
36. Babio, N.; Becerra-Tomás, N.; Martínez-González, M.; Corella, D.; Estruch, R.; Ros, E.; Sayón-Orea, C.; Fitó, M.; Serra-Majem, L.; Arós, F.; et al. Consumption of Yogurt, Low-Fat Milk, and Other Low-Fat Dairy Products Is Associated with Lower Risk of Metabolic Syndrome Incidence in an Elderly Mediterranean Population. *J. Nutr.* **2015** *145*, 2308–2316. [CrossRef] [PubMed]

37. Guasch-Ferré, M.; Bulló, M.; Martínez-González, M.A.; Ros, E.; Corella, D.; Estruch, R.; Fitó, M.; Arós, F.; Wärnberg, J.; Fiol, M.; et al. Frequency of nut consumption and mortality risk in the PREDIMED nutrition intervention trial. *BMC Med.* **2013**, *11*, 164. [CrossRef]
38. Flores-Mateo, G.; Rojas-Rueda, D.; Basora, J.; Ros, E.; Salas-Salvadó, J. Nut intake and adiposity: Meta-analysis of clinical trials. *Am. J. Clin. Nutr.* **2013**, *97*, 1346–1355. [CrossRef] [PubMed]
39. Serra-Majem, L.; Bes-Rastrollo, M.; Román-Viñas, B.; Pfrimer, K.; Sánchez-Villegas, A.; Martínez-González, M.A. Dietary patterns and nutritional adequacy in a Mediterranean country. *Br. J. Nutr.* **2009**, *101* (Suppl. 2), S21–S28. [CrossRef] [PubMed]
40. Sánchez-Tainta, A.; Zazpe, I.; Bes-Rastrollo, M.; Salas-Salvadó, J.; Bullo, M.; Sorlí, J.V.; Corella, D.; Covas, M.I.; Arós, F.; Gutierrez-Bedmar, M.; et al. Nutritional adequacy according to carbohydrates and fat quality. *Eur. J. Nutr.* **2016**, *55*, 93–106. [CrossRef]
41. Smith, J.D.; Hou, T.; Ludwig, D.S.; Rimm, E.B.; Willett, W.; Hu, F.B.; Mozaffarian, D. Changes in intake of protein foods, carbohydrate amount and quality, and long-term weight change: Results from 3 prospective cohorts. *Am. J. Clin. Nutr.* **2015**, *101*, 1216–1224. [CrossRef]
42. Casas-Agustench, P.; López-Uriarte, P.; Bulló, M.; Ros, E.; Gómez-Flores, A.; Salas-Salvadó, J. Acute effects of three high-fat meals with different fat saturations on energy expenditure, substrate oxidation and satiety. *Clin. Nutr.* **2009**, *28*, 39–45. [CrossRef]
43. Camargo, A.; Meneses, M.E.; Perez-Martinez, P.; Delgado-Lista, J.; Jimenez-Gomez, Y.; Cruz-Teno, C.; Tinahones, F.J.; Paniagua, J.A.; Perez-Jimenez, F.; Roche, H.M.; et al. Dietary fat differentially influences the lipids storage on the adipose tissue in metabolic syndrome patients. *Eur. J. Nutr.* **2014**, *53*, 617–626. [CrossRef]
44. Hermsdorff, H.H.; Zulet, M.Á.; Abete, I.; Martínez, J.A. Discriminated benefits of a Mediterranean dietary pattern within a hypocaloric diet program on plasma RBP4 concentrations and other inflammatory markers in obese subjects. *Endocrine* **2009**, *36*, 445–451. [CrossRef]
45. Martínez-Fernández, L.; Laiglesia, L.M.; Huerta, A.E.; Martínez, J.A.; Moreno-Aliaga, M.J. Omega-3 fatty acids and adipose tissue function in obesity and metabolic syndrome. *Prostaglandins Other Lipid Mediat.* **2015**, *121*, 24–41. [CrossRef] [PubMed]
46. Phillips, C.M.; Kesse-Guyot, E.; McManus, R.; Hercberg, S.; Lairon, D.; Planells, R.; Roche, H.M. High dietary saturated fat intake accentuates obesity risk associated with the fat mass and obesity-associated gene in adults. *J. Nutr.* **2012**, *142*, 824–831. [CrossRef] [PubMed]
47. Wehling, H.; Lusher, J. People with a body mass index $\geq$30 under-report their dietary intake: A systematic review. *J. Health Psychol.* **2017**. [CrossRef] [PubMed]
48. Verweij, L.M.; Terwee, C.B.; Proper, K.I.; Hulshof, C.T.; van Mechelen, W. Measurement error of waist circumference: Gaps in knowledge. *Public Health Nutr.* **2013**, *16*, 281–288. [CrossRef] [PubMed]
49. Hu, F.B. *Obesity Epidemiology*; Oxford University Press: New York, NY, USA, 2008.
50. Vittinghoff, E.; Glidden, D.V.; Shiboski, S.C.; McCulloch, C.E. *Regression Methods in Biostatistics: Linear, Logistic, Survival, and Repeated Measures Models*, 2nd ed.; Springer: Boston, MA, USA, 2012; ISBN 978-1-4614-1352-3.
51. Harika, R.K.; Eilander, A.; Alssema, M.; Osendarp, S.J.; Zock, P.L. Intake of fatty acids in general populations worldwide does not meet dietary recommendations to prevent coronary heart disease: A systematic review of data from 40 countries. *Ann. Nutr. Metab.* **2013**, *63*, 229–238. [CrossRef] [PubMed]

15

Possible Role of CYP450 Generated Omega-3/Omega-6 PUFA Metabolites in the Modulation of Blood Pressure and Vascular Function in Obese Children

Sara Bonafini [1], Alice Giontella [1], Angela Tagetti [1], Denise Marcon [1], Martina Montagnana [2], Marco Benati [2], Rossella Gaudino [3], Paolo Cavarzere [3], Mirjam Karber [4], Michael Rothe [5], Pietro Minuz [1], Franco Antoniazzi [3], Claudio Maffeis [3], Wolf Hagen Schunck [6] and Cristiano Fava [1,*]

1 Department of Medicine, University of Verona, 37129 Verona, Italy; bonafinisara@gmail.com (S.B.); alice.giontella@gmail.com (A.G.); angela.tagetti@libero.it (A.T.); denise.m@hotmail.com (D.M.); pietro.minuz@univr.it (P.M.)
2 Department of Neurosciences, Biomedicine and Movement Sciences, University of Verona, 37129 Verona, Italy; martina.montagnana@univr.it (M.M.); marco.benati@univr.it (M.B.)
3 Department of Surgery, Dentistry, Paediatrics and Gynaecology, University of Verona, 37129 Verona, Italy; rossella.gaudino@univr.it (R.G.); paolo.cavarzere@ospedaleuniverona.it (P.C.); franco.antoniazzi@univr.it (F.A.); claudio.maffeis@univr.it (C.M.)
4 Berlin Institute of Health (BIH), 10178 Berlin, Germany; mirjam.karber@charite.de
5 Lipidomix, 13125 Berlin, Germany; michael.rothe@lipidomix.de
6 Max Delbrueck Center for Molecular Medicine, 13092 Berlin, Germany; schunck@mdc-berlin.de
* Correspondence: cristiano.fava@univr.it

Abstract: Obesity is often accompanied by metabolic and haemodynamic disorders such as hypertension, even during childhood. Arachidonic acid (AA) is metabolized by cytochrome P450 (CYP450) enzymes to epoxyeicosatrienoic acids (EETs) and 20-hydroxyeicosatetraenoic acid (20-HETE), vasoactive and natriuretic metabolites that contribute to blood pressure (BP) regulation. Eicosapentaenoic acid (EPA) and docosahexaenoic acid (DHA) omega-3 polyunsaturated fatty acids may compete with AA for CYP450-dependent bioactive lipid mediator formation. We aimed at investigating the role of AA, EPA and DHA and their CYP450-dependent metabolites in BP control and vascular function in 66 overweight/obese children. Fatty acid profile moderately correlated with the corresponding CYP450-derived metabolites but their levels did not differ between children with normal BP (NBP) and high BP (HBP), except for higher EPA-derived epoxyeicosatetraenoic acids (EEQs) and their diols in HBP group, in which also the estimated CYP450-epoxygenase activity was higher. In the HBP group, EPA inversely correlated with BP, EEQs inversely correlated both with systolic BP and carotid Intima-Media Thickness (cIMT). The DHA-derived epoxydocosapentaenoic acids (EDPs) were inversely correlated with diastolic BP. Omega-3 derived epoxymetabolites appeared beneficially associated with BP and vascular structure/function only in obese children with HBP. Further investigations are needed to clarify the role of omega-3/omega-6 epoxymetabolites in children's hemodynamics.

Keywords: CYP450 eicosanoids; omega-3 PUFA; omega-6 PUFA; blood pressure; hemodynamics; children; EETs; EEQs

---

1. Introduction

The prevalence of overweight and obesity in children and adolescents has been increasing in the last few decades worldwide. Childhood obesity can have serious short- and long-term consequences, including metabolic and hemodynamic complications, such as hypertension, insulin resistance and dyslipidaemia [1].

Beside the impact of body mass index (BMI) per se on blood pressure (BP), several mechanisms are implicated in hemodynamic control. Dietary habits, in particular, lipid intake can influence not only body weight but also haemodynamics [2,3]. Indeed, in the last years many studies assessed the role of different polyunsaturated fatty acids (PUFA), such as arachidonic acid (AA), an omega-6 PUFA and eicosapentaenoic acid (EPA) and docosahexaenoic acid (DHA), which belong to omega-3 PUFA family, indicating a beneficial cardiovascular effect of omega-3 PUFA [4,5], whereas it is not clear whether omega-6 PUFA are cardioprotective or not [6,7]. Several trials and meta-analyses indicated a possible beneficial effect of omega-3 PUFA supplementation on BP control, although the effect is modest, and the results of the studies are not always consistent [5,8,9]. Furthermore, omega-3 PUFA may improve vascular function, that is, arterial stiffness and endothelial function, as supported by some studies and meta-analysis [10–12], suggesting a possible, at least partial, BP lowering effect of omega-3 PUFA. We have recently shown, in the same study population, that omega-6 PUFA and in particular AA are inversely associated with several features of the metabolic syndrome in a sample of obese children, suggesting their possible protective role [13].

AA, EPA and DHA can be metabolized via cytochrome P-450 (CYP450) into lipid mediators, which can have profound effects on blood pressure control [2,14], AA can be metabolized by different CYP450 enzymes leading to the formation of several compounds: 5,6-, 8,9-, 11,12-, 14,15-epoxyeicosatrienoic acids (EETs) via epoxygenase and for example, 20-hydroxyeicosatetraenoic acid (20-HETE) via hydroxylases. In general, EETs have been shown to play a protective role in cardiovascular diseases through their anti-inflammatory, vasodilating and sodium excreting effects [15,16]. They are further metabolized by soluble epoxide hydrolase (sEH) to dihydroxyeicosatrienoic acids (DHETs), which are less potent or even inactive compounds. Instead, 20-HETE exerts a natriuretic action at kidney level, but, in the systemic vasculature, it induces vasoconstriction [17,18]. Linoleic acid (LA) is also metabolized by CYP450 epoxygenase to 9,10- and 12,13-epoxyoctadecenoic acids (EpOMEs), which are converted by sEH to 9,10- and 12,13-dihydroxyoctadecenoic acids (DiHOMEs). They have potential toxic cardiovascular effects, probably mediated by mitochondrial dysfunction and may affect the cardiac inotropic response but the evidences are rare and diverging [19,20]. Epoxyeicosatetraenoic acids (EEQs), yielded from EPA, have vasodilating and anti-inflammatory properties and are further metabolized by sEH to diydroxxyeicosatetraenoic acids (DiHETEs) [21–23]. Epoxydocosapentaenoic acids (EDPs), derived from DHA via CYP-epoxygenase, are potent vasodilators [23]; they are hydrolysed by sEH to dihydroxydocosapentaenoic acids (DiHDPAs). Preliminary studies in animal models have shown that the epoxymetabolites derived from EPA and DHA have a vasodilating action that largely exceeds that of the AA-derived epoxides [24,25]. EPA and DHA can also be metabolized by CYP-hydroxylase producing for example, 20-hydroxyeicosapentaenoic acid (20-HEPE) and 22-hydroxydocosahexaenoic acid (22-HDHA) respectively, whose biological activities are still largely unknown.

Thus, the aim of the present study was to evaluate the possible association between the omega-3 and omega-6 PUFA metabolites via CYP450-epoxygenase/sEH in the modulation of haemodynamic parameters and especially BP, in a sample of overweight/obese children.

2. Materials and Methods

2.1. Patients and Study Design

Obese children were recruited consequently from October 2012 to September 2014, coming from the "Paediatric Obesity Outpatients Unit" of the University Hospital of Verona and of the "Local Health Unit n. 20" of Verona. Inclusion criteria were: children and adolescents aged 5–18 years; overweight or obesity (BMI $\geq$ 85th and 95th percentile for sex and age, respectively). We excluded children with hepatic or renal chronic diseases, malignancies, diabetes mellitus, lipid-lowering or antihypertensive therapy, secondary causes of obesity.

The study was conducted according to a cross-sectional observational design.

The study was approved by the Ethical Committee of the University Hospital of Verona (CE n. 2218) and written informed consent was obtained from each participant's parents.

2.2. Anthropometric, Blood Pressure and Vascular Assessments

Each child was evaluated in a single occasion, between 8:00 and 9:00 a.m. A questionnaire was administered to patients and to their parents, dealing with medical history, family history, physiological and pathological information and use of drugs. Then, the participants underwent a physical examination. They were advised not to engage in strenuous exercise and to avoid consuming caffeine containing beverages within 12 h preceding the vascular studies.

During the visit, blood pressure was measured with a semiautomatic oscillometric device (TM-2551, A&D instruments Ltd., Abingdon Oxford, UK) 3 times, 3 min apart with the patient lying supine for at least 10 min before the first measurement in a room with controlled temperature (22–24 °C). The mean value of the 3 clinostatic measurements were calculated and considered for z-score and percentile calculation. Afterward, BP levels were confirmed by a measurement in the sitting position by the oscillometric device and by auscultatory method. Ambulatory blood pressure measurement (ABPM) was recorded with an oscillometric device (Spacelabs 90217; Spacelabs Inc., Issaquah, WA, USA), which measured BP every 15 min during the day and ever 30 min during the night. Children and parents recorded physical activities, resting and sleeping time and symptoms on a dedicated diary. After recording, the daytime and night-time periods (set to default at 7:00 A.M. and 10:00 P.M., respectively) were adapted to "real" awake and sleep times according to what was declared in the activity diary.

All values derived from BP measurements were transformed in z-score and percentile, according to normative values [26–28]. The 95th of office and ambulatory BP measurements was used as cut-off for hypertension, according to current European guidelines [27].

Body weight, height and waist and hip circumferences were measured with the patient wearing light clothes. Body weight was measured by a calibrated balance and height by a calibrated stadiometer.

Body mass index (BMI) calculated as weight in kg divided by the square of height in m; waist/hip ratio was calculated as waist circumference in cm divided by hip circumference in cm and waist/height ratio (WHtR) was calculated as waist circumference in cm divided by height in cm.

Waist circumference was transformed in z-score and percentile according to normative values [29]. Overweight or obesity were defined for BMI $\geq$ 90th and 95th percentile for sex and age, respectively [30]. WHO reference for BMI was used for categorizing children into the overweight and obese groups [31].

Carotid Intima-media Thickness (cIMT) was assessed by ultrasound of carotid arteries (LogiQ P5 Pro) and the cIMT was estimated tracking the artery wall in the last centimetre of the common carotid artery and calculated by a dedicated software (Multimedia Video Engine II (MVE2) DSP Lab., Pisa CNR, Italy). The relative z-score and percentile were calculated according to reference values [32].

Endothelial function was assessed by ultrasound of the brachial artery using the Flow Mediated Dilatation (FMD) technique according to international guidelines and with the aid of a dedicated hardware (Multimedia Video Engine II (MVE2) DSP Lab., Pisa CNR, Italy) [33]. Common carotid artery distensibility (DC) was calculated as: $DC = \Delta A/(A \times \Delta P)$ where A is the diastolic lumen area, ΔA is the stroke change in lumen area and ΔP is pulse pressure (PP). Changes in diameters were detected using ultrasound B-mode image sequences of the right and left common carotid arteries acquired at different steps and analysed by the above-mentioned automatic system [34]. The relative z-score and percentile were calculated according to reference values [32].

2.3. CYP-Derived Eicosanoids Measurement

Plasma samples were subjected to alkaline hydrolysis and subsequent solid phase extraction was performed as described previously [35].

In brief, 500 μL Methanol, 300 μL 10 molar sodium hydroxide and deuterated internal standards were added to 500 μL Plasma. The samples were hydrolysed for 30 min at 60 °C. The solution containing free fatty acids and metabolites were neutralized with acetic acid and adjusted to pH = 6.2.

A solid phase extraction procedure using Agilent Bond-Elut-Certify II was performed as formerly described by Rivera [36].

The LC-ESI-MS/MS method for determination of metabolites was performed by the Lipidomix GmbH, Berlin Germany, as described previously [35]. The plasma levels of individual metabolites are given in ng/mL.

Moreover, biomarkers reflecting the endogenous CYP450 epoxygenase and sEH activities were estimated by calculating the sum of epoxymetabolites plus their corresponding diols or the ratio between diols and epoxymetabolites.

2.4. Red Blood Cell Membrane Fatty Acids Measurement

EDTA-blood tubes were centrifuged, plasma and buffy coat taken off and erythrocytes frozen at −80 °C until analysis. Erythrocyte fatty acid composition was analysed using the HS-Omega-3 Index® methodology as previously described [37,38]. Fatty acid methyl esters were generated from erythrocytes by acid transesterification and analysed by gas chromatography using a GC2010 Gas Chromatograph (Shimadzu, Duisburg, Germany) equipped with a SP2560, 100-m column (Supelco, Bellefonte, PA, USA) using hydrogen as carrier gas. Fatty acids were identified by comparison with a standard mixture of fatty acids characteristic of erythrocytes. A total of 26 fatty acids were identified and quantified.

Results are given as percentage of total identified fatty acids after response factor correction. The coefficient of variation for EPA plus DHA and for most other fatty acids was 4%. Analyses were quality-controlled according to DIN ISO 15189. All fatty acid determinations were performed by Omegametrix GmbH, Munich, Germany.

2.5. Statistics

Data are presented as the median and range unless otherwise stated. The statistical analysis was performed using the software Statistical Package for Social Sciences software (SPSS/PC for Windows version 21.0; IBM, Armonk, New York, NY, USA). Bivariate nonparametric correlations were estimated by Spearman coefficient (r_S).

Differences in the measured parameters between normotensive and hypertensive children were analysed by nonparametric (Wilcoxon-Mann-Witney U) tests. A two-tailed test with a $p < 0.05$ was considered statistically significant. In order to take into account the multiple comparisons, along with original p-values, the false discovery rate (FDR) adjusted *p*-values were also calculated and reported in the tables, where appropriate.

3. Results

3.1. Patient Characteristics

From the whole study consisting of 72 children we included 66 children (females *n*: 28; 42%) with full phenotypic data about eicosanoids, red blood cell membrane FA, ABPM and vascular tests in the present study.

The collection lasted from October 2012 to October 2014 and included children are 5 to 17 years old. Four children were overweight (BMI > 90th) and 62 children were obese (BMI > 95th percentile for sex and age). All children had a central distribution of adiposity (percentile of waist circumference >90th percentile).

On the basis of ABPM, we divided the population in two subgroups: high blood pressure (HBP) (*n*: 17; 26%) and normal blood pressure (NBP) (*n*: 49; 74%). In an exploratory analysis we investigated the correlations of fatty acids and their metabolites with BP and vascular function in each subgroup, in order to check different associations related to the hypertensive status.

General characteristics of the obese children split by gender and NBP and HBP, diagnosed on the basis of ABPM (daytime, night-time or 24-hours systolic BP(SBP) or diastolic BP (DBP) ≥ 95th percentile), are detailed in Table 1. The characteristics of the children divided according to pubertal status are listed in Table S1.

Table 1. General characteristics of the population divided according to gender and blood pressure status.

	Male (*n* = 38)	Female (*n* = 28)		NBP (*n* = 49)	HBP (*n* = 17)	
Variable	**Median (Range)**	**Median (Range)**	***p*-Value ***	**Median (Range)**	**Median (Range)**	***p*-Value ***
Age, years	11.5 (10.0–14.0)	11.0 (9.0–13.0)	0.187	12.0 (10.0–13.5)	11.0 (8.5–12.5)	0.181
BMI, Kg/m^2	28.3 (25.4–31.0)	29.3 (26.1–33.2)	0.392	28.4 (25.7–31.0)	30.4 (26.7–35.3)	0.125
BMI percentile	98.3 (97.2–99.0)	98.7 (97.8–99.3)	0.238	98.0 (97.3–99.0)	99.1 (98.3–99.5)	0.011
Office-SBP, mmHg	119.0 (112.9–125)	116.3 (109.8–129)	0.471	117.0 (110.2–110.2)	123.3 (114.5–133.2)	0.031
Office-SBP percentile	83.1 (64.9–94.8)	79.9 (67.7–96.4)	0.697	77.7 (64.7–93.7)	95.6 (76.7–99.3)	0.012
Office-DBP, mmHg	68.3 (63.3–76.1)	66.7 (64.1–72.7)	0.673	66.7 (63.7–72)	75.0 (63.7–77.3)	0.179
Office-DBP percentile	65.1 (43.9–80.7)	66.1 (50.8–77.9)	0.577	64.3 (46.9–76.2)	83.0 (51.4–87.2)	0.033
24 h-SBP, mmHg	118.0 (114–121)	112.0 (107–116)	0.001 °	114.0 (109–118)	121.0 (118.5–128.0)	<0.001 °
24 h-SBP, percentile	73.7 (50.6–82.6)	54.4 (35.3–79.8)	0.169	51.7 (37.8–74.6)	90.4 (80.0–98.8)	<0.001 °
24 h-DBP, mmHg	68.0 (64.0–70.3)	64.0 (61.3–67.0)	0.001 °	65.0 (62.0–68.5)	70.0 (65.5–74.5)	0.002 °
24 h-DBP, percentile	57.4 (28.5–74.5)	34.5 (18.7–50.6)	0.007	35.1 (20.0–57.4)	69.9 (42.5–94.5)	0.001 °
cIMT, mm	0.46 (0.42–0.51)	0.41 (0.39–0.47)	0.032	0.44 (0.40–0.48)	0.46 (0.42–0.51)	0.179
cIMT, percentile	98.4 (80.3–99.7)	82.3 (60.4–96.7)	0.021	88.2 (59.6–99.1)	96.5 (82.2–99.7)	0.207
cDC, 10^{-3}/Kpa	39.7 (33.5–46.4)	43.8 (34.9–48.3)	0.199	42.0 (34.7–48.5)	37.3 (33.0–42.5)	0.127
cDC, percentile	6.4 (2.4–23.2)	12.8 (2.2–27.0)	0.249	12.3 (2.9–27.0)	4.2 (2.2–13.2)	0.110
Glucose, mg/dL	88.0 (84.0–93.0)	85.0 (79.0–88.0)	0.026	86.0 (83–90)	87.0 (82–93.8)	0.855
Insulin, uU/mL	18.5 (12.4–27.5)	17.8 (13.0–28.2)	0.887	17.7 (11.8–27.6)	24.1 (17.1–30.0)	0.110
Cholesterol, mg/dL	160 (139.9–186.8)	165.0 (134–192)	0.536	165.0 (139–192)	151.5 (132–173.3)	0.297
Triglycerides, mg/dL	79 (55–103.5)	79 (54–100)	0.744	76.5 (54–99.8)	87 (59.5–118)	0.231
FMD, %	7.7 (5.3–10.2)	6.2 (3.4–9.6)	0.403	7.4 (4.2–10.2)	7.6 (3.2–9.8)	0.682
LA, %	11.8 (11.1–12.9)	11.8 (11.1–12.8)	0.841	11.7 (11.0–12.6)	12.4 (11.4–13.1)	0.104
AA, %	16.0 (14.9–17.1)	16.4 (15.8–17.3)	0.082	16.4 (15.6–17.5)	15.5 (14.6–16.6)	0.038
EPA, %	0.4 (0.3–0.5)	0.4 (0.3–0.5)	0.340	0.37 (0.30–0.47)	0.4 (0.3–0.6)	0.127
DHA, %	4.3 (3.8–4.7)	4.4 (3.8–5.0)	0.425	4.4 (3.8–4.8)	4.2 (3.5–4.8)	0.367
Omega-3 Index, %	4.6 (4.1–5.2)	4.6 (4.3–5.5)	0.417	4.6 (4.2–5.3)	4.5 (3.9–5.3)	0.639
EpOMEs, ng/mL	11.2 (8.2–15.9)	10.8 (8.7–15.7)	0.907	11.5 (8.4–15.9)	10.8 (8.3–12.4)	0.613
DiHOMEs, ng/mL	7.2 (5.3–9.7)	6.3 (5.3–8.8)	0.340	6.5 (5.3–9.2)	7.5 (5.6–9.6)	0.363
EpOMEs/DiHOMEs	1.6 (0.9–2.1)	1.6 (1.3–2.4)	0.347	1.7 (1.3–2.3)	1.2 (0.8–1.9)	0.093
EpOMEs+DiHOME	18.6 (14.0–25.7)	18.4 (15.3–22.2)	0.795	19.4 (14.8–23.7)	17.0 (13.4–24.2)	0.634
EETs, ng/mL	7.4 (6.6–8.9)	7.7 (6.8–8.9)	0.460	7.5 (6.6–8.5)	8.4 (7.2–9.2)	0.131
DHETs, ng/mL	4.1 (3.3–4.7)	4.0 (3.5–4.7)	0.726	4.0 (3.4–4.5)	4.0 (3.5–5.1)	0.367
EETs/DHETs	1.9 (1.6–2.4)	2.0 (1.6–1.2)	0.902	1.9 (1.6–2.3)	2.0 (1.6–2.2)	0.814
EETs+DHETs	11.7 (10.1–13.3)	12.1 (10.7–13.2)	0.448	11.8 (10.2–13.0)	12.7 (10.8–14.3)	0.110
EEQs, ng/mL	0.3 (0.2–0.4)	0.4 (0.3–0.5)	0.302	0.3 (0.2–0.5)	0.4 (0.3–0.7)	0.047
DiHETEs, ng/mL	0.9 (0.7–1.3)	0.9 (0.7–1.3)	0.568	0.9 (0.7–1.1)	1.2 (0.9–1.6)	0.021
EEQs/DiHETEs	0.33 (0.31–0.38)	0.42 (0.33–0.54)	0.004 °	0.37 (0.31–0.46)	0.34 (0.31–0.51)	0.872
EEQs+DiHETEs	1.3 (1.0–1.8)	1.3 (0.9–1.8)	0.871	1.2 (1.0–1.5)	1.8 (1.2–2.2)	0.025
EDPs, ng/mL	2.9 (2.4–3.3)	3.2 (2.7–4.2)	0.050	2.9 (2.4–3.3)	3.3 (2.5–3.9)	0.221
DiHDPAs, ng/mL	0.9 (0.8–1.0)	0.9 (0.8–1.1)	0.399	0.9 (0.8–1.1)	0.9 (0.8–1.1)	0.665
EDPs/DiHDPAs	3.3 (2.9–3.6)	3.6 (2.8–4.3)	0.186	3.4 (2.8–3.8)	3.2 (3.0–4.2)	0.878
EDPs+DiHDPAs	3.8 (3.1–4.3)	4.3 (3.5–5.3)	0.044	3.8 (3.3–4.4)	4.3 (3.3–4.9)	0.238
20-HETE	0.74 (0.61–0.86)	0.64 (0.57–0.87)	0.459	0.7 (0.58–0.84)	0.83 (0.53–0.91)	0.553
22-HDHA	0.65 (0.44–0.92)	0.66 (0.41–0.83)	0.721	0.67 (0.42–0.89)	0.64 (0.43–0.91)	0.837

BMI: body mass index, SBP: systolic blood pressure, DBP: diastolic blood pressure, cIMT: carotid intima-media thickness, cDC: carotid distensibility coefficient, FMD: flow-mediated dilation, LA: Linoleic acid, AA: Arachidonic acid, EPA: Eicosapentaenoic acid, DHA: Docosahexaenoic acid, Omega-3 Index: (EPA + DHA)/total FA × 100, EpOME: epoxyoctadecenoic acid, DiHOME: dihydroxyoctadecenoic acid, EET: epoxyeicosatrienoic acid, DHET: dihydroxyeicosatrienoic acid, EEQ: epoxyeicosatetraenoic acid, DiHETE: dihydroxyeicosatetraenoic acid, EDP: epoxydocosapentaenoic acid, DiHDPA: dihydroxydocosapentaenoic acid, 20-HETE: 20-hydroxyeicosatetraenoic acid, 22-HDHA: 22-hydroxydocosahexaenoic acid, HBP: high blood pressure subgroup, NBP: normal blood pressure subgroup, *n*: number. 20-hydroxyeicosapentaenoic acid (20-HEPE) plasma concentration was under the limit of detection. *: Mann-Whitney *U*-Test; °: $p < 0.05$ after False Discovery Rate correction.

Girls showed higher BP at ABPM compared to boys. Omega-3 Index, a marker of dietary intake of long-chain omega-3 PUFA, was 4.61% (2.87–6.61%).

3.2. *Omega-6 PUFA*

3.2.1. LA and CYP450-Derived Eicosanoids

Associations of LA with Clinical Features and with its Metabolites

LA was similarly distributed according to gender and hypertensive status (Table 1 and Figure 1). LA directly correlated with DiHOMEs in the whole population and in particular in HBP children (Table 2 and Figure 2). LA also directly correlates with the estimated CYP450 epoxygenase activity in HBP (Figure S1).

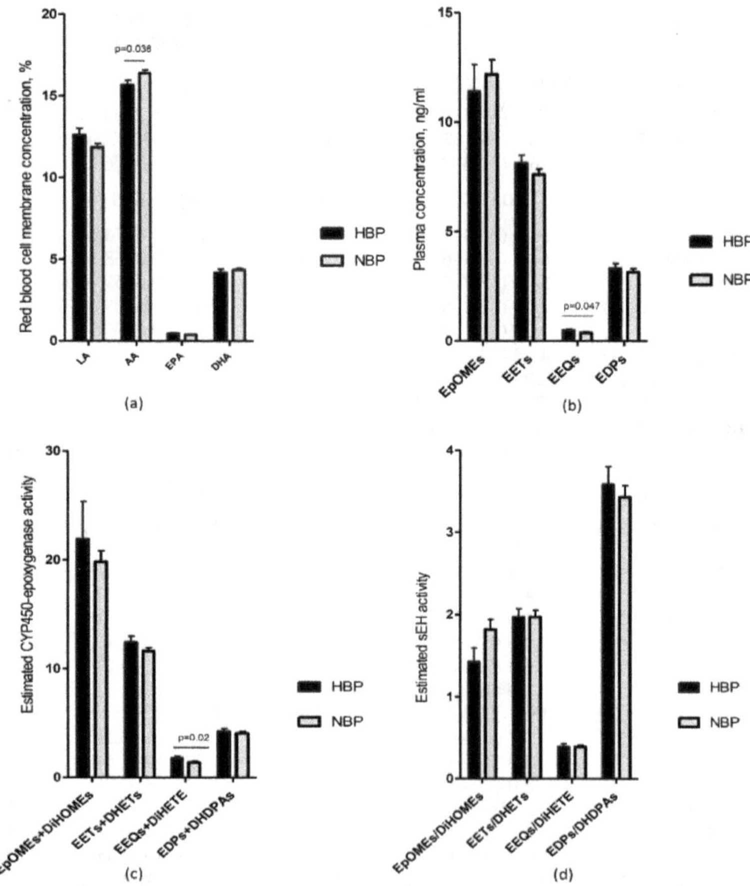

Figure 1. Comparison of fatty acids and their metabolites via CYP450-epoxygenase in HBP and NBP obese children. The histograms represent the comparison between HBP and NBP obese children for: (**a**) concentration of fatty acids in red blood cell membranes, that is, LA, AA, EPA and DHA; (**b**) plasma concentration of the CYP450 epoxygenase generated metabolites, that is, EpOMEs, EETs, EEQs and EDPs; (**c**) the estimated CYP450 epoxygenase activity, calculated as the sum of epoxymetabolites plus their corresponding diols; (**d**) the estimated sEH activity, calculated as the ratio between plasma concentrations (ng/mL) of diols and epoxymetabolites. Data are presented as mean and SEM. LA: Linoleic acid; AA: Arachidonic acid; EPA: Eicosapentaenoic acid; DHA: Docosahexaenoic acid; EpOME: epoxyoctadecenoic acid; DiHOME: dihydroxyoctadecenoic acid; EET: epoxyeicosatrienoic acid; DHET: dihydroxyeicosatrienoic acid; EEQ: epoxyeicosatetraenoic acid; DiHETE: dihydroxyeicosatetraenoic acid; EDP: epoxydocosapentaenoic acid; DiHDPA: dihydroxydocosapentaenoic acid; HBP: high blood pressure subgroup; NBP: normal blood pressure subgroup; sEH: soluble epoxide hydrolase; *p*: *p*-value. Vertical lines represent the standard errors.

Table 2. Correlations between fatty acids (precursors) and the derived eicosanoids via CYP450-epoxygenase/sEH.

	Whole Population	NBP	HBP
	LA		
9,10-EpOME	0.102	0.064	0.434
12,13-EpOME	0.094	0.063	0.465
9,10-DiHOME	0.438 ^	0.311 *	0.674 ^
12,13-DiHOME	0.336 ^	0.265	0.659 ^
EpOME/DiHOME	−0.292 *	−0.172	−0.424
EpOME+DiHOME	0.292 *	0.234	0.718 ^
	AA		
5,6-EET	0.029	0.152	−0.049
8,9-EET	0.061	0.162	−0.064
11,12-EET	0.049	0.096	0.177
14,15-EET	0.040	0.114	0.074
5,6-DHET	0.032	0.196	−0.251
8,9-DHET	0.105	0.201	−0.051
11,12-DHET	0.014	0.166	−0.418
14,15-DHET	0.210	0.218	0.220
EET/DHET	−0.007	−0.053	0.292
EET+DHET	0.051	0.186	−0.081
	EPA		
8,9-EEQ	0.434 ^	0.267 °	0.784 ^,°
11,12-EEQ	0.575 ^	0.482 ^,°	0.794 ^,°
14,15-EEQ	0.641 ^	0.590 ^,°	0.808 ^,°
17,18-EEQ	0.552 ^	0.509 ^,°	0.643 ^,°
5,6-DiHETE	0.512 ^	0.441 ^,°	0.652 ^,°
8,9-DiHETE	0.398 ^	0.337 *,°	0.446
11,12-DiHETE	0.217	0.244	−0.023
14,15-DiHETE	0.464 ^	0.393 ^,°	0.532 *,°
17,18-DiHETE	0.484 ^	0.431 ^	0.440
EEQ/DiHETE	0.228	0.138	0.521 *,°
EEQ+DiHETE	0.605 ^	0.578 ^,°	0.652 ^
	DHA		
7,8-EDP	0.482 ^,°	0.553 ^,°	0.666 ^°
10,11-EDP	0.375 ^,°	0.360 *,°	0.569 *
13,14-EDP	0.467 ^,°	0.515 ^,°	0.563 *
16,17-EDP	0.502 ^,°	0.591 ^,°	0.546 *
19,20-EDP	0.456 ^,°	0.581 ^,°	0.473
7,8-DiHDPA	0.453 ^,°	0.521 ^,°	0.324
10,11-DiHDPA	0.220	0.310 *,°	0.205
13,14-DiHDPA	0.256 *,°	0.325 *,°	0.290
16,17-DiHDPA	0.386 ^,°	0.531 ^,°	0.086
19,20-DiHDPA	0.383 ^,°	0.565 ^,°	0.010
EDP/DiHDPA	0.150	0.072	0.433
EDP+DiHDPA	0.526 *,°	0.617 ^,°	0.575 *

The table shows the coefficients of correlations (r_S) between the fatty acid precursors, namely LA, AA, EPA and DHA and their metabolites via CYP450-epoxygenase/sEH in the whole sample and in the subgroups of HBP and NBP children. The underlined correlations remained significant after adjustment for sex, age, pubertal status and BMI. The sum of epoxymetabolites and corresponding diols estimates the CYP450-epoxygenase activity, whereas their ratio estimates the sEH activity. *: $p < 0.05$; ^: $p < 0.01$; °: $p < 0.05$ after False Discovery Rate correction. NBP: normal blood pressure; HBP high blood pressure; LA: Linoleic acid; AA: Arachidonic acid; EPA: Eicosapentaenoic acid; DHA: Docosahexaenoic acid; EpHOME: epoxyoctadecenoic acid; DiHOME: dihydroxyoctadecenoic acid; EET: epoxyeicosatrienoic acid; DHET: dihydroxyeicosatrienoic acid; EEQ: epoxyeicosatetraenoic acid; DiHETE: dihydroxyeicosatetraenoic acid; EDP: epoxydocosapentaenoic acid; DiHDPA: dihydroxydocosapentaenoic acid.

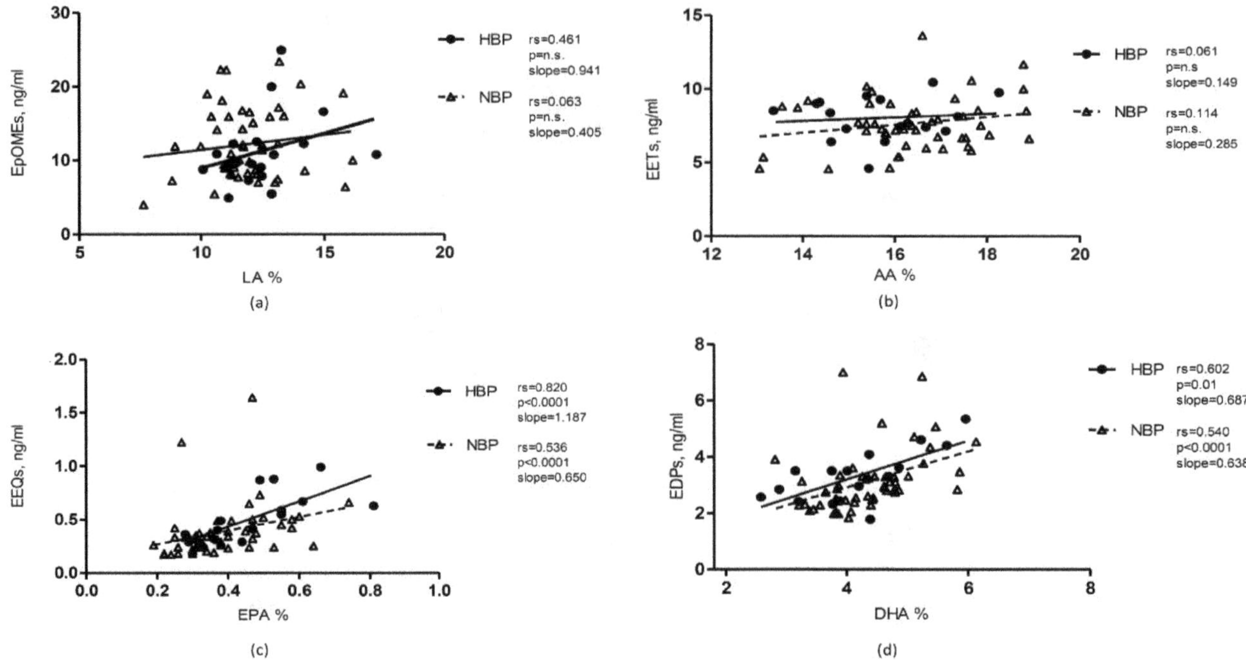

Figure 2. Correlations between fatty acids and their metabolite via CYP450-epoxygenase. The graphs represent the correlations of the fatty acids with their corresponding epoxymetabolites. The two subgroups of obese children with high (HBP) and normal blood pressure (NBP) are differently graphically depicted. The panels represent: (**a**) the correlation of LA with EpOMEs, which was stronger in HBP children; (**b**) the association of AA with EETs; (**c**) the correlation of EPA with EEQs, which was stronger in HBP children; (**d**) the association of DHA with EDPs. LA: Linoleic acid; AA: Arachidonic acid; EPA: Eicosapentaenoic acid; DHA: Docosahexaenoic acid; EpOME: epoxyoctadecenoic acid; EET: epoxyeicosatrienoic acid; EEQ: epoxyeicosatetraenoic acid; EDP:epoxydocosapentaenoic acid; HBP: high blood pressure subgroup; NBP: normal blood pressure subgroup, *p*: *p*-value; r_S: Spearman correlation coefficient; n.s.: not significant.

CYP450-Derived Eicosanoids of LA and Their Associations with Clinical Features

LA did not show any significant correlation with BP (Table 3), whereas DiHOMEs, especially 9,10-DiHOME, directly correlated with DBP in the whole sample and in the NBP subgroup (Table 4). (The associations of the eicosanoids with BP percentiles are reported in Table S2). Vascular tests did not show any significant correlation with LA and its metabolites (Table 5).

Table 3. Correlations between red blood cell membrane fatty acids and BP in the whole study population and in the subgroups of HBP and NBP obese children.

	LA	AA	EPA	DHA
Whole population				
Office-SBP, mmHg	−0.091	−0.070	0.035	0.090
Office-SBP percentile	0.002	0.002	−0.049	−0.094
Office-DBP, mmHg	0.168	−0.130	−0.167	−0.106
Office-DBP percentile	0.217	−0.095	−0.175	−0.210
24 h-SBP, mmHg	0.096	−0.329 ^	0.154	0.016
24 h-SBP percentile	0.229	−0.134	0.014	−0.214
24 h-DBP, mmHg	0.171	−0.222	−0.069	−0.140
24 h-DBP percentile	0.200	−0.176	−0.092	−0.175
Day-time SBP, mmHg	0.070	−0.277 *	0.172	0.043
Day-time SBP, percentile	0.192	−0.129	0.086	−0.132

Table 3. *Cont.*

	LA	AA	EPA	DHA
Whole population				
Day-time DBP, mmHg	0.136	−0.132	−0.075	−0.142
Day-time DBP, percentile	0.136	−0.092	−0.084	−0.142
Night-time SBP, mmHg	0.066	−0.327 ^	0.154	−0.001
Night-time SBP, percentile	0.213	−0.178	0.051	−0.121
Night-time DBP, mmHg	0.145	−0.359 ^	0.014	−0.046
Night-time DBP, percentile	0.159	−0.353 ^	0.043	−0.040
HBP				
Office-SBP, mmHg	0.013	0.088	−0.639 ^	−0.050
Office-SBP percentile	0.017	0.172	−0.609 ^	−0.113
Office-DBP, mmHg	0.206	−0.136	−0.564 *	−0.377
Office-DBP percentile	0.218	0.083	−0.668^	−0.157
24 h-SBP, mmHg	−0.425	0.220	−0.111	0.236
24 h-SBP percentile	−0.279	0.387	−0.043	0.250
24 h-DBP, mmHg	−0.278	−0.205	−0.251	0.010
24 h-DBP percentile	−0.228	−0.184	−0.269	−0.012
Day-time SBP, mmHg	−0.433	0.055	0.013	0.257
Day-time SBP, percentile	−0.277	0.306	0.037	0.257
Day-time DBP, mmHg	−0.263	−0.167	−0.164	0.001
Day-time DBP, percentile	−0.252	−0.142	−0.188	0.015
Night-time SBP, mmHg	−0.413	0.319	−0.225	0.172
Night-time SBP, percentile	−0.193	0.466	−0.029	0.076
Night-time DBP, mmHg	−0.258	−0.182	−0.427	−0.021
Night-time DBP, percentile	−0.228	−0.191	−0.426	−0.049
NBP				
Office-SBP, mmHg	−0.180	−0.034	0.169	0.188
Office-SBP percentile	−0.087	0.042	0.063	−0.050
Office-DBP, mmHg	0.089	−0.144	−0.049	0.025
Office-DBP percentile	0.128	−0.111	−0.079	−0.125
24 h-SBP, mmHg	0.059	−0.325 *	0.060	0.057
24 h-SBP percentile	0.217	−0.037	−0.163	−0.311 *
24 h-DBP, mmHg	0.233	−0.221	−0.131	−0.151
24 h-DBP percentile	0.268	−0.172	−0.159	−0.196
Day-time SBP, mmHg	0.062	−0.268	0.092	0.067
Day-time SBP, percentile	0.184	−0.069	−0.058	−0.160
Day-time DBP, mmHg	0.208	−0.124	−0.136	−0.176
Day-time DBP, percentile	0.209	−0.060	−0.147	−0.176
Night-time SBP, mmHg	0.052	−0.335 *	0.090	0.025
Night-time SBP, percentile	0.249	−0.154	−0.042	−0.212
Night-time DBP, mmHg	0.229	−0.340 *	−0.044	−0.025
Night-time DBP, percentile	0.251	−0.333 *	−0.027	−0.035

The table shows the spearman coefficients of correlations (r_s) between fatty acids (precursors), namely LA, AA, EPA, DHA and office and ambulatory BP in the whole sample and in the subgroups of HBP and NBP children. The underlined correlations remained significant after adjustment for sex, age, pubertal status and BMI. *: $p < 0.05$; ^: $p < 0.01$ after False Discovery Rate correction. NBP: normal blood pressure; HBP high blood pressure; AA: arachidonic acid; DHA: docosahexaenoic acid; DBP: diastolic blood pressure; EPA: eicosapentaenoic acid; LA: linolenic acid; SBP: systolic blood pressure.

Table 4. Correlations of CYP450-epoxygenase/sEH metabolites of LA, AA, EPA and DHA with BP in the whole study population and in the two subgroups of high blood pressure and normal blood pressure obese children.

	Office SBP, mmHg	Office DBP, mmHg	24-h SBP, mmHg	24-h DBP, mmHg	Day-time SBP, mmHg	Day-time DBP, mmHg	Night-time SBP, mmHg	Night-time DBP, mmHg
				Whole population				
EpOMEtot	−0.092	0.070	−0.025	0.069	−0.045	0.073	−0.086	−0.019
DiHOME tot	−0.060	0.279 * 9,10-DiHOME 0.319 ^	0.031	0.149	−0.053	0.052	0.103	0.252 * 9,10-DiHOME 0.256 *
EET tot	0.060	−0.008	0.019	0.037	0.004	0.040	0.017	−0.044
DHET tot	0.142	0.052	0.036	0.006	0.077	0.050	0.012	−0.020
EEQ tot	−0.120	−0.211 8,9-EEQ −0.307 *	0.045	0.030	0.038	0.021	0.052	−0.076
DiHETE tot	−0.069	−0.171	0.117	0.109	0.131	0.058	0.080	0.112
EDP tot	−0.128	−0.180	−0.013	−0.077	0.001	−0.067	−0.076	−0.140
DiHDPA tot	−0.035	−0.077	−0.028	−0.086	0.030	−0.054	−0.161	−0.134
				HBP				
EpOME tot	−0.256	−0.094	−0.315	−0.291	−0.428	−0.380	−0.271	0.068
DiHOME tot	−0.104	0.232	−0.252	−0.098	−0.363	−0.123	−0.266	0.037
EET tot	−0.108	−0.287	−0.211	0.071	−0.087	0.183	−0.311	0.106
DHET tot	−0.016	−0.109	−0.034	−0.050	0.112	0.046	−0.102	−0.047
EEQ tot	−0.539 * 11,12-EEQ −0.694 ^ 17,18-EEQ −0.584 *	−0.299	−0.276 11,12-EEQ −0.492 *	−0.117	−0.080	−0.038	−0.439 11,12-EEQ −0.559 * 17,18-EEQ −0.615 ^	−0.216
DiHETE tot	−0.437 17,18-DiHETE −0.578 *	−0.120	−0.233 17,18-DiHETE −0.512 *	0.142	−0.076	0.205	−0.348 17,18-DiHETE −0.492 *	0.089
EDP tot	−0.229 7,8-EDP −0.574 * 10,11-EDP −0.506 * 16-17-EDP−0.539 *	−0.526*	−0.120	−0.284	−0.010	−0.205	−0.361	−0.240
DiHDPA tot	−0.090	−0.382	0.093	−0.183	0.277	−0.070	−0.195	−0.350
				NBP				
EpOME tot	−0.048	0.148	0.065	0.147	0.070	0.206	−0.049	−0.033
DiHOME tot	−0.094	0.281 9,10-DiHOME 0.319 *	0.027	0.158	−0.054	0.062	0.141	0.313 * 9,10-DiHOME 0.312 *
EET tot	0.057	−0.003	−0.029	−0.076	−0.043	−0.064	−0.121	−0.264 8,9-EET −0.332 *
DHET tot	0.189	0.104	−0.013	0.013	0.025	0.034	−0.071	−0.044
EEQ tot	−0.080	−0.143	−0.073	−0.024	−0.070	−0.013	−0.104	−0.279 14,15-EEQ −0.297 *
DiHETE tot	−0.065	−0.211 11,12-DiHETE −0.339 *	−0.003	−0.018	0.023	−0.089	−0.095	−0.086
EDP tot	−0.156	−0.090	−0.078	−0.084	−0.059	−0.072	−0.251 19,20-EDP −0.303 *	−0.259
DiHDPA tot	−0.018	−0.009	−0.094	−0.068	−0.050	−0.067	−0.280	−0.143

The table shows the coefficients of correlations (rs) between the metabolites of LA, AA, EPA, DHA via CYP450-epoxygenase/sEH and office and ambulatory BP in the whole sample and in the subgroups of HBP and NBP children. The underlined correlations remained significant after adjustment for sex, age, pubertal status and BMI. *: $p < 0.05$; ^: $p < 0.01$. NBP: normal blood pressure; HBP high blood pressure; SBP: systolic blood pressure; DBP: diastolic blood pressure; EpOME: epoxyoctadecenoic acid; DiHOME: dihydroxyoctadecenoic acid; EET: epoxyeicosatrienoic acid; DHET: dihydroxyeicosatrienoic acid; EEQ: epoxyeicosatetraenoic acid; DiHETE: dihydroxyeicosatetraenoic acid; EDP: epoxydocosapentaenoic acid; DiHDPA: dihydroxydocosapentaenoic acid.

Table 5. Correlations of LA, AA, EPA, DHA and the derived CYP450-epoxygenase/sEH metabolites with vascular tests in the whole sample and in the two individual subgroups of HBP and NBP obese children.

	cIMT	**cIMT, (Percentile)**	**DC**	**DC, (Percentile)**	**FMD, %**
		Whole population			
LA	0.112	0.143	0.119	0.094	−0.150
AA	−0.142	−0.097	0.108	0.063	−0.005
EPA	−0.212	−0.305 *	−0.067	−0.015	0.176
DHA	−0.071	−0.170	−0.106	−0.053	0.139
EpOMEs	0.069	0.064	0.120	0.140	−0.141
DiHOMEs	−0.083	−0.077	0.095	0.085	−0.155
EETs	0.093	0.084	0.072	0.073	−0.185
DHETs	−0.070	−0.045	−0.058	−0.052	−0.049
EEQs	−0.184	−0.230 14,15-EEQ −0.279 * 17,18-EEQ −0.263 *	0.069	0.096	−0.008
DiHETEs	0.008	−0.026	0.012	0.024	0.176
EDPs	−0.082	−0.119	0.136	0.147	−0.158
DiHDPAs	−0.171	−0.206	0.091	0.121	−0.101
		HBP			
LA	−0.121	−0.025	0.175	0.207	−0.400
AA	−0.172	−0.174	0.011	−0.039	−0.121
EPA	−0.304	−0.378	0.432	0.407	0.268
DHA	0.027	−0.002	−0.121	−0.136	−0.146
EpOMEs	−0.063	0.034	0.050	0.093	−0.050
DiHOMEs	0.067	0.071	−0.132	−0.132	0.004
EETs	−0.231	−0.061	0.314	0.214	0.118
DHETs	−0.301	−0.273	0.155	0.071	0.296
EEQs	−0.605 * 8;9-EEQ −0.493 * 14;15-EEQ −0.609 ^ 17;18-EEQ −0.615*	−0.620 ^ 8;9-EEQ −0.539 * 14;15-EEQ −0.657 ^ 17;18-EEQ −0.637 ^	0.374 11;12-EEQ 0.575 *	0.388 11;12-EEQ 0.582 *	0.288
DiHETEs	−0.354 5;6-DiHETE −0.559 *	−0.323 5;6-DiHETE −0.577 *	0.290	0.209	0.375 5;6-DiHETE −0.576 *
EDPs	−0.098	0.002	0.312	0.237	−0.220
DiHDPAs	−0.114	−0.104	0.148	0.086	−0.091
		NBP			
LA	0.142	0.181	0.132	0.108	−0.082
AA	−0.067	−0.016	0.088	0.043	0.029
EPA	−0.243	−0.359 *	−0.174	−0.099	0.137
DHA	−0.097	−0.217	−0.137	−0.061	0.248
EpOMEs	0.095	0.078	0.107	0.140	−0.189
DiHOMEs	−0.163	−0.145	0.196	0.186	−0.209
EETs	0.159	0.101	0.032	0.068	−0.272
DHETs	0.010	0.025	−0.103	−0.091	−0.165
EEQs	−0.162	−0.235 14,15-EEQ −0.308 *	0.013	0.046	−0.116
DiHETEs	0.050	−0.014	−0.024	0.019	0.155
EDPs	−0.185	−0.247 19,20-EDP −0.296 *	0.081	0.121	−0.067
DiHDPAs	0.223	0.259	0.195	0.180	−0.095

The table shows the spearman coefficients of correlations (r_S) between LA, AA, EPA, DHA and their metabolites via CYP450-epoxygenase/sEH with the vascular tests and their percentiles for sex and age in the whole sample and in the subgroups of HBP and NBP children. The underlined correlations remained significant after adjustment for sex, age, pubertal status and BMI. * $p< 0.05$; ^ $p < 0.01$. NBP: normal blood pressure; HBP high blood pressure; AA: arachidonic acid; DHA: docosahexaenoic acid; EPA: eicosapentaenoic acid; LA: linolenic acid; EpOME: epoxyoctadecenoic acid; DiHOME: dihydroxyoctadecenoic acid; EET: epoxyeicosatrienoic acid; DHET: dihydroxyeicosatrienoic acid; EEQ: epoxyeicosatetraenoic acid; DiHETE: dihydroxyeicosatetraenoic acid; EDP: epoxydocosapentaenoic acid; DiHDPA: dihydroxydocosapentaenoic acid; cIMT: carotid intima-media thickness; cDC: carotid distensibility; FMD: flow-mediated dilation.

3.2.2. AA and CYP450-Derived Eicosanoids

Associations of AA with Clinical Features and with Its Metabolites

AA was higher in NBP as compared to HBP children (Table 1 and Figure 1). In the whole sample, AA was inversely correlated to ABPM and this inverse association was confirmed in the NBP subgroup (Table 3). No significant correlations were found between AA and vascular features (Table 5).

Considering the metabolic pathway of AA via CYP450 and sEH, AA was not significantly correlated with its metabolites via CYP450/sEH neither in the whole population nor in the subgroups of HBP and NBP children (Table 2 and Figure 2). AA did not show any significant difference also with the estimated CYP450 epoxygenase activity (Figure S1).

CYP450-Derived Eicosanoids of AA and Their Associations with Clinical Features

EETs and DHETs, the epoxymetabolites and the corresponding diols derived from AA respectively, did not show any significant association with BP and vascular function markers (Tables 4 and 5. The associations of the eicosanoids with BP percentiles are detailed in Table S2). Twenty-hydroxyeicosatetraenoiic acid (20-HETE), the hydroxymetabolite of AA, did not differ between HBP and NBP subgroups (Table 1) and did not show any significant correlation with BP and vascular features.

3.3. *Omega-3 PUFA*

3.3.1. EPA and CYP450-Derived Eicosanoids

Associations of EPA with Clinical Features and with Its Metabolites

The amount of EPA in red blood cell membrane was similar in both groups of HBP and NBP obese children (Table 1 and Figure 1). EPA inversely correlated with office BP and with cIMT in the HBP subgroup and the inverse correlation with cIMT was significant also in the whole population (Tables 3 and 5).

EPA was directly correlated with its epoxymetabolites and the corresponding diols, especially the 14,15-isomer, in the whole sample and in both subgroups (Table 2). In the subgroup of HBP children the strength and the slope of the correlations between the precursor and the products were higher and EEQs and DiHETEs were more elevated than in NBP (Figure 2). Moreover, the estimated CYP450 activity (sum of EEQs and DiHETEs) was higher in the HBP than in NBP children (Figure 1 panel (c)) and EPA correlated stronger with the estimated CYP450 activity in the HBP than in NBP subgroup, whereas the estimated sEH activity did not differ between the two groups (Table 2 and Figure S1).

CYP450-Derived Eicosanoids of EPA and Their Associations with Clinical Features

EEQs and DiHETEs inversely correlated with office and ambulatory BP, in particular 11,12-EEQ and 17,18-DiHETE (Table 4 and Figure 3. The associations of the eicosanoids with BP percentiles are reported in Table S2). In the whole sample, only 8,9-EEQ showed an inverse correlation with office DBP (Table 4.). The epoxymetabolites of EPA inversely correlated also with cIMT, in particular 14,15- and 17,18- EEQ (Figure 3) and these associations were more evident in the HBP group, in which also 5,6-DiHETE sowed an inverse correlation with cIMT. In this subgroup 11,12-EEQ was also directly correlated with carotid distensibility (Table 5). Plasma concentration of twenty-hydroxyeicosapentaenoic acid (20-HEPE), the hydroxymetabolite of EPA, was under the limit of detection.

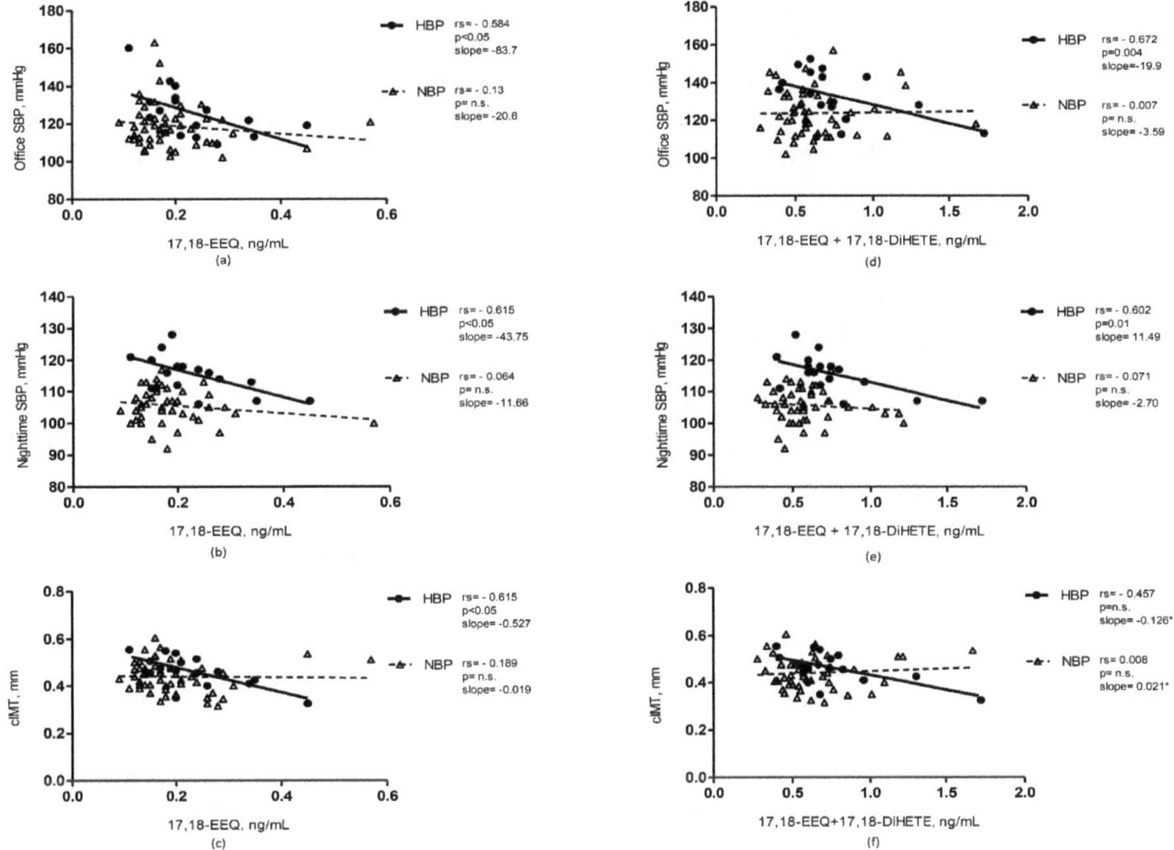

Figure 3. Correlations of EEQ with BP and cIMT in the high blood pressure (HBP) and normal blood pressure (NBP) obese children subgroups. The first column represents the correlation of 17,18-EEQ with: (**a**) office SBP; (**b**) night-time SBP; (**c**) cIMT. The second column represents the correlation of the estimated CYP450 epoxygenase activity, as calculated as the sum of epoxymetabolites plus the corresponding diols, with: (**d**) office SBP; (**e**) night-time SBP; (**f**) cIMT. * there is a significantly difference between the slopes of the two subgroups, $p < 0.05$. The correlations in all panels are stronger in HBP than in NBP children. The two subgroups of obese children with high and normal blood pressure are differently graphically depicted. cIMT: carotid intima-media thickness; EEQ: epoxyeicosatetraenoic acid; DiHETE: dihydroxyeicosatetraenoic acid; HBP: high blood pressure subgroup; NBP: normal blood pressure subgroup; SBP: systolic blood pressure, p: p-value; r_S: Spearman correlation coefficient.

3.3.2. DHA and CYP450-Derived Eicosanoids

Associations of DHA with Clinical Features and with Its Metabolites

DHA had a similar distribution among genders and hypertensive status (Table 1) and was associated neither with BP nor with the main vascular features (Tables 3 and 5).

DHA was directly correlated with its epoxymetabolites, the EDPs, in the whole population and in both subgroups and was directly correlated with DiHDPAs in particular in NBP children (Table 2 and Figure 2). DHA directly correlated with the estimated CYP450 epoxygenase activity in both subgroups (Figure S1).

CYP450-Derived Eicosanoids of EPA and Their Associations with Clinical Features

EDPs and DiHDPAs were not associated with BP and vascular features, except an inverse correlation of most isomers of EDPs with office SBP in HBP children (Table 4. The associations of the eicosanoids with BP percentiles are detailed in Table S2). Plasma concentrations of 22-hydroxydocosahexaenoic acid (22-HDHA) did not differ between HBP and NBP subgroups (Table 1) and did not show any significant correlation with BP and vascular characteristics, except an inverse correlation with cIMT ($r_S = -0.292$, $p < 0.01$) and the relative z-score ($r_S = -0.297$, $p < 0.01$) in the NBP subgroup.

Most of the above-mentioned significant correlations remained significant after adjustment for sex, age and pubertal status, as indicated in the relative tables. After *False Discovery Rate* (FDR) correction only most of the correlations between the precursors and the respective products remained significant.

4. Discussion

Our main hypothesis was that several PUFA, mainly assumed by the diet, could affect hemodynamics and in particular blood pressure, through the formation of specific PUFA-derived lipid mediators generated via the CYP450-epoxygenase/sEH pathway. Scarce is the evidence linking the amount of fatty acids introduced by diet and their metabolites via CYP450/sEH with hemodynamics in humans and, to our knowledge, this is the first study that investigated this link in children. Indeed, red blood cell membrane fatty acids are a reliable marker of dietary intake, especially for essential fatty acids, reflecting the preceding intake of the fatty acid [38].

A complex link between PUFA and BP is supported by the literature, where the putative beneficial effect of omega-3 PUFA on BP and subsequent cardiovascular events is often blurred, being evident in some trials but not in others or in meta-analyses [5,39], with some studies also available in children [40–42]. The underlying mechanisms are multifactorial and may include an improvement in endothelial function and in arterial stiffness [10–12], although the relative effects of omega-3 PUFA and their CYP450 generated metabolites remain not completely understood.

Despite plenty of studies in animal models [43], especially rats, the evidence that EETs could affect BP in humans is scanty. In particular, our group found lower plasma EETs in patients affected by renovascular hypertension as compared to essential hypertension and controls [44] and an augmented production of EETs in plasma and placentas obtained by preeclamptic women [45,46]. Surprisingly, we did not find any association of EETs neither with BP nor vascular function in this sample of obese children.

Little is known about the specific actions of the EPA/DHA-derived metabolites via CYP450/sEH on hemodynamic modulation both in animal models and humans but a few studies support a protective effect on blood pressure, at least for some single isomers [23,25] suggesting that their actions could be even more potent with respect to EETs.

In this study, we found interesting correlations between EPA and DHA and the corresponding metabolites via CYP450-epoxygenase, supporting the hypothesis that a dietary assumption of specific omega-3 PUFA (or at least a higher storage in cellular membranes) drives a higher production of their metabolites. Interestingly, these metabolic steps appear different in HBP and in NBP children. Indeed, the association between precursor and products, especially for EPA metabolism, is stronger and steeper in HBP than in NBP and, moreover, also the estimated CYP450-epoxygenase activity (sum of epoxides and diols) itself is higher in HBP children whereas no difference in the estimated sEH activity (epoxide/diol ratio) was evident between the two subgroups. These data suggest that in HBP obese children the CYP450-epoxygenase, in particular for EPA, might have a different efficacy or regulation as compared to NBP. We could hypothesize that in obese children with HBP is a modulation in CYP450-epoxygenase activity, rather than in sEH activity, leading to an enhanced formation of the epoxymetabolites, which are supposed to have more favourable cardiovascular effects.

Furthermore, the exploratory analyses in the subgroup of HBP children, seems to reveal a potential role of some metabolites (especially EEQs and EDPs) on BP. Especially EEQs and in particular 14,15- and 17,18- EEQ, showed inverse associations with several BP measurements and with the markers of vascular structure and function (namely, cIMT and distensibility) in HBP obese children. Even if this is only an exploratory analysis and should be examined with caution, it is compatible with the hypothesis that the effect of endothelium derived hyperpolarizing factors (such as EETs/EEQs/EDPs) is detectable only in circumstances when the effect of nitric oxide (NO) is altered [47,48]. Indeed, some of the beneficial cardiovascular effects of long-chain omega-3 PUFA and especially EPA, at least those mediated by CYP450/sEH metabolites, could act as compensatory mechanism and thus being more evident in more disadvantageous conditions, that is, obesity together with high blood pressure. Only a few studies addressed this issue: a study in transgenic mice with endothelial expression of the human CYP2J2 and CYP2C8 demonstrated that increased endothelial CYP450 epoxygenase expression reduced BP increase especially when nitric oxide synthase and cyclooxygenase were inhibited [49]. Data from studies in humans also support the hypothesis that the CYP450 pathways compensate the impairment of vasodilation due to classical pathways, like NO, for example in hypertensive patients [47] and in subjects with hyperpathyroidism, which is generally associated with high blood pressure and an increased CV risk [50].

In line with our observations, also some other studies suggest that EPA and DHA exert a stronger effect in hypertensive as compared to normotensive subjects, as suggested also by meta-analyses [5,39,51]. Interestingly, the inverse association of 14,15- and 17,18-EEQ with cIMT, is even stronger in the HBP subgroup compared to the whole group as well.

The observational study design and the exploratory analyses suggest looking at all these associations with caution. Anyhow, we hypothesize that EPA could exert a somehow protective action on blood pressure through their metabolites via CYP450-epoxygenase/sEH, probably mediated by a beneficial influence on vascular structure and function and this effect could be stronger in HBP obese children than in NBP. The stronger correlations of EPA with its metabolites in HBP rather than in NBP children support the hypothesis that their effect becomes more important when BP is higher.

Interestingly, DiHOME, the diols derived from LA via CYP450 and sEH metabolism, showed a direct correlation with diastolic BP in NBP but not in HBP, suggesting that they negatively affect vascular stiffness and BP but only in normotensive obese children. Very little is known about the actions of EpOMEs and DiHOMEs; first data indicated a toxic effect of EpOME and probably of DiHOME that could be dose-dependent; they also could affect cardiac contractility but the results are not always consistent [12,13]. On the other hand, a recent study has proposed a possible protective effect of 12,13-DiHOME on metabolic profile, due to its action on brown adipose tissue uptake of fatty acids [52]. Furthermore, an epoxy-keto derivative of LA has been identified as a possible stimulating factor for aldosterone secretion but its precursor and its metabolic pathway is not known [53]. Furthermore, we found that LA was inversely correlated to BP in HBP subjects, suggesting a possible beneficial effect of LA on BP. These data are not easy to interpret, considering the results of the metabolite of LA, especially the possible positive role of 12,13-DiHOME. Anyhow, it should be considered that from each fatty acid derives a range of lipid mediators, which can have different actions. Moreover, also in a previous animal model a discrepancy has been found regarding the effect of dietary intake of fatty acids, that is, LA and ALA, on the composition of PUFA and their related metabolites [54].

As mentioned above, the present study has limitations: the lack of data about the total food intake of fatty acids and the amount of fatty acids in the diet, the sample size is relatively low, which can primarily expose a problem of statistical power; after statistical adjustment for multiple testing only several correlations remained significant. Thus, considering also the observational design of the study, the results should be regarded as exploratory and need confirmation in new studies. Furthermore, we decided to define hypertension on the basis of a single ABPM registration, considering it being more accurate to establish hypertension based on a single exam. Finally, these results need to be confirmed in other studies analysing also samples of children of different ages and body size, including non-obese children and different ethnic groups.

Anyhow, we obtained also several office BP measurements, both in the supine position and in the recommended sitting position, which strengthened the results derived from ABPM.

Globally, our data suggest that single lipid mediators may exert specific actions in hemodynamic control in obese children, that may be different in hypertensive rather than in normotensive children. What remains to be understood are the regulatory mechanisms that can modulate the metabolic pathways of the fatty acids, leading to the production of specific lipid mediators. Moreover, also the relations, or the competition, between different metabolic pathways might affect the productions of active metabolites, thus influencing the final effect [2]. Furthermore, the omega-3 index of the obese children included in this study was quite low (mean: 4.6%), far below the proposed target of 8% or more, which is suggested as CV protective level by the evaluation of epidemiological and clinical studies [55,56]. Thus, another question that should be addressed by future studies is whether obese children with HBP may benefit from dietary EPA/DHA supplementation.

In conclusion, this study sets out the steps to further investigate, in children as well in adults, the metabolism of dietary fatty acids, especially via CYP450 and their possible influence on hemodynamics and BP control.

Author Contributions: Conceptualization, C.F., W.H.S., C.M., F.A. and S.B.; methodology, C.F., W.H.S., M.M., M.B., M.K., M.R., R.G., P.C., C.M. and F.A.; software, A.G.; formal analysis, S.B., A.G. and M.K.; investigation, S.B., A.T. and D.M.; data curation, S.B., A.G. and A.T.; writing—original draft preparation, S.B.; writing—review and editing, C.F., C.M. and W.H.S.; supervision, P.M.; funding acquisition, C.F.

Acknowledgments: Part of this work was performed in the LURM (Laboratorio Universitario di Ricerca Medica) Research Centre, University of Verona. We acknowledge Sara Raimondi for her support in the statistical analysis.

References

1. Daniels, S.R. Complications of obesity in children and adolescents. *Int. J. Obes.* **2009**, *33* (Suppl. 1), S60–S65. [CrossRef]
2. Bonafini, S.; Fava, C. Omega-3 fatty acids and cytochrome P450-derived eicosanoids in cardiovascular diseases: Which actions and interactions modulate hemodynamics? *Prostaglandins Other Lipid Mediat.* **2017**, *128*, 34–42. [CrossRef] [PubMed]
3. Maffeis, C.; Pinelli, L.; Schutz, Y. Fat intake and adiposity in 8 to 11 year-old obese children. *Int. J. Obes.* **1996**, *20*, 170–174.
4. Anonymous. Dietary supplementation with n-3 polyunsaturated fatty acids and vitamin E after myocardial infarction: Results of the GISSI-Prevenzione trial. Gruppo Italiano per lo Studio della Sopravvivenza nell'Infarto miocardico. *Lancet* **1999**, *354*, 447–455.
5. Miller, P.E.; Van Elswyk, M.; Alexander, D.D. Long-chain omega-3 fatty acids eicosapentaenoic acid and docosahexaenoic acid and blood pressure: A meta-analysis of randomized controlled trials. *Am. J. Hypertens.* **2014**, *27*, 885–896. [CrossRef] [PubMed]
6. Wang, D.D.; Li, Y.; Chiuve, S.E.; Stampfer, M.J.; Manson, J.E.; Rimm, E.B.; Willett, W.C.; Hu, F.B. Association of Specific Dietary Fats with Total and Cause-Specific Mortality. *JAMA Intern. Med.* **2016**, *176*, 1134–1145. [CrossRef] [PubMed]
7. Vanhala, M.; Saltevo, J.; Soininen, P.; Kautiainen, H.; Kangas, A.J.; Ala-Korpela, M.; Mäntyselkä, P. Serum omega-6 polyunsaturated fatty acids and the metabolic syndrome: A longitudinal population-based cohort study. *Am. J. Epidemiol.* **2012**, *176*, 253–260. [CrossRef] [PubMed]
8. Minihane, A.M.; Armah, C.K.; Miles, E.A.; Madden, J.M.; Clark, A.B.; Caslake, M.J.; Packard, C.J.; Kofler, B.M.; Lietz, G.; Curtis, P.J.; et al. Consumption of Fish Oil Providing Amounts of Eicosapentaenoic Acid and Docosahexaenoic Acid That Can Be Obtained from the Diet Reduces Blood Pressure in Adults with Systolic Hypertension: A Retrospective Analysis. *J. Nutr.* **2016**, *146*, 516–523. [CrossRef] [PubMed]
9. Yang, B.; Shi, M.-Q.; Li, Z.-H.; Yang, J.-J.; Li, D. Fish, Long-Chain n-3 PUFA and Incidence of Elevated Blood Pressure: A Meta-Analysis of Prospective Cohort Studies. *Nutrients* **2016**, *8*. [CrossRef] [PubMed]
10. Wang, Q.; Liang, X.; Wang, L.; Lu, X.; Huang, J.; Cao, J.; Li, H.; Gu, D. Effect of omega-3 fatty acids supplementation on endothelial function: A meta-analysis of randomized controlled trials. *Atherosclerosis* **2012**, *221*, 536–543. [CrossRef] [PubMed]

11. Tousoulis, D.; Plastiras, A.; Siasos, G.; Oikonomou, E.; Verveniotis, A.; Kokkou, E.; Maniatis, K.; Gouliopoulos, N.; Miliou, A.; Paraskevopoulos, T.; et al. Omega-3 PUFAs improved endothelial function and arterial stiffness with a parallel antiinflammatory effect in adults with metabolic syndrome. *Atherosclerosis* **2014**, *232*, 10–16. [CrossRef] [PubMed]
12. Pase, M.P.; Grima, N.A.; Sarris, J. Do long-chain n-3 fatty acids reduce arterial stiffness? A meta-analysis of randomised controlled trials. *Br. J. Nutr.* **2011**, *106*, 974–980. [CrossRef] [PubMed]
13. Bonafini, S.; Tagetti, A.; Gaudino, R.; Cavarzere, P.; Montagnana, M.; Danese, E.; Benati, M.; Ramaroli, D.A.D.A.; Raimondi, S.; Giontella, A.; et al. Individual fatty acids in erythrocyte membranes are associated with several features of the metabolic syndrome in obese children. *Eur. J. Nutr.* **2018**. [CrossRef] [PubMed]
14. Schunck, W.-H.; Konkel, A.; Fischer, R.; Weylandt, K.-H. Therapeutic potential of omega-3 fatty acid-derived epoxyeicosanoids in cardiovascular and inflammatory diseases. *Pharmacol. Ther.* **2018**, *183*, 177–204. [CrossRef] [PubMed]
15. Imig, J.D. Epoxide hydrolase and epoxygenase metabolites as therapeutic targets for renal diseases. *Am. J. Physiol. Ren. Physiol.* **2005**, *289*, F496–F503. [CrossRef] [PubMed]
16. Hercule, H.C.; Schunck, W.-H.H.; Gross, V.; Seringer, J.; Leung, F.P.; Weldon, S.M.; da Costa Goncalves, A.C.; Huang, Y.; Luft, F.C.; Gollasch, M. Interaction between P450 eicosanoids and nitric oxide in the control of arterial tone in mice. *Arterioscler. Thromb. Vasc. Biol.* **2009**, *29*, 54–60. [CrossRef] [PubMed]
17. Cheng, J.; Ou, J.-S.; Singh, H.; Falck, J.R.; Narsimhaswamy, D.; Pritchard, K.A.; Schwartzman, M.L. 20-Hydroxyeicosatetraenoic acid causes endothelial dysfunction via eNOS uncoupling. *AJP Heart Circ. Physiol.* **2008**, *294*, H1018–H1026. [CrossRef] [PubMed]
18. Ishizuka, T.; Cheng, J.; Singh, H.; Vitto, M.D.; Manthati, V.L.; Falck, J.R.; Laniado-Schwartzman, M. 20-Hydroxyeicosatetraenoic acid stimulates nuclear factor-kappaB activation and the production of inflammatory cytokines in human endothelial cells. *J. Pharmacol. Exp. Ther.* **2008**, *324*, 103–110. [CrossRef] [PubMed]
19. Mitchell, L.A.; Grant, D.F.; Melchert, R.B.; Petty, N.M.; Kennedy, R.H. Linoleic acid metabolites act to increase contractility in isolated rat heart. *Cardiovasc. Toxicol.* **2002**, *2*, 219–230. [CrossRef] [PubMed]
20. Moran, J.H.; Nowak, G.; Grant, D.F. Analysis of the toxic effects of linoleic acid, 12,13-cis-epoxyoctadecenoic acid, and 12,13-dihydroxyoctadecenoic acid in rabbit renal cortical mitochondria. *Toxicol. Appl. Pharmacol.* **2001**, *172*, 150–161. [CrossRef] [PubMed]
21. López-Vicario, C.; Alcaraz-Quiles, J.; García-Alonso, V.; Rius, B.; Hwang, S.H.; Titos, E.; Lopategi, A.; Hammock, B.D.; Arroyo, V.; Clària, J. Inhibition of soluble epoxide hydrolase modulates inflammation and autophagy in obese adipose tissue and liver: Role for omega-3 epoxides. *Proc. Natl. Acad. Sci. USA* **2015**, *112*, 536–541. [CrossRef] [PubMed]
22. López-vicario, C.; González-Périz, A.; Rius, B.; Morán-Salvador, E.; García-alonso, V.; Lozano, J.J.; Bataller, R.; Kang, J.X.; Arroyo, V.; Clària, J.; et al. Molecular interplay between Δ5/Δ6 desaturases and long-chain fatty acids in the pathogenesis of non-alcoholic steatohepatitis. *Gut* **2014**, *63*, 344–355. [CrossRef] [PubMed]
23. Agbor, L.N.; Walsh, M.T.; Boberg, J.R.; Walker, M.K. Elevated blood pressure in cytochrome P4501A1 knockout mice is associated with reduced vasodilation to omega-3 polyunsaturated fatty acids. *Toxicol. Appl. Pharmacol.* **2012**, *264*, 351–360. [CrossRef] [PubMed]
24. Ye, D.; Zhang, D.; Oltman, C.; Dellsperger, K.; Lee, H.-C.C.; VanRollins, M. Cytochrome p-450 epoxygenase metabolites of docosahexaenoate potently dilate coronary arterioles by activating large-conductance calcium-activated potassium channels. *J. Pharmacol. Exp. Ther.* **2002**, *303*, 768–776. [CrossRef] [PubMed]
25. Ulu, A.; Stephen Lee, K.S.; Miyabe, C.; Yang, J.; Hammock, B.G.; Dong, H.; Hammock, B.D. An omega-3 epoxide of docosahexaenoic acid lowers blood pressure in angiotensin-II-dependent hypertension. *J. Cardiovasc.* **2014**, *64*, 87–99. [CrossRef] [PubMed]
26. Flynn, J.T.; Kaelber, D.C.; Baker-Smith, C.M.; Blowey, D.; Carroll, A.E.; Daniels, S.R.; de Ferranti, S.D.; Dionne, J.M.; Falkner, B.; Flinn, S.K.; et al. Clinical Practice Guideline for Screening and Management of High Blood Pressure in Children and Adolescents. *Pediatrics* **2017**, e20171904. [CrossRef] [PubMed]
27. Lurbe, E.; Agabiti-Rosei, E.; Cruickshank, J.K.; Dominiczak, A.; Erdine, S.; Hirth, A.; Invitti, C.; Litwin, M.; Mancia, G.; Pall, D.; et al. 2016 European Society of Hypertension guidelines for the management of high blood pressure in children and adolescents. *J. Hypertens.* **2016**, *34*, 1887–1920. [CrossRef] [PubMed]

28. Wühl, E.; Witte, K.; Soergel, M.; Mehls, O.; Schaefer, F. Distribution of 24-h ambulatory blood pressure in children: Normalized reference values and role of body dimensions. *J. Hypertens.* **2002**, *20*, 1995–2007. [CrossRef] [PubMed]
29. Sharma, A.K.; Metzger, D.L.; Daymont, C.; Hadjiyannakis, S.; Rodd, C.J. LMS tables for waist-circumference and waist-height ratio Z-scores in children aged 5-19 y in NHANES III: Association with cardio-metabolic risks. *Pediatr. Res.* **2015**, *78*, 1–7. [CrossRef] [PubMed]
30. Barlow, S.E. Expert Committee Expert committee recommendations regarding the prevention, assessment, and treatment of child and adolescent overweight and obesity: Summary report. *Pediatrics* **2007**, *120*, S16–S249. [CrossRef] [PubMed]
31. Cole, T.J.; Bellizzi, M.C.; Flegal, K.M.; Dietz, W.H. Establishing a standard definition for child overweight and obesity worldwide: International survey. *BMJ* **2000**, *320*, 1240–1243. [CrossRef] [PubMed]
32. Doyon, A.; Kracht, D.; Bayazit, A.K.; Deveci, M.; Duzova, A.; Krmar, R.T.; Litwin, M.; Niemirska, A.; Oguz, B.; Schmidt, B.M.W.; et al. 4C Study Consortium Carotid artery intima-media thickness and distensibility in children and adolescents: Reference values and role of body dimensions. *Hypertension* **2013**, *62*, 550–556. [CrossRef] [PubMed]
33. Urbina, E.M.; Williams, R.V.; Alpert, B.S.; Collins, R.T.; Daniels, S.R.; Hayman, L.; Jacobson, M.; Mahoney, L.; Mietus-Snyder, M.; Rocchini, A.; et al. American Heart Association Atherosclerosis, Hypertension, and Obesity in Youth Committee of the Council on Cardiovascular Disease in the Young Noninvasive assessment of subclinical atherosclerosis in children and adolescents: Recommendations for standard assessment for clinical research: A scientific statement from the American Heart Association. *Hypertension* **2009**, *54*, 919–950. [CrossRef] [PubMed]
34. Giannarelli, C.; Bianchini, E.; Bruno, R.M.; Magagna, A.; Landini, L.; Faita, F.; Gemignani, V.; Penno, G.; Taddei, S.; Ghiadoni, L. Local carotid stiffness and intima-media thickness assessment by a novel ultrasound-based system in essential hypertension. *Atherosclerosis* **2012**, *223*, 372–377. [CrossRef] [PubMed]
35. Arnold, C.; Markovic, M.; Blossey, K.; Wallukat, G.; Fischer, R.; Dechend, R.; Konkel, A.; von Schacky, C.; Luft, F.C.; Muller, D.N.; et al. Arachidonic acid-metabolizing cytochrome P450 enzymes are targets of {omega}-3 fatty acids. *J. Biol. Chem.* **2010**, *285*, 32720–32733. [CrossRef] [PubMed]
36. Rivera, J.; Ward, N.; Hodgson, J.; Puddey, I.B.; Falck, J.R.; Croft, K.D. Measurement of 20-hydroxyeicosatetraenoic acid in human urine by gas chromatography-mass spectrometry. *Clin. Chem.* **2004**, *50*. [CrossRef] [PubMed]
37. Von Schacky, C. The Omega-3 Index as a risk factor for cardiovascular diseases. *Prostaglandins Other Lipid Mediat.* **2011**, *96*, 94–98. [CrossRef] [PubMed]
38. Harris, W.S.; Von Schacky, C. The Omega-3 Index: A new risk factor for death from coronary heart disease? *Prev. Med.* **2004**, *39*, 212–220. [CrossRef] [PubMed]
39. Geleijnse, J.M.; Giltay, E.J.; Grobbee, D.E.; Donders, A.R.T.; Kok, F.J. Blood pressure response to fish oil supplementation: Metaregression analysis of randomized trials. *J. Hypertens.* **2002**, *20*, 1493–1499. [CrossRef] [PubMed]
40. Bonafini, S.; Antoniazzi, F.; Maffeis, C.; Minuz, P.; Fava, C. Beneficial effects of ω-3 PUFA in children on cardiovascular risk factors during childhood and adolescence. *Prostaglandins Other Lipid Mediat.* **2015**. [CrossRef] [PubMed]
41. Damsgaard, C.T.; Schack-Nielsen, L.; Michaelsen, K.F.; Fruekilde, M.B.; Hels, O.; Lauritzen, L. Fish oil affects blood pressure and the plasma lipid profile in healthy Danish infants. *J. Nutr.* **2006**, *136*, 94–99. [CrossRef] [PubMed]
42. Damsgaard, C.T.; Eidner, M.B.; Stark, K.D.; Hjorth, M.F.; Sjödin, A.; Andersen, M.R.; Andersen, R.; Tetens, I.; Astrup, A.; Michaelsen, K.F.; Lauritzen, L. Eicosapentaenoic acid and docosahexaenoic acid in whole blood are differentially and sex-specifically associated with cardiometabolic risk markers in 8-11-year-old danish children. *PLoS ONE* **2014**, *9*, e109368. [CrossRef] [PubMed]
43. Capdevila, J.; Wang, W. Role of cytochrome P450 epoxygenase in regulating renal membrane transport and hypertension. *Curr. Opin. Nephrol. Hypertens.* **2013**, *22*, 163–169. [CrossRef] [PubMed]
44. Minuz, P.; Jiang, H.; Fava, C.; Turolo, L.; Tacconelli, S.; Ricci, M.; Patrignani, P.; Morganti, A.; Lechi, A.; McGiff, J.C. Altered release of cytochrome p450 metabolites of arachidonic acid in renovascular disease. *Hypertension* **2008**, *51*, 1379–1385. [CrossRef] [PubMed]

45. Dalle Vedove, F.; Fava, C.; Jiang, H.; Zanconato, G.; Quilley, J.; Brunelli, M.; Guglielmi, V.; Vattemi, G.; Minuz, P. Increased epoxyeicosatrienoic acids and reduced soluble epoxide hydrolase expression in the preeclamptic placenta. *J. Hypertens.* **2016**, *34*, 1364–1370. [CrossRef] [PubMed]
46. Jiang, H.; McGiff, J.C.; Fava, C.; Amen, G.; Nesta, E.; Zanconato, G.; Quilley, J.; Minuz, P. Maternal and fetal epoxyeicosatrienoic acids in normotensive and preeclamptic pregnancies. *Am. J. Hypertens.* **2013**, *26*, 271–278. [CrossRef] [PubMed]
47. Taddei, S.; Versari, D.; Cipriano, A.; Ghiadoni, L.; Galetta, F.; Franzoni, F.; Magagna, A.; Virdis, A.; Salvetti, A. Identification of a cytochrome P450 2C9-derived endothelium-derived hyperpolarizing factor in essential hypertensive patients. *J. Am. Coll. Cardiol.* **2006**, *48*, 508–515. [CrossRef] [PubMed]
48. Halcox, J.P.; Narayanan, S.; Cramer-Joyce, L.; Mincemoyer, R.; Quyyumi, A.A. Characterization of endothelium-derived hyperpolarizing factor in the human forearm microcirculation. *Am. J. Physiol. Heart Circ. Physiol.* **2001**, *280*, H2470–H2477. [CrossRef] [PubMed]
49. Lee, C.R.; Imig, J.D.; Edin, M.L.; Foley, J.; DeGraff, L.M.; Bradbury, J.A.; Graves, J.P.; Lih, F.B.; Clark, J.; Myers, P.; et al. Endothelial expression of human cytochrome P450 epoxygenases lowers blood pressure and attenuates hypertension-induced renal injury in mice. *FASEB J.* **2010**, *24*, 3770–3781. [CrossRef] [PubMed]
50. Virdis, A.; Cetani, F.; Giannarelli, C.; Banti, C.; Ghiadoni, L.; Ambrogini, E.; Carrara, D.; Pinchera, A.; Taddei, S.; Bernini, G.; et al. The Sulfaphenazole-Sensitive Pathway Acts as a Compensatory Mechanism for Impaired Nitric Oxide Availability in Patients with Primary Hyperparathyroidism. Effect of Surgical Treatment. *J. Clin. Endocrinol. Metab.* **2010**, *95*, 920–927. [CrossRef] [PubMed]
51. Morris, M.C.; Sacks, F.; Rosner, B. Does fish oil lower blood pressure? A meta-analysis of controlled trials. *Circulation* **1993**, *88*, 523–533. [CrossRef] [PubMed]
52. Lynes, M.D.; Leiria, L.O.; Lundh, M.; Bartelt, A.; Shamsi, F.; Huang, T.L.; Takahashi, H.; Hirshman, M.F.; Schlein, C.; Lee, A.; et al. The cold-induced lipokine 12,13-diHOME promotes fatty acid transport into brown adipose tissue. *Nat. Med.* **2017**, *23*, 631–637. [CrossRef] [PubMed]
53. Goodfriend, T.L.; Ball, D.L.; Egan, B.M.; Campbell, W.B.; Nithipatikom, K. Epoxy-Keto Derivative of Linoleic Acid Stimulates Aldosterone Secretion. *Hypertension* **2004**, *43*, 358–363. [CrossRef] [PubMed]
54. Caligiuri, S.P.B.; Love, K.; Winter, T.; Gauthier, J.; Taylor, C.G.; Blydt-Hansen, T.; Zahradka, P.; Aukema, H.M. Dietary linoleic acid and α-linolenic acid differentially affect renal oxylipins and phospholipid fatty acids in diet-induced obese rats. *J. Nutr.* **2013**, *143*, 1421–1431. [CrossRef] [PubMed]
55. Hamazaki, K.; Iso, H.; Eshak, E.S.; Ikehara, S.; Ikeda, A.; Iwasaki, M.; Hamazaki, T.; Tsugane, S.; Grp, J.S. Plasma levels of n-3 fatty acids and risk of coronary heart disease among Japanese: The Japan Public Health Center-based (JPHC) study. *Atherosclerosis* **2018**, *272*, 226–232. [CrossRef] [PubMed]
56. Harris, W.S.; Del Gobbo, L.; Tintle, N.L. The Omega-3 Index and relative risk for coronary heart disease mortality: Estimation from 10 cohort studies. *Atherosclerosis* **2017**, *262*, 51–54. [CrossRef] [PubMed]

16

Genome-Wide Association Studies of Estimated Fatty Acid Desaturase Activity in Serum and Adipose Tissue in Elderly Individuals: Associations with Insulin Sensitivity

Matti Marklund [1,2,*], Andrew P. Morris [3], Anubha Mahajan [4], Erik Ingelsson [5,6,7,8], Cecilia M. Lindgren [4,9], Lars Lind [10] and Ulf Risérus [2]

1 The George Institute for Global Health, University of New South Wales, Sydney, NSW 2042, Australia
2 Department of Public Health and Caring Sciences, Clinical Nutrition and Metabolism, Uppsala University, 751 22 Uppsala, Sweden; ulf.riserus@pubcare.uu.se
3 Department of Biostatistics, University of Liverpool, Liverpool L69 3GL, UK; a.p.morris@liverpool.ac.uk
4 The Wellcome Trust Centre for Human Genetics, Oxford OX3 7BN, UK; anubha@well.ox.ac.uk (A.M.); celi@broadinstitute.org (C.M.L.)
5 Department of Medicine, Division of Cardiovascular Medicine, Stanford University School of Medicine, Stanford, CA 94305, USA; eriking@stanford.edu
6 Stanford Cardiovascular Institute, Stanford University, Stanford, CA 94305, USA
7 Stanford Diabetes Research Center, Stanford University, Stanford, CA 94305, USA
8 Department of Medical Sciences, Molecular Epidemiology, Uppsala University, 751 85 Uppsala, Sweden
9 Li Ka Shing Centre for Health Information and Discovery, The Big Data Institute, University of Oxford, Oxford OX3 7LF, UK
10 Department of Medical Sciences, Cardiovascular Epidemiology, Uppsala University, 751 85 Uppsala, Sweden; lars.lind@medsci.uu.se
* Correspondence: mmarklund@georgeinstitute.org.au

Abstract: Fatty acid desaturases (FADS) catalyze the formation of unsaturated fatty acids and have been related to insulin sensitivity (IS). FADS activities differ between tissues and are influenced by genetic factors that may impact the link to IS. Genome-wide association studies of δ-5-desaturase (D5D), δ-6-desaturase (D6D) and stearoyl-CoA desaturase-1 (SCD) activities (estimated by product-to-precursor ratios of fatty acids analyzed by gas chromatography) in serum cholesterol esters (n = 1453) and adipose tissue (n = 783, all men) were performed in two Swedish population-based cohorts. Genome-wide significant associated loci were evaluated for associations with IS measured with a hyperinsulinemic euglycemic clamp (n = 554). Variants at the *FADS1* were strongly associated with D5D in both cholesterol esters ($p = 1.9 \times 10^{-70}$) and adipose tissue ($p = 1.1 \times 10^{-27}$). Variants in three further loci were associated with D6D in cholesterol esters (*FADS2*, $p = 3.0 \times 10^{-67}$; *PDXDCI*, $p = 4.8 \times 10^{-8}$; and near *MC4R*, $p = 3.7 \times 10^{-8}$) but no associations with D6D in adipose tissue attained genome-wide significance. One locus was associated with SCD in adipose tissue (*PKDL1*, $p = 2.2 \times 10^{-19}$). Genetic variants near *MC4R* were associated with IS ($p = 3.8 \times 10^{-3}$). The *FADS* cluster was the main genetic determinant of estimated FADS activity. However, fatty acid (FA) ratios in adipose tissue and cholesterol esters represent FADS activities in separate tissues and are thus influenced by different genetic factors with potential varying effects on IS.

Keywords: fatty acid; desaturase; Genome-wide association study (GWAS); Insulin sensitivity; adipose tissue; cholesterol ester

1. Introduction

Fatty acid desaturases (FADS) catalyze the formation of mono- and polyunsaturated fatty acid and thus influence the fatty acid (FA) composition of the blood stream and in adipose tissue (AT). The major human FADS include δ-5-desaturase (D5D), δ-6-desaturase (D6D) and δ-9-desaturase or stearoyl-CoA desaturase-1 (SCD). While SCD synthesizes monounsaturated FA from saturated FA, D5D and D6D catalyze the formation of polyunsaturated FA. Since in vivo measurement of enzyme activity can be challenging, ratios of substrate and product concentrations are commonly used to estimate activities of SCD, D6D and D5D [1].

Both circulating fatty acid composition and estimated FADS activities have previously been associated with insulin sensitivity (IS) and incidence of type 2 diabetes (T2D), although the mechanisms underlying these relationships have not been fully determined [2]. It has been suggested that the effects of FADS on IS are mediated by alterations in FA compositions. This could lead to effects on cell membranes (influencing insulin receptor binding and affinity, translocation of glucose transporters and intercellular signaling) and altered levels of polyunsaturated fatty acids (PUFA) which function as ligands for a variety of transcription factors [3]. In addition, polymorphisms in the genes encoding for FADS have been was associated with fasting glucose levels and estimated β-cell function in a large-scale meta-analysis of genome-wide association studies (GWAS) [4].

Genome-wide associations of FADS activity estimated in the circulation have been reported previously and demonstrated that not only variants in desaturase encoding genes are associated with estimated FADS activity [5,6]. However, no prior GWAS have reported associations between genotype and activities of SCD, D5D, or D6D estimated in AT. Furthermore, previous studies investigating relationships between *FADS* polymorphisms and IS have relied on indirect measurements (e.g., fasting glucose and insulin) instead of gold standard methodology, such as the hyperinsulinemic euglycemic clamp.

The aim of the present study was to perform GWAS of FA metabolizing enzymes in AT and serum cholesterol esters (CE) in participants of the Uppsala Longitudinal Study of Adult Men (ULSAM) and the Prospective Investigation of the Vasculature in Uppsala Seniors (PIVUS). Subsequently, analyses were performed to investigate relationships between desaturase-associated genetic variants and cardiometabolic risk factors, including IS assessed by hyperinsulinemic euglycemic clamp.

2. Materials and Methods

2.1. Study Samples

Details about The Uppsala Longitudinal Study of Adult Men (ULSAM) are available in previous publications [7] and online at http://www.pubcare.uu.se/ulsam/. In brief, at the first collection time-point, all 50-year-old men living in Uppsala County, Sweden, 1970–74, were invited. The present study includes individuals at the re-examination undertaken from August 1991 to May 1995 at the approximate age of 71 years, where 1221 out of 1681 invited individuals participated (73% of those still alive and living in Uppsala). For the present study, we excluded individuals with missing microarray genotyping data (n = 5), failing sample quality control (QC) (n = 37), or missing all estimates of FADS activity (n = 615, cholesterol esters; n = 396, adipose tissue).

A detailed study description of The Prospective Investigation of the Vasculature in Uppsala Seniors (PIVUS) has been published previously [8] and additional information can be found at http://www.medsci.uu.se/pivus/pivus.htm. In brief, all 70-year-old individuals living in Uppsala County, Sweden, between April 2001 and June 2004 were eligible for the study, out of which 2025 randomly selected subjects were invited. In total, 1016 subjects (50% women) participated and were examined within one month of their 70th birthday to standardize for age. For the present study, we excluded individuals with missing microarray genotyping data (n = 34), failing sample QC (n = 33), or missing all outcome measurements (n = 60).

Both the ULSAM and PIVUS studies were approved by the ethics committee of Uppsala University and all participants provided written informed consent.

2.2. Assessments of Fatty Acid Composition and Enzyme Activities

Procedures for measurements of fatty acid composition in ULSAM and PIVUS have previously been described in detail [9,10]. Briefly, FA were measured in CE from blood samples drawn after an overnight fast, during which both medication and smoking were disallowed. A hexane-isopropanol solution was used to extract serum, from which cholesterol esters were separated by thin-layer chromatography followed by inter-esterification with acidic methanol. Free cholesterol was removed by aluminum oxide to avoid contamination of the column. The relative proportion of methylated FA was determined by gas chromatography (25-m NB-351 silica capillary column) with a coefficient of variation <5.0%. In addition, FA in subcutaneous AT were analyzed in ULSAM as previously described [10]. An estimate of enzyme activity was calculated as the product-to-substrate ratio; 20:4n−6/20:3n−6 for D5D, 18:3n−6/18:2n−6 for D6D and 16:1/16:0 for SCD.

2.3. Assessments of Cardiometabolic Risk Factors

Body mass index (BMI) was calculated as the ratio of body weight (in kg) to height (in m) squared. Concentrations of cholesterol and triglycerides were measured in serum and in isolated lipoprotein fractions by enzymatic techniques utilizing Instrumentation Laboratories (IL) Test Cholesterol Trinders's Method and IL Test enzymatic-colorimetric method for use in a monarch apparatus (Instrumentation Laboratories, Lexington, MA, USA). High-density lipoprotein (HDL) particles were separated by precipitation with magnesium chloride/phosphotungstate. IS was directly measured in the ULSAM cohort using the hyperinsulinemic euglycemic clamp, as previously described [11]. In addition, indices of insulin resistance (HOMA-IR) were assessed in both ULSAM and PIVUS as calculated using fasting concentrations of plasma glucose and insulin.

2.4. Preparation of Genotype Data

Genotyping was performed using the Illumina OmniExpress and Illumina Metabochip in PIVUS and Illumina Omni2.5M and Illumina Metabochip in ULSAM. General sample exclusion criteria included: (1) genotype call rate <95%; (2) heterozygosity >3 SD from mean; (3) gender discordance; (4) duplicated samples; (5) identity-by-descent match; and (6) ethnic outliers. General single nucleotide polymorphism (SNP) exclusion criteria of genotyped data before imputation included: (1) monomorphic SNPs; (2) Hardy-Weinberg equilibrium (HWE) p-value $<1 \times 10^{-6}$; (3) genotype call rate < 99% (SNPs with minor allele frequency (MAF) < 5%) or < 95% (SNPs with MAF $\geq$ 5%); (4) MAF < 1%. In ULSAM, for Omni2.5, further SNP exclusions were made if a SNP had large position disagreements, did not map in the genome, mapped more than once in the genome or had bad probe assays.

In PIVUS, 949 out of 982 samples passed QC for the OmniExpress; and Metabochip with the exclusions listed in Table S1. The genotyped data in PIVUS used in the present study consisted of 738,879 SNPs after QC. In ULSAM, 1179 out of 1216 samples passed QC for the Omni2.5 and Metabochip, with the exclusions listed in Table S1. The genotyped data in ULSAM consisted of 1,621,833 SNPs after QC. Imputation was performed for the quality-controlled genotype data of each cohort with IMPUTE v.2.2.2 using haplotypes from the 1000 Genomes, March 2012 release (multi-ethnic panel on NCBI build 37 (b37)). Population substructures in the genotype data were captured using multidimensional scaling (MDS) of a genetic relationship matrix (genome file) constructed on the basis of linkage disequilibrium (LD)-pruned SNPs in PLINK 1.07 [12].

2.5. Statistical Analysis

Estimated enzyme activity levels were normalized using Blom's inverse normal transformation. Regression analyses of genetic variants and estimated desaturase activities were adjusted for the first two principal components of the MDS analysis. All regression analyses of the autosomes in ULSAM and PIVUS were performed separately in each study and then combined in sample size-weighted Z-score meta-analysis assuming fixed effects in the software METAL. [13] The same settings were used in the analysis of the X-chromosome as for the autosomes, with the exception that the analyses in PIVUS were stratified on gender before combining the results in the meta-analysis.

To identify single common variants associated with the estimated enzyme activity in CE, a genome-wide association analysis was performed using the score-based test in SNPTEST 2.4.1. (manufacturer, city, country) [14] Common variants (MAF $\geq$ 5%) available in both studies and with an information quality metric $\geq$ 0.4 were included in the analyses. A p-value $< 5 \times 10^{-8}$ was considered to be genome-wide significant in these analyses. Further, to identify independent variants in each locus associated with enzyme activity levels, a forward selection conditional analysis was performed, where independent signals were considered down to a p-value of ~1×10^{-5}. In addition, genome-wide association analyses of the estimated enzyme activity in AT were performed in ULSAM only.

A lookup was performed for the significant SNPs in the single variant analyses using literature and publicly available databases including RegulomeDB version 1.1 (http://www.regulomedb.org/) [15], GTEx (http://www.gtexportal.org/home/) [16], Metabolomics GWAS server (http://mips.helmholtz-muenchen.de/proj/GWAS/gwas/) [5,6] and PhenoScanner (http://www.phenoscanner.medschl.cam.ac.uk/phenoscanner) [17].

Associations of identified variants with cardiometabolic risk factors including triglycerides, HDL-C, BMI and HOMA-IR were assessed by linear regression in ULSAM and PIVUS separately and subsequently meta-analyzed using sample size-weighted fixed effects models. Similarly, associations between the same variants and M-value determined by hyperinsulinemic euglycemic clamp were assessed in ULSAM using linear regression models. For these associations between desaturase-associated loci and cardiometabolic risk factors, false discovery rate was used to correct for multiple testing [18].

3. Results

The clinical characteristics of individuals with available genotype and cholesterol ester fatty acid data in ULSAM (n = 564) and PIVUS (n = 889) are shown in Table 1. In addition, a number of men (n = 783) in ULSAM also had data available on genotype and desaturase activity assessed in adipose tissue. The correlation between the estimated enzyme activity in CE and AT was low to moderate for D5D (r = 0.36, p < 0.0001), D6D (r = 0.10, p = 0.098) and SCD (r = 0.40, p < 0.0001).

Table 1. Clinical characteristics of individuals in ULSAM and PIVUS with genotype data and estimated desaturase activity in cholesterol esters. [1]

	ULSAM (n = 564)	PIVUS (n = 889)
Age	71.3 (0.4)	70.2 (0.2)
Women (%)	0	49
BMI (kg/m^2)	26.3 (3.4)	27.0 (4.4)
Antihypertensive treatment (%)	37	31
Total cholesterol (mmol/L)	5.8 (1.0)	5.4 (1.0)
HDL cholesterol (mmol/L)	1.3 (0.3)	1.5 (0.4)
Triglycerides (mmol/L)	1.5 (0.8)	1.3 (0.6)
Lipid lowering treatment (%)	9.4	15.9
Fasting plasma glucose (mmol/L)	5.8 (1.5)	6.0 (1.8)
Glucose disposal, M (mg/kg/min)	5.2 (2.1)	N/A
Diabetes treatment (%)	6.5	6.5
Never smokers (%)	40	48
Previous smokers (%)	40	41
Current smokers (%)	20	11

Values are mean (SD) or percentage. [1] PIVUS, Prospective Investigation of Uppsala Seniors; ULSAM, Uppsala Longitudinal Study of Adult Men; HDL, high-density lipoprotein; BMI, body mass index; M, in vivo insulin-mediated glucose disposal.

3.1. GWAS of Desaturase Activity

Quantile-quantile plots of p-values from the single variant association test of the enzyme activities showed no systematic deviation from the null (data not shown). Variation in one locus (fatty acid desaturase 1, *FADS1*) was associated with D5D and variants in or near three loci were associated with D6D (fatty acid desaturase 2, *FADS2*; pyridoxal-dependent decarboxylase domain containing 1, *PDXDC1*/N-terminal asparagine amidase, *NTAN1*; and near melanocortin 4 receptor, *MC4R*) (Figures S1 and S2). The significant lead variant for CE-D5D was also significant when analyzed in AT (Figure 1), unlike D6D, where no signal could be seen in AT (Table 2). No locus was significantly associated with CE-SCD (Figure S3) but one variant close to *SCD*, in polycystic kidney disease 2-like 1 (*PKD2L1*), was significantly associated with AT-SCD, which was analyzed in ULSAM (Table 2). The same direction of effect was seen for CE-SCD, though the association was weaker ($P = 1.6 \times 10^{-4}$).

By conditional association tests of the *FADS1-FADS2-FADS3* region, in a forward selection approach, two SNPs (rs174549, rs968567) were independently associated with CE-D5D and two SNPs (rs138194593, rs2072113) were independently associated with CE-D6D (Table S2). The four SNPs were not in strong LD ($R2 \leq 0.40$) with each other.

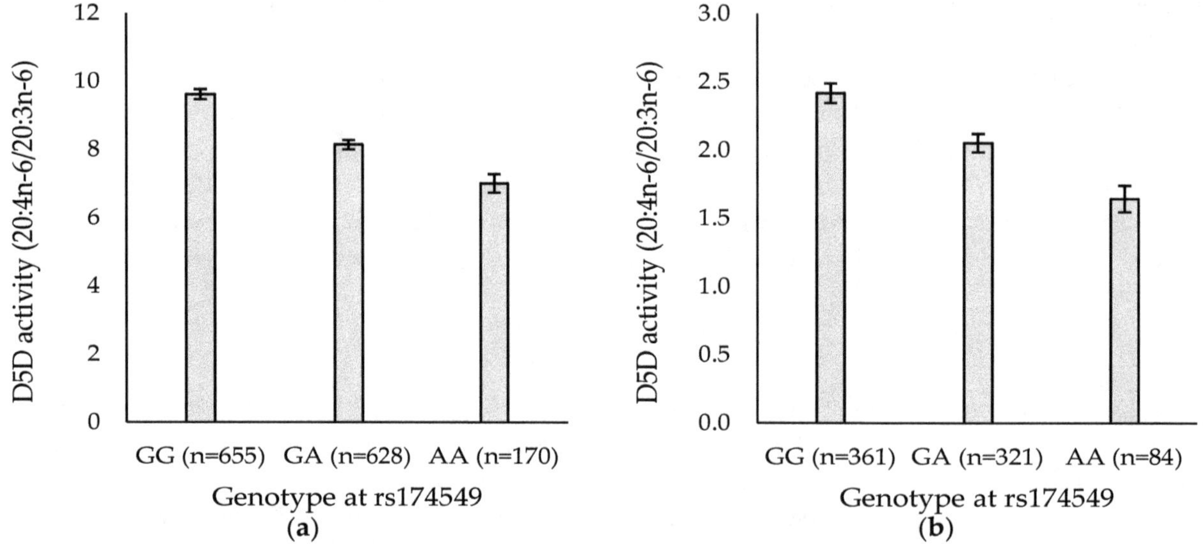

Figure 1. Estimated δ-5-desaturase (D5D) activity in cholesterol esters (**a**) and adipose tissue (**b**) by genotype at rs174549. Values are means and error bars represent 95% confidence intervals of means. D5D activity was estimated as the ratio of arachidonic acid (20:4n−6) and dihomo-gamma-linolenic acid (20:3n−6).

3.2. SNP Lookup

Database searches revealed that the variants independently associated with D5D activity are located in transcription factor binding regions (cited in RegulomeDB [15]) and have been associated with expression of *FADS1* and *FADS2* in diverse tissues (cited in GTEx [16]). In previous GWAS, the two SNPs independently associated with D5D (or variants in full LD) have been linked to circulating polyunsaturated fatty acids [6,19–22]. In studies utilizing candidate SNP approaches, the same SNPs have been associated with FA and ratios thereof in circulation and tissue [23–27].

The lead variant associated with estimated D6D activity, rs138194593, is located in an intronic region of the *FADS2* gene and has been associated with *FADS2* expression in blood from Estonian coronary artery disease patients [28]. The second independent D6D-associated SNP in the *FADS2* gene, rs2072113, or proxies in full LD have been associated to *FADS* expression (as cited in GTEx [16]) and been linked to circulating PUFA in previous GWAS [5,6,19,21]. Another variant linked with D6D activity, rs6498540, is located in *PDXDC1* and has been associated with circulating PUFA and FA ratios [6,21].

Table 2. Common variants (MAF $\geq$ 5%) with $p < 1 \times 10^{-8}$. [a]

Desaturase	Gene	Lead SNP	Chr:Position (b37)	EAF	Effect Allele/ Other Allele	Serum			Adipose Tissue		
						Direction	*p*	*n*	Direction	*p*	*n*
D5D	*FADS1*	rs174549	11:61571382	0.33	A/G	–	1.9×10^{-70}	1448	–	1.1×10^{-27}	766
D6D	*FADS2*	rs138194593	11:61620703	0.63	CTCTT/C	+	3.0×10^{-67}	1448	–	7.9×10^{-1}	611
D6D	*PDXDC1*	rs6498540	16:15130594	0.71	A/G	+	4.8×10^{-8}	1448	–	2.9×10^{-1}	611
D6D	near *MC4R*	rs9957425	18:57462103	0.61	T/C	+	3.7×10^{-8}	1448	–	9.0×10^{-1}	611
SCD	*PKD2L1*	rs603424	10:102075479	0.14	A/G	–	1.6×10^{-4}	1453	–	2.2×10^{-19}	783

[a] A, adenine; C, cytosine; Chr, chromosome; b37, NCBI build 37; D5D, δ-5-desaturase; D6D, δ-6-desaturase; EAF, effect allele frequency; *FADS1*, fatty acid desaturase 1; *FADS2*, fatty acid desaturase 2; G, guanine; *MC4R*, melanocortin 4 receptor; *PDXDC1*, pyridoxal-dependent decarboxylase domain containing 1; *PKD2L1*, polycystic kidney disease 2-like 1; SCD, Stearoyl-CoA desaturase; T, thymine.

In addition, rs6498540 is in perfect LD with rs4500751, a SNP in a transcription binding region (as cited in RegulomeDB [15]) close to *PDXDC1* and *NTAN1* that has been associated with circulating PUFA and ratios thereof in previous GWAS [5,6,29]. This SNP is also located 300 kb from *PLAG10*, a gene involved in phospholipid metabolism, possibly with a fatty-acid specific mechanism [29]. The top SNP of the third locus associated with D6D activity, rs9957425, is not in strong LD with other SNPs ($r^2 < 0.32$) and is not likely in a transcript factor binding region but may affect epigenetic modifications (as cited in RegulomeDB [15]). It has not yet been associated with circulating FA or FA ratios and has not been strongly associated ($p \geq 0.02$) with any traits in the GWAS included in the Metabolomic GWAS scanner [5,6] or PhenoScanner [17]. The variant is located 576 kb downstream of *MC4R*, in close proximity to a region strongly associated with diabetes and related traits.

The variant associated with AT-SCD, rs603424 in the *PKLD1* gene, is located 31 kb from the SCD gene [29] and has previously been associated with adipose SCD expression and circulating saturated fatty acids, monounsaturated fatty acids and ratios thereof [5,29,30].

3.3. Associations of Identified Loci with Metabolic Traits

After correcting for multiple testing, the lead SNP at one of the loci significantly associated with estimated D6D activity, rs9957425, was associated with BMI ($p = 7.4 \times 10^{-4}$) and plasma triglycerides ($p = 2.1 \times 10^{-3}$) in a meta-analysis of ULSAM and PIVUS data (Table 3). The same locus was also associated to M-value in ULSAM ($p = 3.8 \times 10^{-3}$). Associations of the other loci with BMI, HOMA-IR, M-value plasma HDL, triglycerides, or M-value were not evident after correcting for multiple testing (Table 3). All significant loci from the single variant analysis, except rs603424 (*PKD2L1*, close to *SCD*), were associated with HDL cholesterol or triglycerides ($p < 0.05$) in a large meta-analysis of lipid values (Table S3) [31]. In additional lookups of published data, no significant associations were seen for HOMA-IR [4] and only rs6498540 showed some evidence of association for BMI [32].

Table 3. Associations of significant desaturase loci with BMI and metabolic traits. [a]

Gene	rs ID [b]	Chr:Position (b37)	Effect Allele	EAF	ULSAM + PIVUS Meta-Analysis (n = 1453)								ULSAM (n = 564)	
					HDL Cholesterol		Triglycerides		BMI		HOMA-IR		M-Value	
					Direction	p	Direction	p	Direction	p	Direction	p	Direction	p
FADS1	rs174549	11:61571382	A	0.33	−	2.0×10^{-2}	+	1.8×10^{-1}	+	5.4×10^{-1}	+	6.9×10^{-1}	−	7.6×10^{-1}
FADS2	rs968567	11:61595564	T	0.15	−	2.4×10^{-1}	+	5.5×10^{-1}	+	1.1×10^{-1}	+	5.6×10^{-2}	−	2.1×10^{-1}
FADS2	rs138194593	11:61620703	CTCTT	0.63	+	9.3×10^{-3}	−	4.2×10^{-1}	−	1.8×10^{-1}	−	7.9×10^{-1}	+	5.3×10^{-1}
FADS2	rs2072113	11:61604967	T	0.17	−	7.6×10^{-2}	+	3.9×10^{-1}	−	7.3×10^{-1}	−	2.5×10^{-1}	+	5.8×10^{-1}
PDXDC1	rs6498540	16:15130594	A	0.71	+	7.8×10^{-1}	−	8.5×10^{-1}	−	4.2×10^{-1}	+	3.7×10^{-1}	+	7.6×10^{-1}
near *MC4R*	rs9957425	18:57462103	T	0.61	−	2.2×10^{-1}	+ [c]	2.1×10^{-3}	+ [c]	7.4×10^{-4}	+	7.1×10^{-2}	− [c]	3.8×10^{-3}
PKD2L1	rs603424	10:102075479	A	0.14	+	8.4×10^{-1}	+	5.2×10^{-1}	+	8.8×10^{-1}	+	8.8×10^{-1}	−	7.6×10^{-2}

[a] Chr, chromosome; b37, NCBI build 37; EAF, effect allele frequency; *FADS1*, fatty acid desaturase 1; *FADS2*, fatty acid desaturase 2; *PDXDC1*, pyridoxal-dependent decarboxylase domain containing 1; *MC4R*, melanocortin 4 receptor; *PKD2L1*, polycystic kidney disease 2-like 1; PIVUS, Prospective Investigation of Uppsala Seniors; ULSAM, Uppsala Longitudinal Study of Adult Men; HDL, high-density lipoprotein; BMI, body mass index; HOMA-IR, homeostasis model assessment of insulin resistance. [b] Reference SNP ID number. [c] Significant association after adjustment for multiple testing.

4. Discussion

In the present study, five loci were associated at a genome-wide significant level with estimated activities of D5D, D6D, or SCD in the two population-based Swedish cohort studies ULSAM and PIVUS. One of these loci, downstream of *MC4R*, was additionally associated to BMI and triglycerides in the combined study populations; and to M-value in ULSAM, after correcting for multiple testing.

Most variants identified in the present study or proxies in perfect LD have been associated with circulating FAs, ratios thereof or *FADS* gene expression in previous GWAS [5,6,19–22,28–30]. However, one novel variant near the *MC4R* gene was identified. Polymorphisms downstream of the *MC4R* gene are among the strongest genetic determinants of BMI and they have been associated with food preference, IS and HDL [33]. Estimated D6D activity has likewise previously been positively associated to obesity [34,35] and it can be speculated that the observed associations of rs9957425 with desaturase activity, BMI and IS are due to MC4R-mediated effects on food and fatty acid intake, which could influence FA proportions and thereby the FA ratio used for estimating D6D activity.

As expected, the strongest associations with estimated D5D and D6D activities in ULSAM and PIVUS were observed with variants mapped to the *FADS* cluster, which supports the use of FA ratios as estimates of desaturase activity. Polymorphism in FADS encoding genes may be directly linked to IS and T2D [36]; however, identification of such associations could be hampered by high LD in the *FADS* region and pleiotropy of the *FADS* genes. Most genetic variants associated with FADS activity were linked to blood lipid levels in meta-analysis of published GWAS [31], supporting the relationships between FADS activity and development of metabolic syndrome [37]. Thus, it is a challenge to disentangle the potential direct role of *FADS* gene variants on IS, from that of closely related metabolic disorders such as triglycerides and HDL.

The correlations between the estimated enzyme activities in CE and AT observed in the present study confirm results from a previous study in which activities of D5D and SCD in AT and serum were correlated in Swedish men and women [35]. In that study, D6D activity estimated in AT was correlated with that estimated in phospholipids but not non-esterified serum FA. Another study reported that estimated enzyme activities of D5D, D6D and SCD in serum (calculated from total FA in serum) were highly correlated with corresponding activities in liver tissue but not in AT [38]. Similarly, enzyme activities of fatty acid desaturases estimated in different plasma lipid fractions are not ubiquitously correlated, though enzyme activities estimated in cholesteryl esters used in the present study are considered to reflect hepatic fatty acid desaturation [35,39].

Associations between gene expression and enzyme activity of SCD have been observed in liver [40], AT [41] and brain [42]. It should be noted that SCD gene expression may differ in different adipose tissue depots and we have reported that SCD gene expression was correlated with estimated SCD activity in subcutaneous but not in visceral adipose tissue [43].

Similar associations for D5D have been observed in brain [42] and for D6D in liver [40]. Although product-to-substrate ratios are indirect measurements of enzyme activity and their accuracy has been questioned [44,45], FA ratios correlate with direct enzyme activity measurements (by isotope tracer) [46]. The FA composition of CE is regulated in the liver and plasma, while the composition in AT is influenced by adipose metabolism [47]. For example, FA are released from AT by lipase-catalyzed lipolysis and diverse mobilization of individual FA from AT that could affect the ability of FA ratios to estimate enzyme activity in AT [48]. Hence, as FA ratios in CE and AT represent desaturase activities in various tissues (i.e., liver, plasma and adipocytes) they may be affected by diverse genetic determinants.

A major strength of the present study is the availability of data on FADS activity estimated in both AT and serum and to our knowledge this is the first GWAS of adipose FADS activity. Furthermore,

IS was assessed both by the gold standard methodology hyperinsulinemic euglycemic clamp and calculated using HOMA-IR. The combination of the two cohorts, ULSAM and PIVUS resulted in dataset consisting of men and women with measured FA composition.

The relatively small sample size of the two cohorts utilized is a limitation of the present study. Also, data on adipose FADS activity and M-value were only available in one of the cohorts, ULSAM. As the two cohorts consist of individuals from the same geographical location, there is a possibility that the two study population are too homogeneous and thus the possibility to identify associations between genes and fatty acid metabolism are hampered by low genetic variation. Further, the generalizability to other ethnicities is unknown.

Our findings have implications for future research. First, our findings support the use of FA ratios as indirect estimates of desaturase activity, given that the variants most strongly associated with FA ratios were located in or near desaturase encoding genes. However, certain lipid fractions may be less suitable to assess desaturase activity by FA ratios as suggested by the inconsistency in loci associated with D6D and SCD in different fractions. In addition, our findings warrant further evaluation of rs9957425, associated with both desaturase activity and cardiometabolic traits.

5. Conclusions

In conclusion, the activities of FADS estimated in CE and AT were associated with variants in or near five independent loci (*FADS1*, *FADS2*, *MC4R*, *PDKL1* and *PDXDC1*). One of the loci (*FADS1*) was associated with FADS activity in both CE and AT. One variant associated with estimated D6D activity (rs9957425 near *MC4R*) was additionally was associated to BMI, TG and intravenously assessed IS. Activities of D5D and SCD estimated in CE and AT were correlated, while no correlation was observed for D6D activity estimated in the different tissues.

Author Contributions: Conceptualization, M.M., E.I. and U.R.; formal analysis, A.M.; investigation, M.M. and A.M.; resources, L.L. and U.R.; writing—original draft preparation, M.M.; writing—review and editing, M.M., A.P.M., A.M., E.I., C.M.L., L.L. and U.R.; visualization, M.M.; supervision, U.R.; funding acquisition, M.M., U.R. and C.M.L.

Acknowledgments: We thank Mohammed Bajahzer for assistance in graphical presentation and we acknowledge the participants of PIVUS and ULSAM.

References

1. Warensjö, E.; Risérus, U.; Gustafsson, I.-B.; Mohsen, R.; Cederholm, T.; Vessby, B. Effects of saturated and unsaturated fatty acids on estimated desaturase activities during a controlled dietary intervention. *Nutr. Metab. Cardiovasc. Dis.* **2008**, *18*, 683–690. [CrossRef] [PubMed]
2. Vessby, B.; Gustafsson, I.B.; Tengblad, S.; Boberg, M.; Andersson, A. Desaturation and elongation of Fatty acids and insulin action. *Ann. N. Y. Acad. Sci.* **2002**, *967*, 183–195. [CrossRef] [PubMed]
3. Kroger, J.; Schulze, M.B. Recent insights into the relation of Delta5 desaturase and Delta6 desaturase activity to the development of type 2 diabetes. *Curr. Opin. Lipidol.* **2012**, *23*, 4–10. [CrossRef] [PubMed]

4. Dupuis, J.; Langenberg, C.; Prokopenko, I.; Saxena, R.; Soranzo, N.; Jackson, A.U.; Wheeler, E.; Glazer, N.L.; Bouatia-Naji, N.; Gloyn, A.L.; et al. New genetic loci implicated in fasting glucose homeostasis and their impact on type 2 diabetes risk. *Nat. Genet.* **2010**, *42*, 105–116. [CrossRef] [PubMed]
5. Suhre, K.; Shin, S.Y.; Petersen, A.K.; Mohney, R.P.; Meredith, D.; Wagele, B.; Altmaier, E.; Deloukas, P.; Erdmann, J.; Grundberg, E.; et al. Human metabolic individuality in biomedical and pharmaceutical research. *Nature* **2011**, *477*, 54–60. [CrossRef] [PubMed]
6. Shin, S.Y.; Fauman, E.B.; Petersen, A.K.; Krumsiek, J.; Santos, R.; Huang, J.; Arnold, M.; Erte, I.; Forgetta, V.; Yang, T.P.; et al. An atlas of genetic influences on human blood metabolites. *Nat. Genet.* **2014**, *46*, 543–550. [CrossRef] [PubMed]
7. Hedstrand, H. A study of middle-aged men with particular reference to risk factors for cardiovascular disease. *Upsala J. Med. Sci. Suppl.* **1975**, *19*, 1–61.
8. Lind, L.; Fors, N.; Hall, J.; Marttala, K.; Stenborg, A. A comparison of three different methods to evaluate endothelium-dependent vasodilation in the elderly: The Prospective Investigation of the Vasculature in Uppsala Seniors (PIVUS) study. *Arterioscler. Thromb. Vasc. Biol.* **2005**, *25*, 2368–2375. [CrossRef] [PubMed]
9. Rosqvist, F.; Bjermo, H.; Kullberg, J.; Johansson, L.; Michaëlsson, K.; Ahlström, H.; Lind, L.; Risérus, U. Fatty acid composition in serum cholesterol esters and phospholipids is linked to visceral and subcutaneous adipose tissue content in elderly individuals: A cross-sectional study. *Lipids Health Dis.* **2017**, *16*, 68. [CrossRef] [PubMed]
10. Iggman, D.; Arnlov, J.; Cederholm, T.; Riserus, U. Association of Adipose Tissue Fatty Acids with Cardiovascular and All-Cause Mortality in Elderly Men. *JAMA Cardiol.* **2016**, *1*, 745–753. [CrossRef] [PubMed]
11. Nerpin, E.; Riserus, U.; Ingelsson, E.; Sundstrom, J.; Jobs, M.; Larsson, A.; Basu, S.; Arnlov, J. Insulin sensitivity measured with euglycemic clamp is independently associated with glomerular filtration rate in a community-based cohort. *Diabetes Care* **2008**, *31*, 1550–1555. [CrossRef] [PubMed]
12. Purcell, S.; Neale, B.; Todd-Brown, K.; Thomas, L.; Ferreira, M.A.; Bender, D.; Maller, J.; Sklar, P.; de Bakker, P.I.; Daly, M.J.; et al. PLINK: A tool set for whole-genome association and population-based linkage analyses. *Am. J. Hum. Genet.* **2007**, *81*, 559–575. [CrossRef] [PubMed]
13. Willer, C.J.; Li, Y.; Abecasis, G.R. METAL: Fast and efficient meta-analysis of genomewide association scans. *Bioinformatics* **2010**, *26*, 2190–2191. [CrossRef] [PubMed]
14. Marchini, J.; Howie, B. Genotype imputation for genome-wide association studies. *Nat. Rev. Genet.* **2010**, *11*, 499–511. [CrossRef] [PubMed]
15. Boyle, A.P.; Hong, E.L.; Hariharan, M.; Cheng, Y.; Schaub, M.A.; Kasowski, M.; Karczewski, K.J.; Park, J.; Hitz, B.C.; Weng, S.; et al. Annotation of functional variation in personal genomes using RegulomeDB. *Genome Res.* **2012**, *22*, 1790–1797. [CrossRef] [PubMed]
16. The Genotype-Tissue Expression (GTEx) project. *Nat. Genet.* **2013**, *45*, 580–585. [CrossRef] [PubMed]
17. Staley, J.R.; Blackshaw, J.; Kamat, M.A.; Ellis, S.; Surendran, P.; Sun, B.B.; Paul, D.S.; Freitag, D.; Burgess, S.; Danesh, J.; et al. PhenoScanner: A database of human genotype-phenotype associations. *Bioinformatics* **2016**, *32*, 3207–3209. [CrossRef] [PubMed]
18. Benjamini, Y.; Hochberg, Y. Controlling the false discovery rate: A practical and powerful approach to multiple testing. *J. R. Stat. Soc. Ser. B Methodol.* **1995**, *57*, 289–300.
19. Lemaitre, R.N.; Tanaka, T.; Tang, W.; Manichaikul, A.; Foy, M.; Kabagambe, E.K.; Nettleton, J.A.; King, I.B.; Weng, L.C.; Bhattacharya, S.; et al. Genetic loci associated with plasma phospholipid n-3 fatty acids: A meta-analysis of genome-wide association studies from the CHARGE Consortium. *PLoS Genet.* **2011**, *7*, e1002193. [CrossRef] [PubMed]
20. Voruganti, V.S.; Higgins, P.B.; Ebbesson, S.O.; kennish, J.; Goring, H.H.; Haack, K.; Laston, S.; Drigalenko, E.; Wenger, C.R.; Harris, W.; et al. Variants in CPT1A, FADS1, and FADS2 are associated with higher levels of estimated plasma and erythrocyte delta 5 desaturases in Alaskan Eskimos. *Front. Genet.* **2012**, *3*. [CrossRef] [PubMed]
21. Kettunen, J.; Tukiainen, T.; Sarin, A.P.; Ortega-Alonso, A.; Tikkanen, E.; Lyytikainen, L.P.; Kangas, A.J.; Soininen, P.; Wurtz, P.; Silander, K.; et al. Genome-wide association study identifies multiple loci influencing human serum metabolite levels. *Nat. Genet.* **2012**, *44*, 269–276. [CrossRef] [PubMed]

22. Guan, W.; Steffen, B.T.; Lemaitre, R.N.; Wu, J.H.; Tanaka, T.; Manichaikul, A.; Foy, M.; Rich, S.S.; Wang, L.; Nettleton, J.A.; et al. Genome-wide association study of plasma N6 polyunsaturated fatty acids within the cohorts for heart and aging research in genomic epidemiology consortium. *Circ. Cardiovasc. Genet.* **2014**, *7*, 321–331. [CrossRef] [PubMed]
23. Bokor, S.; Dumont, J.; Spinneker, A.; Gonzalez-Gross, M.; Nova, E.; Widhalm, K.; Moschonis, G.; Stehle, P.; Amouyel, P.; De Henauw, S.; et al. Single nucleotide polymorphisms in the FADS gene cluster are associated with delta-5 and delta-6 desaturase activities estimated by serum fatty acid ratios. *J. Lipid Res.* **2010**, *51*, 2325–2333. [CrossRef] [PubMed]
24. Koletzko, B.; Lattka, E.; Zeilinger, S.; Illig, T.; Steer, C. Genetic variants of the fatty acid desaturase gene cluster predict amounts of red blood cell docosahexaenoic and other polyunsaturated fatty acids in pregnant women: Findings from the Avon Longitudinal Study of Parents and Children. *Am. J. Clin. Nutr.* **2011**, *93*, 211–219. [CrossRef] [PubMed]
25. Merino, D.M.; Johnston, H.; Clarke, S.; Roke, K.; Nielsen, D.; Badawi, A.; El-Sohemy, A.; Ma, D.W.; Mutch, D.M. Polymorphisms in FADS1 and FADS2 alter desaturase activity in young Caucasian and Asian adults. *Mol. Genet. Metab.* **2011**, *103*, 171–178. [CrossRef] [PubMed]
26. Aslibekyan, S.; Jensen, M.K.; Campos, H.; Linkletter, C.D.; Loucks, E.B.; Ordovas, J.M.; Deka, R.; Rimm, E.B.; Baylin, A. Fatty Acid desaturase gene variants, cardiovascular risk factors, and myocardial infarction in the costa rica study. *Front. Genet.* **2012**, *3*, 72. [CrossRef] [PubMed]
27. Freemantle, E.; Lalovic, A.; Mechawar, N.; Turecki, G. Age and Haplotype Variations within FADS1 Interact and Associate with Alterations in Fatty Acid Composition in Human Male Cortical Brain Tissue. *PLoS ONE* **2012**, *7*. [CrossRef] [PubMed]
28. Franzén, O.; Ermel, R.; Cohain, A.; Akers, N.K.; Di Narzo, A.; Talukdar, H.A.; Foroughi-Asl, H.; Giambartolomei, C.; Fullard, J.F.; Sukhavasi, K.; et al. Cardiometabolic risk loci share downstream cis- and trans-gene regulation across tissues and diseases. *Science* **2016**, *353*, 827–830. [CrossRef] [PubMed]
29. Demirkan, A.; van Duijn, C.M.; Ugocsai, P.; Isaacs, A.; Pramstaller, P.P.; Liebisch, G.; Wilson, J.F.; Johansson, A.; Rudan, I.; Aulchenko, Y.S.; et al. Genome-wide association study identifies novel loci associated with circulating phospho- and sphingolipid concentrations. *PLoS Genet.* **2012**, *8*, e1002490. [CrossRef] [PubMed]
30. Wu, J.H.; Lemaitre, R.N.; Manichaikul, A.; Guan, W.; Tanaka, T.; Foy, M.; Kabagambe, E.K.; Djousse, L.; Siscovick, D.; Fretts, A.M.; et al. Genome-wide association study identifies novel loci associated with concentrations of four plasma phospholipid fatty acids in the de novo lipogenesis pathway: Results from the Cohorts for Heart and Aging Research in Genomic Epidemiology (CHARGE) consortium. *Circ. Cardiovasc. Genet.* **2013**, *6*, 171–183. [CrossRef] [PubMed]
31. Willer, C.J.; Schmidt, E.M.; Sengupta, S.; Peloso, G.M.; Gustafsson, S.; Kanoni, S.; Ganna, A.; Chen, J.; Buchkovich, M.L.; Mora, S.; et al. Discovery and refinement of loci associated with lipid levels. *Nat. Genet.* **2013**, *45*, 1274–1283. [CrossRef] [PubMed]
32. Locke, A.E.; Kahali, B.; Berndt, S.I.; Justice, A.E.; Pers, T.H.; Day, F.R.; Powell, C.; Vedantam, S.; Buchkovich, M.L.; Yang, J.; et al. Genetic studies of body mass index yield new insights for obesity biology. *Nature* **2015**, *518*, 197–206. [CrossRef] [PubMed]
33. Loos, R.J.; Lindgren, C.M.; Li, S.; Wheeler, E.; Zhao, J.H.; Prokopenko, I.; Inouye, M.; Freathy, R.M.; Attwood, A.P.; Beckmann, J.S.; et al. Common variants near MC4R are associated with fat mass, weight and risk of obesity. *Nat. Genet.* **2008**, *40*, 768–775. [CrossRef] [PubMed]
34. Warensjo, E.; Ohrvall, M.; Vessby, B. Fatty acid composition and estimated desaturase activities are associated with obesity and lifestyle variables in men and women. *Nutr. Metab. Cardiovasc. Dis.* **2006**, *16*, 128–136. [CrossRef] [PubMed]
35. Warensjo, E.; Rosell, M.; Hellenius, M.L.; Vessby, B.; De Faire, U.; Riserus, U. Associations between estimated fatty acid desaturase activities in serum lipids and adipose tissue in humans: Links to obesity and insulin resistance. *Lipids Health Dis.* **2009**, *8*, 37. [CrossRef] [PubMed]
36. Kroger, J.; Zietemann, V.; Enzenbach, C.; Weikert, C.; Jansen, E.H.; Doring, F.; Joost, H.G.; Boeing, H.; Schulze, M.B. Erythrocyte membrane phospholipid fatty acids, desaturase activity, and dietary fatty acids in relation to risk of type 2 diabetes in the European Prospective Investigation into Cancer and Nutrition (EPIC)-Potsdam Study. *Am. J. Clin. Nutr.* **2011**, *93*, 127–142. [CrossRef] [PubMed]

37. Warensjo, E.; Riserus, U.; Vessby, B. Fatty acid composition of serum lipids predicts the development of the metabolic syndrome in men. *Diabetologia* **2005**, *48*, 1999–2005. [CrossRef] [PubMed]
38. Kotronen, A.; Seppanen-Laakso, T.; Westerbacka, J.; Kiviluoto, T.; Arola, J.; Ruskeepaa, A.L.; Yki-Jarvinen, H.; Oresic, M. Comparison of lipid and fatty acid composition of the liver, subcutaneous and intra-abdominal adipose tissue, and serum. *Obesity (Silver Spring)* **2010**, *18*, 937–944. [CrossRef] [PubMed]
39. Gray, R.G.; Kousta, E.; McCarthy, M.I.; Godsland, I.F.; Venkatesan, S.; Anyaoku, V.; Johnston, D.G. Ethnic variation in the activity of lipid desaturases and their relationships with cardiovascular risk factors in control women and an at-risk group with previous gestational diabetes mellitus: A cross-sectional study. *Lipids Health Dis.* **2013**, *12*. [CrossRef] [PubMed]
40. Peter, A.; Cegan, A.; Wagner, S.; Lehmann, R.; Stefan, N.; Konigsrainer, A.; Konigsrainer, I.; Haring, H.U.; Schleicher, E. Hepatic lipid composition and stearoyl-coenzyme A desaturase 1 mRNA expression can be estimated from plasma VLDL fatty acid ratios. *Clin. Chem.* **2009**, *55*, 2113–2120. [CrossRef] [PubMed]
41. Sjogren, P.; Sierra-Johnson, J.; Gertow, K.; Rosell, M.; Vessby, B.; de Faire, U.; Hamsten, A.; Hellenius, M.L.; Fisher, R.M. Fatty acid desaturases in human adipose tissue: Relationships between gene expression, desaturation indexes and insulin resistance. *Diabetologia* **2008**, *51*, 328–335. [CrossRef] [PubMed]
42. McNamara, R.K.; Liu, Y.; Jandacek, R.; Rider, T.; Tso, P. The aging human orbitofrontal cortex: Decreasing polyunsaturated fatty acid composition and associated increases in lipogenic gene expression and stearoyl-CoA desaturase activity. *Prostaglandins Leukot. Essent. Fatty Acids* **2008**, *78*, 293–304. [CrossRef] [PubMed]
43. Petrus, P.; Edholm, D.; Rosqvist, F.; Dahlman, I.; Sundbom, M.; Arner, P.; Ryden, M.; Riserus, U. Depot-specific differences in fatty acid composition and distinct associations with lipogenic gene expression in abdominal adipose tissue of obese women. *Int. J. Obes. (Lond.)* **2017**, *41*, 1295–1298. [CrossRef] [PubMed]
44. Poisson, J.P.G.; Cunnane, S.C. Long-Chain Fatty-Acid Metabolism in Fasting And Diabetes—Relation between Altered Desaturase Activity and Fatty-Acid Composition. *J. Nutr. Biochem.* **1991**, *2*, 60–70. [CrossRef]
45. Brown, J.E. A critical review of methods used to estimate linoleic acid Delta 6-desaturation ex vivo and in vivo. *Eur. J. Lipid Sci. Technol.* **2005**, *107*, 119–134. [CrossRef]
46. Gillingham, L.G.; Harding, S.V.; Rideout, T.C.; Yurkova, N.; Cunnane, S.C.; Eck, P.K.; Jones, P.J. Dietary oils and FADS1-FADS2 genetic variants modulate [13C]alpha-linolenic acid metabolism and plasma fatty acid composition. *Am. J. Clin. Nutr.* **2013**, *97*, 195–207. [CrossRef] [PubMed]
47. Hodson, L.; Skeaff, C.M.; Fielding, B.A. Fatty acid composition of adipose tissue and blood in humans and its use as a biomarker of dietary intake. *Prog. Lipid Res.* **2008**, *47*, 348–380. [CrossRef] [PubMed]
48. Connor, W.E.; Lin, D.S.; Colvis, C. Differential mobilization of fatty acids from adipose tissue. *J. Lipid Res.* **1996**, *37*, 290–298.

Permissions

All chapters in this book were first published by MDPI; hereby published with permission under the Creative Commons Attribution License or equivalent. Every chapter published in this book has been scrutinized by our experts. Their significance has been extensively debated. The topics covered herein carry significant findings which will fuel the growth of the discipline. They may even be implemented as practical applications or may be referred to as a beginning point for another development.

The contributors of this book come from diverse backgrounds, making this book a truly international effort. This book will bring forth new frontiers with its revolutionizing research information and detailed analysis of the nascent developments around the world.

We would like to thank all the contributing authors for lending their expertise to make the book truly unique. They have played a crucial role in the development of this book. Without their invaluable contributions this book wouldn't have been possible. They have made vital efforts to compile up to date information on the varied aspects of this subject to make this book a valuable addition to the collection of many professionals and students.

This book was conceptualized with the vision of imparting up-to-date information and advanced data in this field. To ensure the same, a matchless editorial board was set up. Every individual on the board went through rigorous rounds of assessment to prove their worth. After which they invested a large part of their time researching and compiling the most relevant data for our readers.

The editorial board has been involved in producing this book since its inception. They have spent rigorous hours researching and exploring the diverse topics which have resulted in the successful publishing of this book. They have passed on their knowledge of decades through this book. To expedite this challenging task, the publisher supported the team at every step. A small team of assistant editors was also appointed to further simplify the editing procedure and attain best results for the readers.

Apart from the editorial board, the designing team has also invested a significant amount of their time in understanding the subject and creating the most relevant covers. They scrutinized every image to scout for the most suitable representation of the subject and create an appropriate cover for the book.

The publishing team has been an ardent support to the editorial, designing and production team. Their endless efforts to recruit the best for this project, has resulted in the accomplishment of this book. They are a veteran in the field of academics and their pool of knowledge is as vast as their experience in printing. Their expertise and guidance has proved useful at every step. Their uncompromising quality standards have made this book an exceptional effort. Their encouragement from time to time has been an inspiration for everyone.

The publisher and the editorial board hope that this book will prove to be a valuable piece of knowledge for researchers, students, practitioners and scholars across the globe.

List of Contributors

Shengyan Sun
Institute of Physical Education, Huzhou University, Huzhou 313000, China
Faculty of Education, University of Macau, Macao 999078, China

Zhaowei Kong, Mingzhu Hu and Di Zhang
Faculty of Education, University of Macau, Macao 999078, China

Qingde Shi and Jinlei Nie
School of Health Sciences and Sports, Macao Polytechnic Institute, Macao 999078, China

Haifeng Zhang
School of Health Sciences and Sports, Macao Polytechnic Institute, Macao 999078, China

Vasanti S. Malik
Department of Nutritional Sciences, Faculty of Medicine, University of Toronto, 1 King's College Circle, Toronto, ON M5S 1A8, Canada
Department of Nutrition, Harvard T.H. Chan School of Public Health, 665 Huntington Avenue, Boston, MA 02115, USA

Frank B. Hu
Department of Nutrition, Harvard T.H. Chan School of Public Health, 665 Huntington Avenue, Boston, MA 02115, USA
Department of Epidemiology, Harvard T.H. School of Public Health, Boston, MA 02115, USA
Channing Division of Network Medicine, Brigham and Women's Hospital and Harvard Medical School, Boston, MA 02115, USA

John W. Apolzan, Robbie A. Beyl, Corby K. Martin, Frank L. Greenway and Ursula White
Pennington Biomedical Research Center, Louisiana State University System, Baton Rouge, LA 70808, USA

Alex Pizzini, Thomas Sonnweber, Guenter Weiss and Ivan Tancevski
Department of Internal Medicine II, Infectious Diseases, Pneumology, Rheumatology, Medical University of Innsbruck, 6020 Innsbruck, Austria

Lukas Lunger
Department of Urology, Klinikum rechts der Isar, Technische Universität München, 81675 Munich, Germany
Nini H. Sissener, Robin Ørnsrud, Monica Sanden, Livar Frøyland, Sofie Remø and Anne-Katrine Lundebye
Institute of Marine Research, Nordnes, N-5817 Bergen, Norway

Maria Lankinen and Matti Uusitupa
Institute of Public Health and Clinical Nutrition, University of Eastern Finland, 70211 Kuopio, Finland

Ursula Schwab
Institute of Public Health and Clinical Nutrition, University of Eastern Finland, 70211 Kuopio, Finland
Department of Medicine, Endocrinology and Clinical Nutrition, Kuopio University Hospital, 70210 Kuopio, Finland

Juan S. Henao Agudelo, Milene S. Ormanji, Amandda R. P. Santos and Ita P. Heilberg
Division of Nephrology, Federal University of São Paulo (UNIFESP), Rua Botucatu 740, 04023-900 São Paulo, Brazil

Leandro C. Baia
Division of Nephrology, Federal University of São Paulo (UNIFESP), Rua Botucatu 740, 04023-900 São Paulo, Brazil
Division of Nephrology, University of Groningen, University Medical Centre Groningen (UMCG), 9700 RB Groningen, The Netherlands

Juliana R. Machado
Tropical Medicine & Public Health, Federal University of Goiás (UFG), Rua 235 s/n-University Sector, 74605-050 Goiânia, Brazil

Niels O. Saraiva Câmara
Division of Nephrology, Federal University of São Paulo (UNIFESP), Rua Botucatu 740, 04023-900 São Paulo, Brazil
Department of Immunology, Institute of Biomedical Sciences, University of São Paulo (USP), Av. Prof. Lineu Prestes 1730, ICB IV, Sala 238, 05508-000 São Paulo, Brazil

Gerjan J. Navis and Martin H. de Borst
Division of Nephrology, University of Groningen, University Medical Centre Groningen (UMCG), 9700 RB Groningen, The Netherlands

William S. Harris
Department of Internal Medicine, Sanford School of Medicine, University of South Dakota, Vermillion, SD 57069, USA
Omega Quant Analytics, LLC, Sioux Falls, SD 57106, USA

Nathan L. Tintle
Department of Mathematics & Statistics, Dordt College, Sioux Center, IA 51250, USA

Vasan S. Ramachandran
National Heart Lung and Blood Institute's and Boston University's Framingham Heart Study, Framingham, MA 02118, USA
Departments of Cardiology and Preventive Medicine, Department of Medicine, Boston University School of Medicine, Boston, MA 02118, USA
Department of Biostatistics, Boston University School of Public Health, Boston, MA 02118, USA

Jenny E. Kanter, Leela Goodspeed, Shari Wang, Farah Kramer, Diego Gomes-Kjerulf, Savitha Subramanian, Laura J. den Hartigh, Tomasz Wietecha and Kevin D. O'Brien
Department of Medicine, Division of Metabolism, Endocrinology and Nutrition, University of Washington Medicine Diabetes Institute, University of Washington, 750 Republican Street, Seattle, WA 98109, USA

Ming-Hua Sung and Fang-Hsuean Liao
School of Nutrition and Health Sciences, Taipei Medical University, Taipei 11031, Taiwan

Yi-Wen Chien
School of Nutrition and Health Sciences, Taipei Medical University, Taipei 11031, Taiwan Research Center of Geriatric Nutrition, College of Nutrition, Taipei Medical University, Taipei 11031, Taiwan
Graduate Institute of Metabolism and Obesity Sciences, Taipei Medical University, Taipei 11031, Taiwan

Hayley E. Billingsley and Salvatore Carbone
Pauley Heart Center, Virginia Commonwealth University, Richmond, VA, 23298, USA

Carl J. Lavie
John Ochsner Heart and Vascular Institute, Ochsner Clinical School, University of Queensland School of Medicine, New Orleans, LA 70121, USA

Kelei Li and Feng Zhao
Institute of Nutrition and Health, Qingdao University, Qingdao 266021, China

Andrew J. Sinclair
Faculty of Health, Deakin University, Locked Bag 20000, Geelong, VIC 3220, Australia
Department of Nutrition, Dietetics and Food, Monash University, Notting Hill, VIC 3168, Australia

Duo Li
Institute of Nutrition and Health, Qingdao University, Qingdao 266021, China
Department of Nutrition, Dietetics and Food, Monash University, Notting Hill, VIC 3168, Australia

Julia K. Bird and Manfred Eggersdorfer
DSM Nutritional Products, 4303 Kaiseraugst, Switzerland

Philip C. Calder
Human Development and Health Academic Unit, Faculty of Medicine, University of Southampton, Southampton SO16 6YD, UK
NIHR Southampton Biomedical Research Centre, University Hospital Southampton NHS Foundation Trust and University of Southampton, Southampton SO16 6YD, UK

Yvette Beulen and Ondine van de Rest
Division of Human Nutrition, Wageningen University, 6708 Wageningen, The Netherlands

Miguel A. Martínez-González
Department of Preventive Medicine & Public Health, University of Navarra, 31008 Pamplona, Spain
CIBER Fisiopatología de la Obesidad y Nutrición (CIBEROBN), Instituto de Salud Carlos III (ISCIII), Spanish Government, 28029 Madrid, Spain

Jordi Salas-Salvadó and Nerea Becerra-Tomas
CIBER Fisiopatología de la Obesidad y Nutrición (CIBEROBN), Instituto de Salud Carlos III (ISCIII), Spanish Government, 28029 Madrid, Spain
Human Nutrition Unit, Faculty of Medicine and Health Sciences, Pere Virgili Health Research Institute, Rovira i Virgili University, 43002 Reus, Spain

José V. Sorlí and José I. González
CIBER Fisiopatología de la Obesidad y Nutrición (CIBEROBN), Instituto de Salud Carlos III (ISCIII), Spanish Government, 28029 Madrid, Spain
Department of Preventive Medicine, University of Valencia, 46010 Valencia, Spain

Enrique Gómez-Gracia
Department of Preventive Medicine, University of Málaga, 29016 Málaga, Spain

Miquel Fiol
CIBER Fisiopatología de la Obesidad y Nutrición (CIBEROBN), Instituto de Salud Carlos III (ISCIII), Spanish Government, 28029 Madrid, Spain
Institute of Health Sciences IUNICS, University of Balearic Islands and Hospital Son Espases, 07010 Palma de Mallorca, Spain

Ramón Estruch
CIBER Fisiopatología de la Obesidad y Nutrición (CIBEROBN), Instituto de Salud Carlos III (ISCIII), Spanish Government, 28029 Madrid, Spain
Department of Internal Medicine, Department of Endocrinology and Nutrition Biomedical Research Institute August Pi Sunyer (IDI- BAPS), Hospital Clinic, University of Barcelona, 08036 Barcelona, Spain

José M. Santos-Lozano
CIBER Fisiopatología de la Obesidad y Nutrición (CIBEROBN), Instituto de Salud Carlos III (ISCIII), Spanish Government, 28029 Madrid, Spain
Department of Family Medicine, Research Unit, Distrito Sanitario Atención Primaria Sevilla, Centro de Salud Universitario San Pablo, 41013 Sevilla, Spain

Helmut Schröder
Cardiovascular and Nutrition Research Group (Regicor Study Group), Hospital del Mar Research Institute (IMIM), 08003 Barcelona, Spain
CIBER Epidemiología y Salud Pública (CIBERESP), Instituto de Salud Carlos III (ISCIII), Spanish Government, 28029 Madrid, Spain

Angel Alonso-Gómez
CIBER Fisiopatología de la Obesidad y Nutrición (CIBEROBN), Instituto de Salud Carlos III (ISCIII), Spanish Government, 28029 Madrid, Spain
Department of Cardiology, University Hospital of Alava, 48940 Vitoria, Spain

Luis Serra-Majem
CIBER Fisiopatología de la Obesidad y Nutrición (CIBEROBN), Instituto de Salud Carlos III (ISCIII), Spanish Government, 28029 Madrid, Spain
Research Institute of Biomedical and Health Sciences (IUIBS), University of Las Palmas de Gran Canaria and Service of Preventive Medicine, Complejo Hospitalario Universitario Insular Materno Infantil (CHUIMI), Canary Health Service, 35016 Las Palmas de Gran Canaria, Spain

Xavier Pintó
CIBER Fisiopatología de la Obesidad y Nutrición (CIBEROBN), Instituto de Salud Carlos III (ISCIII), Spanish Government, 28029 Madrid, Spain
Lipids and Vascular Risk Unit, Internal Medicine, Hospital Universitario de Bellvitge, Hospitalet de Llobregat, 08907 Barcelona, Spain

Emilio Ros
CIBER Fisiopatología de la Obesidad y Nutrición (CIBEROBN), Instituto de Salud Carlos III (ISCIII), Spanish Government, 28029 Madrid, Spain
Lipid Clinic, Department of Endocrinology and Nutrition Biomedical Research Institute August Pi Sunyer (IDIBAPS), Hospital Clinic, University of Barcelona, 08036 Barcelona, Spain

Montserrat Fitó
CIBER Fisiopatología de la Obesidad y Nutrición (CIBEROBN), Instituto de Salud Carlos III (ISCIII), Spanish Government, 28029 Madrid, Spain
Cardiovascular and Nutrition Research Group (Regicor Study Group), Hospital del Mar Research Institute (IMIM), 08003 Barcelona, Spain

J. Alfredo. Martínez
CIBER Fisiopatología de la Obesidad y Nutrición (CIBEROBN), Instituto de Salud Carlos III (ISCIII), Spanish Government, 28029 Madrid, Spain
Department of Nutrition and Food Sciences and Physiology, University of Navarra, 31008 Pamplona, Spain

Alfredo Gea
Department of Preventive Medicine & Public Health, University of Navarra, 31008 Pamplona, Spain

Sara Bonafini, Alice Giontella, Angela Tagetti, Denise Marcon, Pietro Minuz and Cristiano Fava
Department of Medicine, University of Verona, 37129 Verona, Italy

Rossella Gaudino, Paolo Cavarzere, Franco Antoniazzi and Claudio Maffeis
Department of Surgery, Dentistry, Paediatrics and Gynaecology, University of Verona, 37129 Verona, Italy

Mirjam Karber
Berlin Institute of Health (BIH), 10178 Berlin, Germany

Michael Rothe
Lipidomix, 13125 Berlin, Germany

Wolf Hagen Schunck
Max Delbrueck Center for Molecular Medicine, 13092 Berlin, Germany

Martina Montagnana and Marco Benati
Department of Neurosciences, Biomedicine and Movement Sciences, University of Verona, 37129 Verona, Italy

Matti Marklund
The George Institute for Global Health, University of New South Wales, Sydney, NSW 2042, Australia
Department of Public Health and Caring Sciences, Clinical Nutrition and Metabolism, Uppsala University, 751 22 Uppsala, Sweden

Andrew P. Morris
Department of Biostatistics, University of Liverpool, Liverpool L69 3GL, UK

Anubha Mahajan
The Wellcome Trust Centre for Human Genetics, Oxford OX3 7BN, UK

Erik Ingelsson
Department of Medicine, Division of Cardiovascular Medicine, Stanford University School of Medicine, Stanford, CA 94305, USA
Stanford Cardiovascular Institute, Stanford University, Stanford, CA 94305, USA
Stanford Diabetes Research Center, Stanford University, Stanford, CA 94305, USA
Department of Medical Sciences, Molecular Epidemiology, Uppsala University, 751 85 Uppsala, Sweden

Cecilia M. Lindgren
The Wellcome Trust Centre for Human Genetics, Oxford OX3 7BN, UK
Li Ka Shing Centre for Health Information and Discovery, The Big Data Institute, University of Oxford, Oxford OX3 7LF, UK

Lars Lind
Department of Medical Sciences, Cardiovascular Epidemiology, Uppsala University, 751 85 Uppsala, Sweden

Ulf Risérus
Department of Public Health and Caring Sciences, Clinical Nutrition and Metabolism, Uppsala University, 751 22 Uppsala, Sweden

Index

Printed in the USA
CPSIA information can be obtained
at www.ICGtesting.com
JSHW051404091023
49903JS00006B/270